DNA- AND M-RNA-BASED VACCINES

An Immunotherapeutic Approach to Cancer

DNA- AND M-RNA-BASED VACCINES

An Immunotherapeutic Approach to Cancer

by

Sonali Sundram

Rishabha Malviya

AAP | APPLE ACADEMIC PRESS

First edition published 2026

Apple Academic Press Inc.
1265 Goldenrod Circle, NE,
Palm Bay, FL 32905 USA

760 Laurentian Drive, Unit 19,
Burlington, ON L7N 0A4, Canada

CRC Press
2385 NW Executive Center Drive,
Suite 320, Boca Raton FL 33431

4 Park Square, Milton Park,
Abingdon, Oxon, OX14 4RN, UK

Apple Academic Press exclusively co-publishes with CRC Press, an imprint of Taylor & Francis Group, LLC

Library and Archives Canada Cataloguing in Publication

CIP data on file with Canada Library and Archives

Library of Congress Cataloging-in-Publication Data

CIP data on file with US Library of Congress

ISBN: 978-1-77491-960-6 (hbk)
ISBN: 978-1-77491-961-3 (ebk)
DOI: 10.1201/9781774919613

About the Authors

Sonali Sundram, MPharm
Assistant Professor, School of Medical & Allied Sciences, Galgotias University, Greater Noida, Uttar Pradesh India

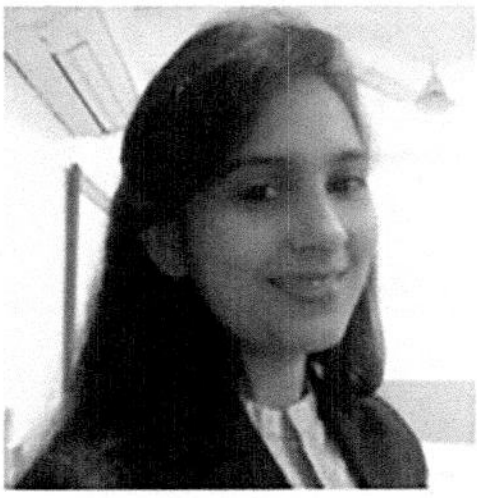

Prof. Sonali Sundram completed her BPharm and MPharm (Pharmacology) from AKTU, Lucknow, India. She has worked as a research scientist on a project of the Indian Council of Medical Research at King George's Medical University, Lucknow, and after that, she joined the Babu Banarasi Das Northern India Institute of Technology (BBDNIIT). Currently, she is working at the School of Medical & Allied Sciences of Galgotias University, Greater Noida, Uttar Pradesh, India. Her PhD (Pharmacy) work was in the area of neurodegeneration and nanoformulation. Her areas of interest are neurodegeneration, clinical research, and artificial intelligence. She has authored/edited/editing more than 20 books (Wiley, CRC Press/Taylor and Francis, IOP Publishing, Apple Academic Press/ Taylor and Francis, Springer, and River Publisher). She has attended as well as organized more than 15 national and international seminars, conferences, and workshops. She has more than eight patents national and international to her credit. She has published six SCI-indexed papers (cumulative impact factor: 20.71) with reputed international publishers. She has presented papers in international conferences organized in different European countries.

Rishabha Malviya, PhD
Professor, Department of Pharmacy, School of Medical and Allied Sciences, Galgotias University, India

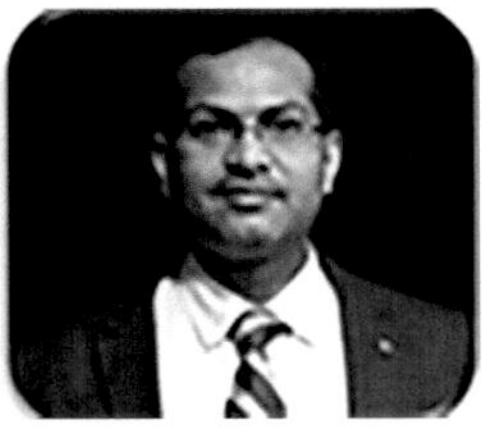

Dr. Rishabha Malviya completed his BPharm from Uttar Pradesh Technical University and MPharm (Pharmaceutics) from Gautam Buddha Technical University, Lucknow, Uttar Pradesh, India. His PhD (Pharmacy) work was in the area of novel formulation development techniques. He has 15 years of research experience and is presently working as a Professor in the Department of Pharmacy, School of Medical and Allied Sciences, Galgotias University, India, for the last eight years. His areas of interest include formulation optimization, nanoformulation, targeted drug delivery, localized drug delivery, and characterization of natural polymers as pharmaceutical excipients. He has authored more than 300 research and review papers for national and international journals of repute, with a total of more than 350 cumulative impact factors. He has 58 patents (19 grants, 38 published, one filed). He has also received an Outstanding Reviewer Award from Elsevier. He has authored and edited over 110 books (Wiley, CRC Press/Taylor and Francis, Springer, River Publisher, IOP Publishing, and OMICS Publishing Group) and authored 170 book chapters. His name has been included in the world's top 2% of scientists list for the years 2020, 2021, 2022, 2023 and 2024, compiled by Elsevier BV and Stanford University. He is a reviewer, editor, and editorial board member of more than 50 national and international journals of repute. He has been invited as the author for *Atlas of Science* and a pharma magazine dealing with industry (B2B), *Ingredient South Asia.*

Contents

Foreword

Cancer is a formidable challenge in the field of medical research, which has impacted millions of lives. It is matter of huge concern. For years, we have been searching for new approaches to combat this difficult and fatal disease. This book, DNA- and m-RNA-Based Vaccines: An Immunotherapeutic Approach to Cancer, by Sonali Sundram and Dr. Rishabha Malviya, will provide very useful scientific literature for newer therapies for cancer.

A pioneer in the field of cancer research and immunotherapy, Sonali Sundram and Dr. Rishabha Malviya have put together an extensive book that explores the cutting-edge application of messenger RNA (m-RNA) and DNA vaccines to target and eradicate cancer. This book is a collection of contemporary scientific studies on relevant topics that can be very useful to the scientists working in these areas for future strategies and be an invaluable source of motivation for everyone involved in the battle against cancer.

The idea of cancer immunotherapy has completely changed the way we treat this illness. Today, we are using the immune system's strength to attack cancer at its source rather than only depending on conventional therapies. In this field, DNA and m-RNA vaccines provide a fresh and exciting approach that has the potential to revolutionize how we think about cancer treatment.

This book is a result of a collaborative effort to investigate and comprehend the possibilities of m-RNA and DNA-based cancer vaccines. Every chapter advances knowledge on the topic, revealing new information on anything from the intricacies of tumor angiogenesis to the significance of noncoding RNAs in treatment resistance.

Let us approach the world of DNA- and m-RNA-based cancer vaccines with optimism, dedication, and a regenerated devotion to the fight against cancer. The findings in the book provide clarity for the route ahead, and it is up to all to keep pushing the boundaries of science and medicine in order to create a future in which cancer is no longer a permanent challenge.

—Roop Krishen Khar
Director, B. S. Anangpuria Educational Institutes.
Ballabgarh Sohna Road, Alampur, Faridabad;
Director, Formulators Koncept Pvt. Ltd.;
Director, Unicure India Ltd
Former Dean & HOD, Jamia Hamdard, New Delhi, India

Preface

Scientific discovery is a never-ending adventure that presents fresh perspectives on the most important issues of our day, challenges long-standing paradigms, and opens up fresh possibilities. The combination of DNA and messenger RNA (m-RNA) vaccines has become a novel and promising strategy in medical research and the fight against cancer. This book, *DNA- and m-RNA-Based Vaccines: An Immunotherapeutic Approach to Cancer*, explores this novel and fascinating area of cancer immunotherapy in great detail.

Cancer continues to be one of the most deadly enemies of contemporary medicine, taking the lives of countless people and their families. Because of the disease's intricacy, effective treatment require innovative and inventive approaches. The development of vaccines based on DNA and m-RNA has revolutionized our understanding of how to direct the immune system of the body to specifically target and eliminate cancer cells. With the goal of comprehending, enhancing, and utilizing the power of genetic material in the battle against cancer, we set out on a trip across the pages of this book to investigate the many aspects of this ground-breaking strategy.

Each chapter offers a unique perspective on a different facet of DNA- and mRNA-based cancer vaccines. This book offers a thorough overview of the constantly changing field of cancer immunotherapy, from comprehending the unique aspects of tumor angiogenesis and the part noncoding RNAs play in treatment resistance, to investigating the most recent developments in gene therapy and splicing control.

The enormous promise of DNA- and m-RNA-based vaccines as immunotherapeutic agents against cancer will become clear to us as we go through the chapters of this book. The book explores the therapeutic uses, biological processes, and difficulties related to this novel strategy. It also looks at this fascinating field's future potential, giving cancer patients hope for less intrusive and more effective therapies.

For researchers, physicians, students, and everyone else interested in the most recent advancements in cancer therapy and vaccination technology, we believe that this book will be an invaluable resource. Our objective is to stimulate fresh research, promote teamwork, and eventually develop cancer immunotherapy.

The fight against cancer is a team effort, and with every new finding and advancement, we get closer to a day when the disease will no longer be a deadly force. We really hope that the knowledge offered on these pages advances the continuing fight against this terrible illness.

CHAPTER 1

Various Prospects of Tumor Angiogenesis

ABSTRACT

The ramifications of cancer vascularization are influenced by a range of factors, such as anatomical site and tumor classification. The aforementioned process takes place simultaneously inside the malignant tissue via many discrete biological processes. A diverse array of chemicals is produced, accompanied by signaling systems that play a crucial role in coordinating these processes. Moreover, it is noteworthy to mention that several cell types, including progenitor cells and cancer stem cells, in addition to specialized endothelium cells, may potentially contribute to these physiological processes. Various antiangiogenic interventions, such as the use of antibodies or tyrosine-kinase inhibitors, have shown considerable effectiveness in the therapeutic management of many cancer variants. Certain people have shown a notable absence of response, while others have displayed a degree of resistance to the drug that was given. The growing awareness of the difficulties involved with hindering the infiltration of tumors into the bloodstream is becoming more evident. When doing a comparative analysis across various subtypes of cancer, it becomes apparent that there is a substantial variation in both tumor vascular function and gene expression. Furthermore, it is crucial to acknowledge that the phenotypic of a certain cancer might display a significant variety. This review examines recent advancements in the field of cellular and molecular processes, with a special emphasis on elucidating the fundamental mechanisms involved in tumor angiogenesis. Furthermore, this

DNA- and m-RNA-Based Vaccines: An Immunotherapeutic Approach to Cancer.

Sonali Sundram and Rishabha Malviya (Authors)

DOI: 10.1201/9781774919613-1

chapter provides a critical evaluation of the possible benefits and drawbacks linked to vascular-targeting treatment.

1.1 INTRODUCTION

Cancer cells can only survive and spread if they have access to blood arteries, which provide nourishment and oxygen to every cell in the body. It was postulated that the initiation of tumor angiogenesis is a crucial factor in facilitating proliferation of tumors, as evidenced by the observation that rapidly growing tumors exhibit significant vascularization, while dormant tumors do not [1]. Angiogenesis has been seen in cancer cells, and Folkman suggested that inhibiting angiogenic signaling pathways might prevent new vessels from forming and hence prevent tumor dormancy [2]. Due to the captivating nature of this notion, numerous endeavors have been undertaken to discern the pro-antigenic substances generated by tumors and then trace the signals they emit [3]. In a clinical experiment conducted in 2003, it was shown that humanized antibodies targeting antivascular endothelial growth factor exhibited efficacy in patients diagnosed with metastatic colorectal cancer. The trial results indicated better survival rates, so providing evidence supporting the effectiveness of antiangiogenic therapy [4]. Furthermore, the Food and Drug Administration (FDA) has granted authorization to a number of cancer medications that specifically target pro-angiogenic signaling pathways. Despite the continuously increasing range of drugs that have received approval from the FDA, the effectiveness of antiangiogenic treatment in suppressing tumor growth has been limited, as resistance tends to develop shortly after treatment initiation. Consequently, the observed improvements in survival time have been very modest. The lack of efficiency can be attributed to various variables, including the utilization of alternative angiogenesis pathways by tumors and the emergence of resistance mechanisms, among other contributing factors. Furthermore, numerous types of cancer have the ability to bypass the requirement for tumor angiogenesis by employing vascular co-option [5]. Tumor angiogenesis and its molecular and functional heterogeneities, as well as developing approaches for vascular targeting during cancer treatment, are discussed in detail in this chapter.

1.2 THE COMMENCEMENT OF TUMOR ANGIOGENESIS: THE ACTIVATION OF THE ANGIOGENESIS SWITCHES

During the initial stages of constructing multistage carcinoma models, which involve the use of human tissue and genetically modified animals, the tumors generally exhibit limited size and inactivity, lacking any indications of actively initiating angiogenesis. One common consequence associated with the progression of tumors is the development of additional blood capillaries, indicating that malignant cells necessitate a continuous supply of oxygenated blood in order to proliferate. In the subsequent discussion, an in-depth analysis will be provided about various molecular and cellular pathways that play a crucial role in facilitating tumor vascularization [5]. These processes can either utilize the existing tumor vasculature or facilitate the development of new blood supply pathways for the tumor. The regulation of the angiogenic process is governed by both pro-angiogenic and antiangiogenic factors. The proliferation of endocrine cells is inhibited when these factors achieve equilibrium within the vasculature. The phenomenon known as the "angiogenic switch" has been identified by researchers in the field of oncology as the mechanism responsible for initiating the process of blood vessel formation [6]. Upon the emergence of neovascularization, tumors undergo a reactivation process, transitioning from a dormant state to a rapid growth phase. The advancement of genetically modified mice that effectively replicate various tumor stages has greatly enhanced research on the angiogenic switch. Besides the RIP1-Tag2 pancreas insulinoma model developed by the research team led by Douglas Hanahan, various other models of insulinoma have been subject to intensive investigation [7, 8]. Nonangiogenic clusters of dysplastic cells in mice expressing the transgene initially develop into small angiogenic tumors, which have the potential to progress into larger vascularized tumors capable of metastasizing to the lungs. This study, along with other animal tumor models, has identified various factors and biological pathways that can potentially induce tumor vascular growth. These findings have been further supported by contemporary *in vivo* and *in vitro* angiogenesis models [8]. Tumor-associated inflammation and immune cell recruitment can activate the angiogenic switch, or additional genetic abnormalities in cancer cells, such as enhanced proliferation and hypoxia, can do the same.

1.3 FORMATION OF VASCULAR PATHWAYS ASSOCIATED WITH MALIGNANCY

The fundamental functions of the circulatory system encompass the preservation of homeostasis, the provision of nutrients, and the supply of chemicals to various tissues. The circulatory system facilitates the transportation of blood throughout the human body and uses a complex network of blood vessels such as the aorta, arteries, capillaries, and veins. Oxygenated blood is ejected from the heart and distributed to the various tissues of the body via the arterial system. The capillary walls play a critical role in facilitating the flow of gases from the blood to the tissues. The heart facilitates the conversion of carbon dioxide, which has been expelled from the tissues, into oxygen as it is transported by the blood. The postcapillary venules serve as a conduit through which immune cells are able to infiltrate various tissues. The structure of the capillary wall consists of endothelial cells (ECs), two layers of basement membrane, and a framework of pericytes [9]. Tumor growth and metastasis require angiogenesis, which occurs mostly in capillaries. Here, a few of the biological mechanisms have been addressed which could set in motion the growth of tumor blood vessels, as seen schematically in Figure 1.1.

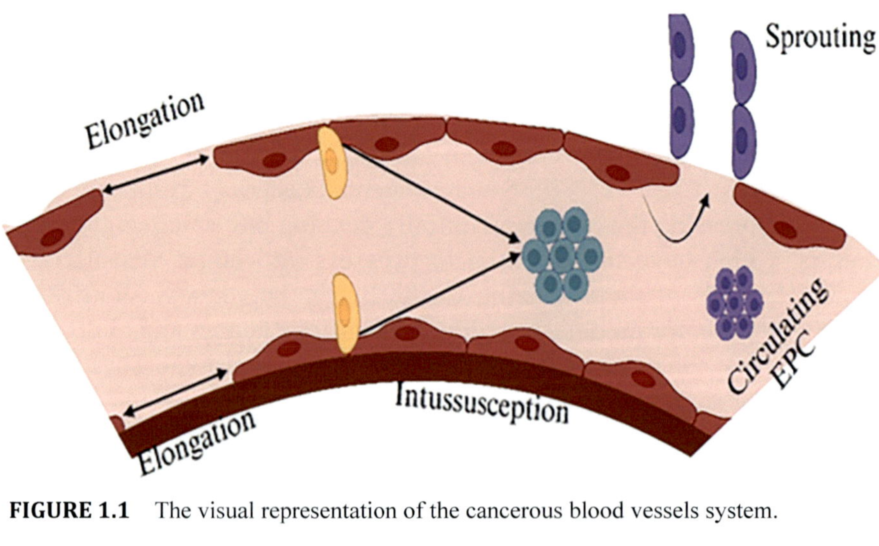

FIGURE 1.1 The visual representation of the cancerous blood vessels system.

1.4 A SURGE IN ANGIOGENESIS

The process of multistep sprouting angiogenesis facilitates the emergence of new capillaries through the branching out of established blood vessels. In order for the initiation of a sprout, a parent vascular cell assumes the role of a migratory leading cell and employs a mechanism known as lateral inhibition to prevent adjacent cells from undergoing the same process. The stem cells that migrate alongside the sprout over its entire length exhibit chemotaxis, and the fusion of the sprout's luminal space with the parent channel results in the formation of a lumen. The sprout undergoes a biological phenomenon known as anastomosis, which involves the formation of novel connections between blood vessels.

Chemical substances such as vascular endothelial growth factor (VEGF) have the ability to stimulate the proliferation of ECs and trigger the activation of dormant angiogenesis. The regulation of tip and stalk cell development is governed by the interactions between the VEGF and the Delta-like ligand 4 (Dll4)/Notch signaling pathways [9]. Because of VEGF, TIP cells release DLL4 ligand, platelet-derived growth factor B (PDGF-B), vascular endothelial growth factor receptor-2 (VEGFR-2), and VEGFR-3/flt-4 [10–12]. There is evidence that VEGF, or VEGF, blocks Notch signaling and promotes tip cell sprouting, branching, migration, and the creation of filopodia [13]. By upregulating VEGFR1 (a VEGF decoy) and decreasing VEGFR2 and VEGFR3 expression [14–17], DLL4-releasing tip cells inhibit the development of neighboring tip cells. Damage-inducing proteins, which are released by vascular tip cells, direct angiogenesis along a VEGF gradient [18]. Neuropilins, a kind of nontyrosine kinase receptors, have been found to enhance the signaling of VEGFR2 and VEGFR3, leading to the activation of tip cells [19, 20]. After the tip cells have undergone branching from the parent artery, it is the task of the stalk cells to generate the vascular lumen and create junctional connections with the sprout. The protein Notch, which is distinguished by its ankyrin repeats, elicits a notable augmentation in cellular proliferation while concurrently diminishing the quantity of filopodia in tip cells [21]. A head-to-head anastomosis is when two new blood vessels are joined together, while head-to-side anastomosis connects a single new blood artery to an existing one. Zebrafish cell connection formation is extremely stereotyped, as shown by live imaging investigations [21–24]. During cell migration, filopodia located in close proximity to the leading edge of cells are responsible for the production of junctional proteins, including VE-cadherin [25, 26]. The initial stages of contact development involve the repeated formation and dissolution of connections between the filopodia of adjacent tip cells. This process leads to the accumulation of VE-cadherin and the formation of a circular junction at the site of filopodia contact, resulting in the formation of a small luminal pocket [27]. The presence of more filopodia is withdrawn, and apical markers, such as podocalyxin and junctional molecules, are observed [25]. Betz et al. [28] provide a comprehensive description of two distinct types of anastomosis, referred to as types I and II, based on the development of the lumen and perfused tubes.

1.5 ANGIOGENESIS IN CONJUNCTION WITH INTUSSUSCEPTION

The phenomenon known as neo-angiogenesis refers to the development of novel blood vessels that integrate with preexisting vessels through a process referred to as "intussusception" [29, 30]. The aforementioned mechanism was initially documented in the restructuring of pulmonary capillaries. The promotion of angiogenesis can be facilitated by growth factors such as erythropoietin, PDGF, and VEGF [31–33]. However, the specific molecular processes underlying this process are yet unknown. Cancers such as skin cancer, colorectal cancer, glioblastoma, and breast tumors have all demonstrated the presence of indurated angiogenesis. The generation of VEGF in melanoma is associated with the presence of intraluminal tissue folds and angiogenesis [34]. Human adenocarcinoma xenografts employ intussuscepted angiogenesis as a mechanism to efficiently restructure blood vessels and sustain adequate blood circulation within tumors [35, 36]. It is postulated that the augmentation of tumor-associated microvascular structures, both in terms of complexity and number, may play a role in facilitating tumor progression through a mechanism referred to as intussusceptive angiogenesis [37].

1.6 VASCULARIZATION AND ENDOTHELIUM PRECURSOR CELLS ENGRAFTMENT

Vasculogenesis refers to the biological mechanism via which endothelial progenitor cells (EPCs) facilitate the formation and proliferation of nascent blood arteries over the course of embryonic development [38, 39]. The process of cellular differentiation and aggregation into blood islands commences in mice at the embryonic stage between days 6.5 and 7. The equatorial areas of blood islands are responsible for the production of hematopoietic cells, whereas the polar regions are responsible for the production of angioblasts, which are a type of EC. The proliferation and differentiation of angioblasts inside the paraxial mesoderm of mice results in the formation of a plexus rich in endocardial tubules. The procedure in question gives rise to the embryo's aorta, cardinal vein, and vascular networks. In order to cater to the heightened requirement for oxygen and nutrient transportation, a novel process of neo-vascularization within tumors has been discovered in the adult population. This process involves vasculogenesis occurring during the formation of capillaries subsequent to ischemia [40, 41]. The process of vasculogenesis, rather than angiogenesis, is accountable for the revascularization observed in recurrent gliomas subsequent to radiation therapy [42, 43]. EPCs, also known as bone marrow-derived hematopoietic cells, have been suggested as a potential contributor to cancer vasculogenesis, which refers to the formation of new blood vessels that provide nourishment to growing tumors [44, 45]. EPCs, a kind of adult stem cell characterized by their ability to undergo self-renewal through division, have been observed to play a role in the process of neovascularization [46, 47]. EPCs express tyrosine kinase receptors, namely CD34, Nanog, Octamer-4 (Oct-4), and Tie-2 (VEGFR 1) [48, 49]. Various types of cells can be utilized to generate EPCs, such as stem cells, myeloid cells, mature ECs, and other cell types [46, 50]. A variety of growth factors, cytokines, and signaling pathways that are associated with hypoxia play a crucial role in guiding bone marrow-derived EPCs toward sites of injury. Once at these locations, the EPCs undergo differentiation into ECs and actively contribute to the process of neovascularization [41, 51]. The process of tumor vasculogenesis is initiated through the interaction between EPCs derived from the bone marrow and tumor cells. EPCs have been observed to be liberated by VEGF within the bone marrow. The expression of VEGFR2 is a distinguishing feature of these EPCs, which have been linked to the development of malignant conditions [52–54]. Chemokines, namely CCL2, CCL5, adiponectin, and CXCL12 (sometimes referred to as SDF-1), are released by tumors in response to hypoxia [55–57].

1.7 RESEMBLANCE TO THE CARDIOVASCULAR SYSTEM

Tumor cells during active division have the ability to generate vascular-like structures, a process referred to as vascular mimicry. Tumor cells are capable of acquiring the necessary blood supply and nutrients from these structures, even in the absence of ECs. Vascular mimicry has been observed in various types of cancer, such as melanomas [58], gliomas [59], head and neck cancers [60], lung cancers [61], colorectal cancers [62], and prostate cancers [63]. Initially, there was scepticism about the concept of vascular mimicry. However, further research has provided evidence supporting its presence and relative importance [64]. Immunohistochemistry utilizing periodic acid-Schiff (PAS) markers and CD31 can be employed to identify tumor tissues that exhibit structures resembling blood vessels [65, 66]. The cancer cells have the ability to secrete a variety of substances that facilitate the formation and sustenance of tubular structures [67]. Tissue transglutaminase antigen 2, as well as collagens IV and VI, serve as illustrative instances of such molecular entities. Tumor cells exhibiting vascular mimicry in uveal melanoma have been found to express CD271, and these particular cells demonstrate characteristics reminiscent of stem cells [68]. Distinguishing between the fibrovascular septa and vascular mimicry of melanoma stroma can be achieved by analyzing their distinct thicknesses and lamination structures [69].

The aggressiveness and metastatic potential of cancer are influenced by various factors, one of which is the disease's ability to imitate blood arteries. The enhancement of vascular mimicry in melanoma is attributed, at least in part, to the activation of the Met proto-oncogene by hypoxia-reactive oxygen species generated by mitochondria [70]. This phenomenon promotes the infiltration of tumor cells into distant anatomical sites and facilitates the process of metastasis. There have been documented instances of heightened vascular mimicry observed in gliomas subsequent to the administration of antiangiogenic treatment [71]. This observation suggests that the tumor may have adopted an alternative mechanism of tumor neovascularization in order to adapt to the treatment and counteract the hypoxic conditions. Cancers that have vascular mimicry are generally correlated with a more unfavorable outcome [62, 72]. The lack of precise methodologies for distinguishing between these processes is a challenge in investigating the comparative significance of vascular mimicry and regular EC lining.

1.8 THE METAMORPHOSIS OF CANCEROUS PRECURSOR CELLS

There is evidence to suggest that various types of tumors exhibit indications of neovascularization, a process that is thought to be initiated by the differentiation of cancer stem cells into endothelial and vascular smooth muscle-like cells [59, 73–76]. Previous studies [59, 73] have demonstrated that the ECs within tumors have somatic mutations that are also present in the cancer cells of the same tumors. *In vitro*, glioma cancer stem cells demonstrated the ability to undergo trans-differentiation into vascular cells by the promotion of EC growth, tubular structure formation, and proliferation. The expression of CD34, CD144, and VEGFR2 has been seen in tumor vascular ECs in the context of human glioma stem cells employed as *in vivo* xenografts [77]. The researchers ascertained that ECs derived from glioma stem cells played a role in the vascularization of glioblastoma by specifically targeting tumor cells expressing the integrin Tie-2. Previous investigations have not shown any genetic alterations in ECs within human glioblastoma [78, 79]; however, this absence of evidence should not be misconstrued as evidence of absence. ECs, together with pro-angiogenic monocytes and pericytes, demonstrate elevated expression of Tie-2 [80]. Despite the absence of conclusive evidence regarding the differentiation of glioma stem cells into ECs, a recent investigation utilizing fluorescent reporters capable of identifying distinct lineages has shown that targeted reduction of pericytes selectively impeded tumor vasculature and hindered tumor progression. The transdifferentiation of glioma cancer stem cells into pericytes was facilitated by TGF. Subsequently, these pericytes were attracted to ECs through the signaling pathway involving CXCL12/CXCR4 [81].

1.9 TUMOR VASCULAR ARTERY TRAITS: MOLECULAR AND OPERATIONAL CHARACTERISTICS

The uncontrolled proliferation of tumor blood vessels persists due to the presence of pro-angiogenic substances inside the tumor microenvironment. The vascular system, comprising veins, capillaries, venules, arteries, and arterioles, is divided into segments to facilitate proper circulation of blood. The development of vascular networks may be hindered from reaching full maturity and undergo pruning due to the continuous presence of pro-angiogenic signals within the tumor. Consequently, this phenomenon may impede the formation of arterioles, capillaries, and venules, resulting in a diverse range of vessel diameter sizes and disorganized blood flow [82, 83]. The outcome of this phenomenon could potentially lead to the presence of localized areas characterized by either continuous or sporadic oxygen deficiency inside the tumor tissue [84, 85]. The elevation in interstitial fluid pressure occurs as a consequence of the disruption of endothelial junctions in tumor arteries, leading to increased permeability [86]. The efficacy of cancer treatment may be compromised due to the stenosis of tumor arteries and insufficient vascular perfusion [87]. The occurrence of bleeding is more prevalent in tumor arteries as a result of the uneven organization of pericytes and ECs within the basement membrane [88–90]. The tumor microenvironment experiences significant changes when there is a disruption in vascular function and integrity (see Figure 1.2). The vascular structure of tumors exhibits significant heterogeneity in terms of structural and functional problems, which can differ not only between tumors of different types and locations, but also within tumors of the same kind and location.

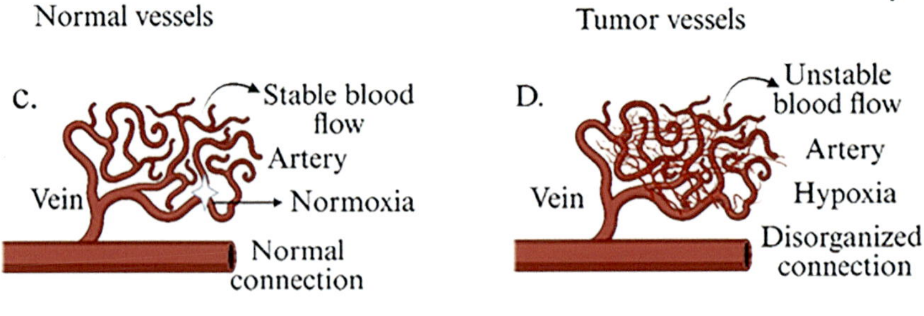

FIGURE 1.2 Tumor vessel structure and function in comparison to normal vessels.

The molecular characteristics of blood vessels in tumors differ from those of normal blood vessels due to the transcriptional regulation of gene expression in response to environmental stimuli [91–99], hence establishing a distinct identity for tumor vessels. For instance, it has been observed that the transcriptional signatures of tumor ECs might vary based on factors such as their location, kind, and malignant grade. In contrast, it is common for tumor vasculature to upregulate the transcription of certain sets of genes that are active in both developmental processes and naturally occurring angiogenesis [100]. Gene expression study revealed the identification of crucial regulators involved in the pro-angiogenic signaling pathways of VEGF and angiopoietin. Notably, VEGFR2, TIE1, and TIE2 were among the key regulators discovered by this analysis. The tumor angiogenesis core gene signature consisted of CLEC14A and CD93, together with endosialin and thrombomodulin [95, 101–106]. The overexpression of the C-type lectin protein family in tumor blood vessels is a commonly observed phenomenon. Multimerin-2, an extracellular matrix protein that is released, has been found to possess binding partners such as CLEC14A, CD93, and endosialin. The regulation of glioma angiogenesis is influenced by the interplay between CD93, MMRN2, and endosialin [107, 108]. Endosialin, which is abundantly expressed in pericytes and acts as a deterrent to fibrosis, potentially contributes to the modulation of the extracellular matrix [105, 109]. Nevertheless, the generation of endosialin by pericytes amplifies the intravasation of tumor cells and facilitates metastasis, indicating that these two phenomena play contrasting roles in the control of vascular integrity. In contrast, there exists a correlation between CD93 deficiency and heightened permeability [104, 110]. The unique transcriptional response of tumor ECs has the potential to impact both endothelial activation and leukocyte recruitment. The reduction in pro-angiogenic signaling is accompanied by a decrease in the responsiveness of chemokines and adhesion molecules, which are essential for trans-endothelial migration and leukocyte capture [111–114]. The immunological suppression is facilitated by the upregulation of FASL in tumor arteries, which induces apoptosis in cytotoxic T-lymphocytes [115]. The synthesis of Endothelin B in the vasculature of ovarian cancer tumors has been found to hinder the homing of T cells, as has been documented in previous studies [116]. The potential therapeutic efficacy of modulated gene expression in ECs is prompted by the tumor microenvironment, specifically in cerebral malignancies. The expression of a specific collection of genes in ECs of WNT-medulloblastoma tumors leads to an enhanced vulnerability of the tumor to therapy, as well as a weaker blood–brain barrier [117]. Variable proteins have the capacity to modify vascular function and hence hold promise as possible therapeutic targets, given their increased presence in tumor vasculature.

1.10 TUMOR PROLIFERATION VIA GROWTH FACTOR AND CHEMOTHERAPY SIGNALING

The creation of tumor vasculature is induced by a variety of pro-angiogenic chemicals and their corresponding receptors. These substances include VEGF, fibroblast growth factor 2 (FGF-2), chemokines, apelin (APLN), ephrins, PDGF, and angiopoietins. The growth factors that are encompassed within this category are PDGF, FGF-2, and VEGF. In numerous instances, these factors effectively collaborate at different stages of tumor angiogenesis. In this analysis, we will investigate many key pro-angiogenic factors of significant importance.

The placental growth factor (PGF), VEGF-A, VEGF-B, VEGF-C, and other members of the VEGF family are secreted proteins.

1.10.1 ANGIOGENESIS AND ENDOTHELIAL GROWTH FACTORS

Although previously referred to as VPF, VEGF is currently recognized as a potent inducer of angiogenesis. Tumor cells and their adjacent stromal tissues secrete VEGF, a key factor implicated in various aspects of tumorigenesis, including tumor progression, angiogenesis, invasiveness, metastasis, and recurrence [118, 119].

The activation of VEGFR-2 through the EC mechanism under hypoxic conditions plays a critical role in the formation of neovascularization [120]. VEGFR-2 activation induces alterations in endothelial function, including several processes such as survival, proliferation, migration, invasion, permeability, and inflammation. The successful formation of new blood vessels requires precise regulation of cellular processes [121]. Tumor cells have been seen to release VEGF, which triggers the survival and proliferation of ECs through the activation of signaling pathways, including ERK and PI3K/Akt [122, 123]. Various processes, such as the activation of PI3K and Rho GTPases, are triggered in response to VEGFR2, leading to the migration of ECs [124]. Urokinase plasminogen activator, matrix metalloproteinases 2 and 9, and membrane type (MT)-matrix metalloproteinases (MMPs) are synthesized in response to VEGF [123,

125], and they collectively promote cell invasion in the presence of VEGF stimulation. The formation of capillary sprouts during EC migration is facilitated by the action of enzymes, which degrade the basal membrane and extracellular matrix.

In order for VEGF-induced angiogenesis to take place, it is imperative that vascular permeability is elevated, as this process is crucial for the maintenance of proper tissue function. Multiple mechanisms are involved in this process, including junctional remodeling, fenestrae formation, and the activation of vesicula-vascular organelles (VVOs) by VEGF, resulting in an increase in vascular permeability [126]. Dysregulation of interstitial pressure and impaired treatment delivery might directly impact the tumor microenvironment in pathological situations such as cancer [127, 128]. The presence of blood vessels with compromised integrity can potentially facilitate the dissemination of tumor cells through the circulatory system, hence enabling their metastasis to distant organs.

The permeability of blood arteries is closely linked to the occurrence of vascular inflammation. The activation of the transcription factor NFAT in ECs can potentially occur through the PLC/calcineurin pathway when stimulated by VEGF. However, it is important to note that VEGF is not classified as an inflammatory cytokine [129]. This study investigates the impact of IL-1 on the modulation of gene expression related to inflammatory processes. The available evidence indicates that the activation of the inflammasome leads to the activation of NF-kB downstream of Akt, which plays a role in the process of angiogenesis [123].

The degree to which PlGF, a member of the VEGF family, exerts an impact on tumor angiogenesis is a subject of ongoing scholarly discussion. The promotion of pathological angiogenesis can be attributed to PlGF through the cross-talk between VEGFR-1 and VEGFR-2, as has been documented in previous research [130]. However, it is worth noting that some investigations have suggested that PlGF has antiangiogenic effects [131]. The efficacy of anti-PlGF treatment in lowering angiogenesis and inhibiting tumor development has yielded inconsistent results in preclinical tumor models [132, 133].

1.10.2 FIBEROBLAST GROWTH FACTOR-2

The mammalian FGF family consists of a total of 22 members, of which 18 have been found to exhibit a strong binding affinity toward the Fgfr1-4,

Fgfr2, Fgfr3, and Fgfr4 receptors [134]. Cells secrete and deposit a distinct category of glycoproteins that facilitate the release of FGFs into the adjacent extracellular environment. Heparinases, proteases, or specific FGF-binding proteins have the ability to liberate FGFs from the extracellular matrix. The stability of the FGF-FGFR interaction is maintained by the subsequent binding of these FGFs to heparan sulfate proteoglycans (HPSGs) on the surface of the cell [135].

The presence of FGFs and their corresponding receptors (FGFRs) can potentially impact both tumor cells and the surrounding stromal tissue. One of the observed outcomes is an increase in metastasis and angiogenesis (source: Reference [134]). Cell growth and resistance to apoptosis are two more factors to consider. Extensive research has been conducted on both benign and malignant disorders in order to gain a deeper understanding of pro-angiogenic mediators, including fibroblast growth factor 2 (bFGF) [136, 137]. Paracrine signaling between tumor and stromal cells has the potential to exert an influence on ECs. Two potential mechanisms for this phenomenon are the stimulation of the extracellular matrix and the release of FGF-2. MMPs, such as plasminogen activator protein and collagenase, have been observed to facilitate the process of angiogenesis through the involvement of FGF-2 [134]. VEGF is among the other MMPs. The formation, proliferation, and migration of blood and lymphatic vessels are regulated by FGF signaling, which is dependent on the presence of MYC [138]. The expression of FGF is significantly elevated within the tumor, which increases the likelihood of developing resistance to antiangiogenic therapy. Cancer cells have the ability to evade VEGF-targeted treatment by activating the pro-angiogenic FGF signaling pathway. In preclinical studies using animal models of breast cancer, the inhibition of FGF receptors was found to result in a reduction in the number of blood vessels within tumors, hence enhancing the vulnerability of the tumors to anti-VEGF therapy [139].

1.10.3 PLATELET-DERIVED GROWTH FACTOR (PDGF)

There exist a collective of four constituents within the PDGF family, each of which possesses a shared characteristic of being capable of binding heparin. When activated, platelets, ECs, epithelial cells, and glial cells release PDGF. Subsequently, this cytokine exerts its effects on several cell types, such as fibroblasts, pericytes, smooth muscles, glia, and mesangial cells [140]. In addition to several biological activities, such as angiogenesis, the tyrosine kinase receptors PDGFR and PDGFR contribute to the enhancement of vascular maturation and pericyte recruitment through their interaction with PDGF [141]. The study conducted on the angiogenic functions of the PDGF family in living organisms has predominantly centered around the PDGF-B/PDGFR axis. The study revealed that mice lacking the components of the PDGF-B/PDGFR pathway exhibited vascular leakage and micro-hemorrhage [142], ultimately resulting in mortality. This underscores the importance of PDGF in maintaining proper artery function.

The promotion of cancer is facilitated by both the autocrine and paracrine effects of PDGF and PDGFR on malignant cells as well as the supportive stromal cells. The augmentation in the quantity of ECs associated with tumors resulted in the stimulation of VEGF production and facilitated angiogenesis in a murine model of glioma. This was achieved by the attraction of pericytes to the newly formed blood vessels [143].

1.10.4 BLOOD VESSEL-FORMING PROTEINS (ANGIOPOIETINS)

Crucial regulators of malignant tumors and the following process of angiogenesis are angiogenesis-related growth factors (ANGPTs). The ligands for the three primary human angiopoietins are ANGPT-1, ANGPT-2, and ANGPT-4 [144, 145]. TIE-2 is the more extensively investigated of the two TIEs involved in the mediation of angiopoietin signaling [146].

While both ANGPT-1 and ANGPT-2 have binding affinity toward TIE-2, it is conceivable that their individual mechanisms of action may differ. The presence of ANGPT-1 facilitates the Akt/survivin pathway, which plays a crucial role in the maintenance and maturation of recently developed blood vessels. Nevertheless, there is evidence linking ANGPT-2 to vascular instability and angiogenesis [147]. In response to hypoxia and VEGF, activated ECs and the tumor-associated vasculature in several types of patient malignancies have exhibited increased levels of ANGPT-2 [147]. The autocrine regulation of the inflammatory response in ECs is enhanced by ANGPT-2, leading to an increase in adhesion molecules and rendering them more susceptible to tumor necrosis factor (TNF), as exemplified by previous studies [148].

According to a study, individuals diagnosed with glioblastoma who exhibit elevated levels of ANGPT-2 expression demonstrate reduced efficacy of anti-VEGF medicine and an increased propensity for treatment resistance [149]. Preclinical experiments have demonstrated that the simultaneous suppression of ANGPT-2 and VEGFR2 yields favorable outcomes in tumor development. In experimental studies involving mice with gliomas, it has been observed that the concurrent inhibition of ANGPT-2 and VEGFR2 leads to tumor shrinkage, preservation of normal arteries, and prevention of macrophage recruitment. These combined effects have been associated with enhanced survival outcomes [150, 151]. Several mouse tumors of various sorts have exhibited encouraging outcomes when the combination of the medication [152] and the targeting of ANGPT-2/VEGFR2 is employed.

1.10.5 PHRIN-MEDIATED SIGNALING AND EPHRINS

The human Eph superfamily receptor tyrosine kinases consist of a total of 14 distinct types of transmembrane proteins. The Eph proteins, namely EphA and EphB, can be categorized into two distinct categories based on their sequence homologies and their ability to interact with their ephrin-binding ligands. The EphA subgroup consists of 10 members, namely EphA1–A10, while the EphB subgroup has five members, specifically EphB1–A5 (including EphB1-B4, B6) [153]. Ephs have a distinctive characteristic among tyrosine kinases due to their ligands being associated with the cell membrane. Moreover, these ligands can be categorized into two distinct types based on their specific mechanisms of attachment to the plasma membrane. The glycosylphosphatidylinositol (GPI) domain connects the six ephrin-A (A1–A6) proteins together. Ephrins B1–B3 are classified under this subclass due to their shared characteristics as type 1 transmembrane proteins, which necessitate a single translocation event across the cellular membrane.

The reciprocal communication between Eph receptors and their ligands, which are anchored to the cell membrane, can function as a bidirectional signaling mechanism between neighboring cells, regulating determinations regarding the cellular destiny. The term "forward signal" refers to the result of transduction in cells that possess receptor-binding capabilities, whereas the concept of a "reverse signal" is elucidated in Reference [153] and pertains to the transduction process occurring in cells expressing the ligands upon interaction with receptors.

Ephrins and Eph receptors are involved in various processes during embryogenesis, such as axon guidance, tissue differentiation, angiogenesis, and cell migration [154, 155]. The Eph/ephrins system has been demonstrated to have a pivotal role in the context of pathogenic disorders such as cancer [156, 157]. Various types of human cancer, such as melanoma, breast, colon, liver, brain, and prostate tumors, have been documented to exhibit elevated levels of Ephrins and Eph receptors. The downregulation of Eph receptors has been observed to be linked with an elevated occurrence of metastasis in various types of malignancies, such as colorectal cancer, prostate carcinoma, and melanoma [158, 159].

Numerous studies have provided evidence supporting the involvement of the Eph/ephrins pathway in the process of tumor angiogenesis. The initial demonstration of EphA2 and ephrinA1 expression in the vasculature of tumors established preclinical models for breast cancer and Kaposi's sarcoma [160]. The inhibition of tumor angiogenesis can be achieved through the elevation of serum EphA receptor levels, hence impeding tumor formation and cell proliferation [161–163].

The signaling pathway involving EphB4-ephrinB2 has been associated with heightened tumor angiogenesis, tumor development, and enhanced resistance to antiangiogenic therapy [164, 165]. The preclinical examination of glioma demonstrated a correlation between the upregulation of EphB4 and alterations in vascular morphogenesis, pericyte coverage, cellular proliferation, and apoptosis. These modifications collectively contributed to the development of a treatment-resistant vascular phenotype. According to recent studies, it has been discovered that the perivascular invasion and proliferation of glioblastoma stem-like cells are regulated by ephrinB2 [166].

Another noteworthy discovery pertains to the interconnectedness between ephrins and VEGF signaling. Furthermore, previous studies have demonstrated that ephrin-B2 has the potential to impede VEGF signaling through the augmentation of VEGFR2 and VEGFR3 internalization in both healthy tissues and malignant tumors [167, 168].

1.10.6 PHRINS AND EPHRINS ARE INVOLVED IN THE SIGNALING PROCESS

APLN has been identified as one of the endogenous peptide ligands for G protein-coupled receptors [169]. The APLN/APLNR signaling system is hypothesized to exert influence on embryonic angiogenesis, as evidenced by the particular expression of APLNR in ECs and the involvement of

APLN in the regulation of vascular patterning [170–172]. The APLN/APLNR signaling system is of significant importance in multiple physiological processes, including but not limited to heart function, angiogenesis, metabolic regulation, and fluid balance maintenance [173].

Moreover, the upregulation of APLN levels leads to the activation of the APLN/APLNR pathway, which not only promotes the proliferation of cancer cells and tumor endothelium cells, but also results in unfavorable clinical outcomes [174–179]. Prior research has presented empirical support for the proposition that hypoxia has a stimulating impact on the growth of tumors through various pathways, while also affecting the expression of APLN within cancer cells. The presence of APLN directly facilitates the processes of cancer cell proliferation, migration, and metastasis. The identified effects of APLN include the enhancement of tumor development through its promotion of neoangiogenesis and microvascular proliferation within the tumor [180–183].

The efficacy of cancer therapy targeting the APLN/APLNR pathway is dependent on the specific tumor being treated [184]. The function of APLN in breast and lung cancers has been associated with its capacity to suppress tumor growth and metastasis, while also improving vascular function, via antiangiogenic therapy [185]. The augmentation of tumor cell invasiveness in glioma model organisms was seen following the targeted modulation of APLN, specifically in tumor cells that had positive APLNR expression. The simultaneous targeting of VEGFR2 and APLN in mice with gliomas led to an improved survival rate, as reported in a study [186]. Prior research has established that the suppression of APLNR by the use of competitive antagonists results in a decrease in tumor growth in mouse models [187]. In a specific subgroup of patients, the examination of renal cell carcinoma found a negative relationship between APLNR expression and tumor PD-L1 expression [175]. This observation suggests that the signaling pathway including APLN/APLNR may have a substantial impact on the regulation of immunological processes, therefore justifying the need for additional research.

1.10.7 CHEMICAL MESSENGERS (CHEMOKINES)

G-protein-coupled chemokine receptors are a diverse group of tiny secreted proteins within the family of proteins. The receptors exhibit seven discrete transmembrane topologies and possess conserved cysteine residues. The four subclasses of chemokines are CC, CXC, XC, and CX3C, which are categorized based on the number of amino acids present between each cysteine residue that forms the fundamental structural disulfide linkages [188]. Both the ELR-positive (ELR+) and ELR-negative (ELR–) subgroups of CXC chemokines possess a conserved Glu-Leu-Arg motif situated in the N-terminus, just preceding the initial cysteine residue. This motif plays a crucial role in regulating chemotaxis across the endothelium. Chemokines facilitate the migration of progenitor cells and leukocytes expressing chemokine receptors to precise anatomical locations. Chemokines play a role in cancer angiogenesis by either directly binding to EC receptors or indirectly recruiting inflammatory cells and progenitors to the tumor site.

The chemokines CXCL1, CXCL2, and CXCL8, along with ELR, induce angiogenesis through their interaction with CXCR2 receptors [189]. The presence of CXCR2 expression on tumor vasculature has been documented in several types of malignancies [190, 191]. The cancers encompassed in this category are breast, lung, and prostate cancers. The inhibition of CXCR2 in a murine model of hereditary pancreatic ductal adenocarcinoma resulted in a deceleration of tumor growth and angiogenesis, as reported in a previous study [192]. The researchers noticed that excessive activation of CXCR2 led to an increase in VEGF synthesis, subsequently resulting in heightened angiogenesis in human ovarian cancer cells (CXCR2 [193]). Neutrophils, due to their potential expression of CXCR2 and involvement in leukocyte arrest prior to trans-endothelial migration, may indirectly promote angiogenesis through the stimulation of ELR+ chemokines [194]. Previous studies have demonstrated the significance of CXCL8 in the process of angiogenesis in various types of tumors [195, 196]. Based on available data, it has been observed that ECs secrete VEGF, matrix MMP-2, and MMP-9 in order to facilitate the process of angiogenesis [196]. When neutrophils are recruited, the chemokine CXCL8 induces a respiratory burst.

In the context of CXC ELR-chemokines, it is noteworthy that only CXCL12/SDF1, which exhibits binding affinity toward CXCR4, demonstrates angiostatic properties. In the context of comparing tumor tip cells and their associated vasculature, it has been observed that CXCR4 is notably overrepresented, as indicated by a study with a sample size [197].

1.11 CONCLUSION

Due to the hostile environment created by tumor arteries that are typically anergic and dysfunctional in the presence of inflammatory stimuli, cancer growth and treatment methods are made more difficult. Angiogenesis-inducing signaling pathways are the focus of current vascular targeting methods. While various antiangiogenic medications have been licensed, their effectiveness is limited by innate and acquired resistance to treatment. To overcome the challenges that hinder effective management of the angiogenic response to cancer treatment, a greater understanding of the vascular character of tumors and the processes involved in treatment response and resistance is required. Vascular targeting, on the other hand, needs improvement so that new, nontraditional approaches can be used to attack tumor blood vessels. It is possible that antiangiogenic medication will need to be adjusted or that new medicines will need to be created to better suit the current cancer treatment, directly target tumor vasculature, or enhance their functionality.

KEYWORDS

- **angiogenesis**
- **carcinoma**
- **neovascularization**
- **tumors**
- **vascular mimicry**
- **vascularization**

REFERENCES

1. Newport, E., Pedrosa, A. R., Lees, D., Dukinfield, M., Carter, E., Gomez-Escudero, J., ... & Hodivala-Dilke, K. (2022). Elucidating the role of the kinase activity of endothelial cell focal adhesion kinase in angiocrine signalling and tumor growth. *The Journal of Pathology, 256*(2), 235–247.
2. Folkman, J. (1971). Isolation of a tumor factor responsible for angiogenesis. *Journal of Experimental Medicine, 133*(2), 275–288.

3. Abou-Fadel, J., Vasquez, M., Grajeda, B., Ellis, C., & Zhang, J. (2019). Systems-wide analysis unravels the new roles of CCM signal complex (CSC). *Heliyon, 5*(12).
4. Hsu, J. Y., & Wakelee, H. A. (2009). Monoclonal antibodies targeting vascular endothelial growth factor: Current status and future challenges in cancer therapy. *BioDrugs, 23*, 289–304.
5. Qian, C. N., Tan, M. H., Yang, J. P., & Cao, Y. (2016). Revisiting tumor angiogenesis: Vessel co-option, vessel remodeling, and cancer cell-derived vasculature formation. *Chinese Journal of Cancer, 35*, 1–6.
6. Shchors, K., & Evan, G. (2007). Tumor angiogenesis: cause or consequence of cancer?. *Cancer Research, 67*(15), 7059–7061.
7. Hunter, K. E., Quick, M. L., Sadanandam, A., Hanahan, D., & Joyce, J. A. (2013). Identification and characterization of poorly differentiated invasive carcinomas in a mouse model of pancreatic neuroendocrine tumorigenesis. *PLoS One, 8*(5), e64472.
8. Buicko, J. L., Finnerty, B. M., Zhang, T., Kim, B. J., Fahey III, T. J., & Du, Y. C. (2019). Insights into the biology and treatment strategies of pancreatic neuroendocrine tumors. *Annals of Pancreatic Cancer, 2*.
9. Frank, R. N., Turczyn, T. J., & Das, A. (1990). Pericyte coverage of retinal and cerebral capillaries. *Investigative Ophthalmology & Visual Science, 31*(6), 999–1007.
10. Tammela, T. (2008). Blocking VEGFR-3 suppresses angiogenic sprouting and vascular network formation. *Nature, 454*(7204), 656–660.
11. Strasser, G. A., Kaminker, J. S., & Tessier-Lavigne, M. (2010). Microarray analysis of retinal endothelial tip cells identifies CXCR11 as a mediator of tip cell morphology and branching. *Blood, 115*(24), 5102–5110.
12. Shawber, C. J. (2007). Notch alters VEGF responsiveness in human and murine endothelial cells by direct regulation of VEGFR-3 expression. *Journal of Clinical Investigation, 117*(11), 3369–3382.
13. Jakobsson, L. (2010). Endothelial cells dynamically compete for the tip cell position during angiogenic sprouting. *Nature Cell Biology, 12*(10), 943–953.
14. Hellstrom, M. (2007). Dll4 signalling through Notch1 regulates formation of tip cells during angiogenesis. *Nature, 445*(7129), 776–780.
15. Lobov, I. B. (2007). Delta-like ligand 4 (Dll4) is induced by VEGF as a negative regulator of angiogenic sprouting. *Proceedings of the National Academy of Science of the United States of America, 104*(9), 3219–3224.
16. Harrington, L. S. (2008). Regulation of multiple angiogenic pathways by Dll4 and Notch in human umbilical vein endothelial cells. *Microvascular Research, 75*(2), 144–154.
17. Funahashi, Y. (2010). Notch regulates the angiogenic response via induction of VEGFR-1. *Journal of Angiogenes Research, 2*(1), 3
18. Gerhardt, H. (2003). VEGF guides angiogenic sprouting utilizing endothelial tip cell flopodia. *Journal of Cell Biology, 161*(6), 1163–1177.
19. Zhao, L., Chen, H., Lu, L., Wang, L., Zhang, X., & Guo, X. (2021). New insights into the role of co-receptor neuropilins in tumour angiogenesis and lymphangiogenesis and targeted therapy strategies. *Journal of Drug Targeting, 29*(2), 155–167.
20. Kofler, N. M., & Simons, M. (2015). Angiogenesis versus arteriogenesis: Neuropilin 1 modulation of VEGF signaling. *F1000prime Reports, 7*, 26.

21. Siebel, C., & Lendahl, U. (2017). Notch signaling in development, tissue homeostasis, and disease. *Physiological Reviews, 97*(4), 1235–1294.
22. Herwig, L. (2011). Distinct cellular mechanisms of blood vessel fusion in the zebrafish embryo. *Current Biology, 21*(22), 1942–1948.
23. Kochhan, E. (2013). Blood fow changes coincide with cellular rearrangements during blood vessel pruning in zebrafsh embryos. *PLoS One, 8*(10), e75060.
24. Lenard, A. (2015). Endothelial cell self-fusion during vascular pruning. *PLoS Biology, 13*(4), e1002126.
25. Hoelzle, M. K., & Svitkina, T. (2012). The cytoskeletal mechanisms of cell–cell junction formation in endothelial cells. *Molecular Biology of the Cell, 23*(2), 310–323.
26. Harris, E. S., & Nelson, W. J. (2010). VE-cadherin: At the front, center, and sides of endothelial cell organization and function. *Current Opinion in Cell Biology*, *22*(5), 651–658.
27. Blum, Y. (2008). Complex cell rearrangements during intersegmental vessel sprouting and vessel fusion in the zebrafsh embryo. *Developmental Biology, 316*(2), 312–322.
28. Betz, C., & et al. (2016). Cell behaviors and dynamics during angiogenesis. *Development, 143*(13), 2249–2260.
29. Patan, S. (1992). Intussusceptive microvascular growth: A common alternative to capillary sprouting. *Archives of Histology and Cytology*, *55*(Suppl), 65–75.
30. Burri, P. H., & Tarek, M. R. (1990). A novel mechanism of capillary growth in the rat pulmonary microcirculation. *The Anatomical Record*, *228*(1), 35–45.
31. Appelmann, I., Liersch, R., Kessler, T., Mesters, R. M., & Berdel, W. E. (2010). Angiogenesis inhibition in cancer therapy: Platelet-derived growth factor (PDGF) and vascular endothelial growth factor (VEGF) and their receptors: Biological functions and role in malignancy. *Angiogenesis Inhibition,* 51–81.
32. Kunze, R., & Marti, H. H. (2019). Angioneurins–key regulators of blood–brain barrier integrity during hypoxic and ischemic brain injury. *Progress in Neurobiology, 178*, 101611.
33. Tomanek, R. J. (2012). *Coronary vasculature: Development, structure-function, and adaptations* (p 19). Springer Science & Business Media.
34. Ribatti, D. (2005). Microvascular density, vascular endothelial growth factor immunoreactivity in tumor cells, vessel diameter and intussusceptive microvascular growth in primary melanoma. *Oncology Reports, 14*(1), 81–84.
35. Nico, B. (2010). Intussusceptive microvascular growth in human glioma. *Clinical and Experimental Medicine, 10*(2), 93–98.
36. Saravanan, S., Vimalraj, S., Pavani, K., Nikarika, R., & Sumantran, V. N. (2020). Intussusceptive angiogenesis as a key therapeutic target for cancer therapy. *Life Sciences, 252*, 117670.
37. Djonov, V. (2001). MMP-19: Cellular localization of a novel metalloproteinase within normal breast tissue and mammary gland tumours. *Journal of Pathology, 195*(2), 147–155.
38. Naito, H., Iba, T., & Takakura, N. (2020). Mechanisms of new blood-vessel formation and proliferative heterogeneity of endothelial cells. *International Immunology, 32*(5), 295–305.

39. Reale, A., Melaccio, A., Lamanuzzi, A., Saltarella, I., Dammacco, F., Vacca, A., & Ria, R. (2016). Functional and biological role of endothelial precursor cells in tumour progression: A new potential therapeutic target in haematological malignancies. *Stem Cells International, 2016*, 7954580.
40 Tepper, O. M., Capla, J. M., Galiano, R. D., Ceradini, D. J., Callaghan, M. J., Kleinman, M. E., & Gurtner, G. C. (2005). Adult vasculogenesis occurs through in situ recruitment, proliferation, and tubulization of circulating bone marrow–derived cells. *Blood, 105*(3), 1068–1077.
41. Tomanek, R. J., & Schatteman, G. C. (2000). Angiogenesis: New insights and therapeutic potential. *The Anatomical Record, 261*(3), 126–135.
42. Bussolati, B., Grange, C., & Camussi, G. (2011). Tumor exploits alternative strategies to achieve vascularization. *FASEB Journal, 25*(9), 2874–2882.
43. Kioi, M. (2010). Inhibition of vasculogenesis, but not angiogenesis, prevents the recurrence of glioblastoma after irradiation in mice. *Journal of Clinical Investigation, 120*(3), 694–705.
44. Ahn, J. B. (2010). Circulating endothelial progenitor cells (EPC) for tumor vasculogenesis in gastric cancer patients. *Cancer Letter, 288*(1), 124–132.
45. Greenfeld, J. P., Cobb, W. S., & Lyden, D. (2010). Resisting arrest: A switch from angiogenesis to vasculogenesis in recurrent malignant gliomas. *Journal of Clinical Investigation, 120*(3), 663–667.
46. Chopra, H. (2018). Insights into endothelial progenitor cells: Origin, classifcation, potentials, and prospects. *Stem Cells International, 2018*, 9847015.
47. Schmidt, A., Brixius, K., & Bloch, W. (2007). Endothelial precursor cell migration during vasculogenesis. *Circulation Research, 101*(2), 125–136.
48. Romagnani, P. (2005). CD14 + CD34low cells with stem cell phenotypic and functional features are the major source of circulating endothelial progenitors. *Circulation Research, 97*(4), 314–322.
49. Shin, J. W. (2005). Isolation of endothelial progenitor cells from cord blood and induction of diferentiation by ex vivo expansion. *Yonsei Medical Journal, 46*(2), 260–267.
50. Urbich, C., & Dimmeler, S. (2004). Endothelial progenitor cells: Characterization and role in vascular biology. *Circulation Research, 95*(4), 343–353.
51. Reale, A. (2016). Functional and biological role of endothelial precursor cells in tumour progression: A new potential therapeutic target in haematological malignancies. *Stem Cells International, 2016*, 7954580.
52. Moschetta, M., Mishima, Y., Sahin, I., Manier, S., Glavey, S., Vacca, A., Roccaro, A. M., & Ghobrial, I. M. (2014). Role of endothelial progenitor cells in cancer progression. *Biochimica et Biophysica Acta (BBA)-Reviews on Cancer, 1846*(1), 26–39.
53. Miller-Kasprzak, E., & Jagodziński, P. P. (2007). Endothelial progenitor cells as a new agent contributing to vascular repair. *Archivum Immunologiae et Therapiae Experimentalis, 55*, 247–259.
54. Ribatti, D. (2004). The involvement of endothelial progenitor cells in tumor angiogenesis. *Journal of Cellular and Molecular Medicine, 8*(3), 294–300.
55. Chang, E. I. (2007). Hypoxia, hormones, and endothelial progenitor cells in hemangioma. *Lymphatic Research and Biology, 5*(4), 237–243.

56. Spring, H. (2005). Chemokines direct endothelial progenitors into tumor neovessels. *Proceedings of the National Academy of Sciences of the United States of America, 102*(50), 18111–18116.
57. Nakamura, N. (2009). Adiponectin promotes migration activities of endothelial progenitor cells via Cdc42/Rac1. *FEBS Letter, 583*(15), 2457–2463.
58. Luo, Q., Wang, J., Zhao, W., Peng, Z., Liu, X., Li, B., Zhang, H., Shan, B., Zhang, C., & Duan, C. (2020). Vasculogenic mimicry in carcinogenesis and clinical applications. *Journal of Hematology & Oncology, 13*, 1–5.
59. Zhang, X., Zhang, J., Zhou, H., Fan, G., & Li, Q. (2019). Molecular mechanisms and anticancer therapeutic strategies in vasculogenic mimicry. *Journal of Cancer, 10*(25), 6327.
60. Lugano, R., Ramachandran, M., & Dimberg, A. (2020). Tumor angiogenesis: Causes, consequences, challenges and opportunities. *Cellular and Molecular Life Sciences, 77*, 1745–1770.
61. Fan, Y. L., Zheng, M., Tang, Y. L., & Liang, X. H. (2013). A new perspective of vasculogenic mimicry: EMT and cancer stem cells. *Oncology Letters, 6*(5), 1174–1180.
62. Delgado-Bellido, D., Serrano-Saenz, S., Fernández-Cortés, M., & Oliver, F. J. (2017). Vasculogenic mimicry signaling revisited: Focus on non-vascular VE-cadherin. *Molecular Cancer, 16*(1), 1–4.
63. Giordo, R., Wehbe, Z., Paliogiannis, P., Eid, A. H., Mangoni, A. A., & Pintus, G. (2022). Nano-targeting vascular remodeling in cancer: Recent developments and future directions. *Seminars in Cancer Biology, 86*, 784–804.
64. Fausto, N. (2000). Vasculogenic mimicry in tumors. Fact or artifact? *The American Journal of Pathology, 156*(2), 359.
65. Liu, T. J., Sun, B. C., Zhao, X. L., Zhao, X. M., Sun, T., Gu, Q., Yao, Z., Dong, X. Y., Zhao, N., & Liu, N. (2013). CD133+ cells with cancer stem cell characteristics associates with vasculogenic mimicry in triple-negative breast cancer. *Oncogene, 32*(5), 544–553.
66. Imani, S., Liu, S., Maghsoudloo, M., & Wen, Q. (2022). Histochemical staining of vasculogenic mimicry. *Vasculogenic Mimicry: Methods and Protocols, 1*, 107–120.
67. Angara, K., Borin, T. F., & Arbab, A. S. (2017). Vascular mimicry: A novel neovascularization mechanism driving anti-angiogenic therapy (AAT) resistance in glioblastoma. *Translational Oncology, 10*(4), 650–660.
68. Valyi-Nagy, K. (2012). Stem cell marker CD271 is expressed by vasculogenic mimicry-forming uveal melanoma cells in threedimensional cultures. *Molecular Vision, 18*, 588–592.
69. Lin, A. Y. (2005). Distinguishing fibrovascular septa from vasculogenic mimicry patterns. *Archives of Pathology and Laboratory Medicine, 129*(7), 884–892.
70. Comito, G. (2011). HIF-1alpha stabilization by mitochondrial ROS promotes Met-dependent invasive growth and vasculogenic mimicry in melanoma cells. *Free Radical Biology and Medicine, 51*(4), 893–904.
71. Angara, K. (2017). Vascular mimicry in glioblastoma following anti-angiogenic and anti-20-HETE therapies. *Histology and Histopathology, 32*(9), 917–928.
72. Li, M. (2010). Vasculogenic mimicry: A new prognostic sign of gastric adenocarcinoma. *Pathology and Oncology Research, 16*(2), 259–266.

73. Ping, Y. F., & Bian, X. W. (2011). Concise review: Contribution of cancer stem cells to neovascularization. *Stem Cells, 29*(6), 888–894.
74. Cheung, C., & Sinha, S. (2011). Human embryonic stem cell-derived vascular smooth muscle cells in therapeutic neovascularisation. *Journal of Molecular and Cellular Cardiology, 51*(5), 651–64.
75. Kotiyal, S., & Bhattacharya, S. (2015). Epithelial mesenchymal transition and vascular mimicry in breast cancer stem cells. *Critical Review in Eukaryotic Gene Expression, 25*(3), 269–280.
76. Cao, Y. (2020) Neural is fundamental: Neural stemness as the ground state of cell tumorigenicity and differentiation potential. *Stem Cell Reviews and Reports, 7*, 1–9.
77. Zhao, Y. (2010). Endothelial cell transdifferentiation of human glioma stem progenitor cells in vitro. *Brain Research Bulletin, 82*(5–6), 308–312.
78. Sattiraju, A., Sai, K. K., & Mintz, A. (2017). Glioblastoma stem cells and their microenvironment. *Advances in Experimental Medicine and Biology, 1041*, 119–40.
79. Plate, K. H., Scholz, A., & Dumont, D. J. (2012). Tumor angiogenesis and anti-angiogenic therapy in malignant gliomas revisited. *Acta Neuropathologica, 124*, 763-775.
80. De Palma, M. (2005). Tie2 identifes a hematopoietic lineage of proangiogenic monocytes required for tumor vessel formation and a mesenchymal population of pericyte progenitors. *Cancer Cell, 8*(3), 211–226.
81. Würth, R., Bajetto, A., Harrison, J. K., Barbieri, F., & Florio, T. (2014). CXCL12 modulation of CXCR4 and CXCR7 activity in human glioblastoma stem-like cells and regulation of the tumor microenvironment. *Frontiers in Cellular Neuroscience, 28*(8), 144.
82. Pearce, J. A., & Thomsen, S. L. (2000). Blood vessel architectural features and their effects on thermal phenomena. In *Matching the Energy Source to the Clinical Need: A Critical Review* (Vol. 10297, pp. 122–168).
83. Baluk, P., Hashizume, H., & McDonald, D. M. (2005). Cellular abnormalities of blood vessels as targets in cancer. *Current Opinion in Genetics & Development, 15*(1), 102–111.
84. Kimura, H. (1996). Fluctuations in red cell fux in tumor microvessels can lead to transient hypoxia and reoxygenation in tumor parenchyma. *Cancer Research, 56*(23), 5522–5528.
85. Bennewith, K. L., & Durand, R. E. (2004). Quantifying transient hypoxia in human tumor xenografts by flow cytometry. *Cancer Research, 64*(17), 6183–6189.
86. Hashizume, H. (2000). Openings between defective endothelial cells explain tumor vessel leakiness. *The American Journal of Patholology, 156*(4), 1363–1380.
87. Padera, T. P. (2004). Pathology: Cancer cells compress intratumour vessels. *Nature, 427*(6976), 695.
88. Abramsson, A. (2002). Analysis of mural cell recruitment to tumor vessels. *Circulation, 105*(1), 112–117.
89. Morikawa, S. (2002). Abnormalities in pericytes on blood vessels and endothelial sprouts in tumors. *American Journal of Pathology, 160*(3), 985–1000.
90. Baluk, P. (2003). Abnormalities of basement membrane on blood vessels and endothelial sprouts in tumors. *American Journal of Pathology, 163*(5), 1801–1815.

91. Fukumura, D., Jain, R. K. (2007). Tumor microenvironment abnormalities: Causes, consequences, and strategies to normalize. *Journal of Cellular Biochemistry, 101*(4), 937–949.
92. Conway, E. M., Collen, D., & Carmeliet, P. (2001). Molecular mechanisms of blood vessel growth. *Cardiovascular Research, 49*(3), 507–521.
93. Herbert, S. P., & Stainier, D. Y. (2011). Molecular control of endothelial cell behaviour during blood vessel morphogenesis. *Nature Reviews Molecular Cell Biology, 12*(9), 551–564.
94. Brown, J. M., & Giaccia, A. J. (1998). The unique physiology of solid tumors: Opportunities (and problems) for cancer therapy. *Cancer Research, 58*(7), 1408–1416.
95. Rensen, S. S., Doevendans, P. A., & Van Eys, G. J. (2007). Regulation and characteristics of vascular smooth muscle cell phenotypic diversity. *Netherlands Heart Journal, 15*, 100–108.
96. Ruhrberg, C., Gerhardt, H., Golding, M., Watson, R., Ioannidou, S., Fujisawa, H., Betsholtz, C., & Shima, D. T. (2002). Spatially restricted patterning cues provided by heparin-binding VEGF-A control blood vessel branching morphogenesis. *Genes & Development, 16*(20), 2684–2698.
97. Zhao, Q. (2018). Single-cell transcriptome analyses reveal endothelial cell heterogeneity in tumors and changes following antiangiogenic treatment. *Cancer Research, 78*(9), 2370–2382.
98. Buckanovich, R. J. (2007). Tumor vascular proteins as biomarkers in ovarian cancer. *Journal of Clinical Oncology, 25*(7), 852–861.
99. Zhang, L. (2018). IDH mutation status is associated with distinct vascular gene expression signatures in lower-grade gliomas. *Neuro Oncology, 20*(11), 1505–1516.
100. Masiero, M. (2013). A core human primary tumor angiogenesis signature identifes the endothelial orphan receptor ELTD1 as a key regulator of angiogenesis. *Cancer Cell, 24*(2), 229–241.
101. Hanly, A. M., & Winter, D. C. (2007). The role of thrombomodulin in malignancy. *Seminars in Thrombosis and Hemostasis, 33*(7), 673–679.
102. Maruno, M. (1994). Expression of thrombomodulin in astrocytomas of various malignancy and in gliotic and normal brains. *Journal of Neurooncology, 19*(2), 155–160.
103. Mura, M. (2012). Identification and angiogenic role of the novel tumor endothelial marker CLEC14A. *Oncogene, 31*(3), 293–305.
104. Langenkamp, E. (2015). Elevated expression of the C-type lectin CD93 in the glioblastoma vasculature regulates cytoskeletal rearrangements that enhance vessel function and reduce host survival. *Cancer Research, 75*(21), 4504–4516.
105. Lugano, R. (2018). CD93 promotes beta1 integrin activation and fbronectin fbrillogenesis during tumor angiogenesis. *Journal of Clinical Investigation, 128*(8), 3280–3297.
106. Christian, S. (2008). Endosialin (Tem1) is a marker of tumorassociated myofbroblasts and tumor vessel-associated mural cells. *The American Journal of Pathology, 172*(2), 486–494.
107. Khan, K. A. (2017). Multimerin-2 is a ligand for group 14 family C-type lectins CLEC14A, CD93 and CD248 spanning the endothelial pericyte interface. *Oncogene, 36*(44), 6097–6108.

108. Galvagni, F. (2017). Dissecting the CD93-Multimerin 2 interaction involved in cell adhesion and migration of the activated endothelium. *Matrix Biology, 64*, 112–127.
109. Mogler, C. (2015). Hepatic stellate cell-expressed endosialin balances fbrogenesis and hepatocyte proliferation during liver damage. *EMBO Molecular Medicine, 7*(3), 332–338.
110. Viski, C. (2016). Endosialin-expressing pericytes promote metastatic dissemination. *Cancer Resarch, 76*(18), 5313–5325.
111. Lugano, R., Ramachandran, M., & Dimberg, A. (2020). Tumor angiogenesis: Causes, consequences, challenges and opportunities. *Cellular and Molecular Life Sciences, 77*, 1745–1770.
112. Zhao, Y., Ting, K. K., Coleman, P., Qi, Y., Chen, J., Vadas, M., & Gamble, J. (2021). The tumour vasculature as a target to modulate leucocyte trafficking. *Cancers, 13*(7), 1724.
113. Lecuyer, M. A., Kebir, H., & Prat, A. (2016). Glial influences on BBB functions and molecular players in immune cell trafficking. *Biochimica et Biophysica Acta (BBA)-Molecular Basis of Disease, 1862*(3), 472–482.
114. Dzobo, K. E., Hanford, K. M., & Kroon, J. (2021). Vascular metabolism as driver of atherosclerosis: Linking endothelial metabolism to inflammation. *Immunometabolism, 3*(3), e210020.
115. Kyaw, T., Peter, K., Li, Y., Tipping, P., Toh, B. H., & Bobik, A. (2017). Cytotoxic lymphocytes and atherosclerosis: Significance, mechanisms and therapeutic challenges. *British Journal of Pharmacology, 174*(22), 3956–3972.
116. Kandalaft, L. E., Facciabene, A., Buckanovich, R. J., & Coukos, G. (2019). Endothelin B receptor, a new target in cancer immune therapy. *Clinical Cancer Research, 15*(14), 4521–4528.
117. Phoenix, T. N. (2016). Medulloblastoma genotype dictates blood brain barrier phenotype. *Cancer Cell, 29*(4), 508–522.
118. Zhao, Y., & Adjei, A. A. (2015). Targeting angiogenesis in cancer therapy: Moving beyond vascular endothelial growth factor. *The Oncologist, 20*(6), 660–673.
119. Jiang, X., Wang. J., Deng, X., Xiong, F., Zhang, S., Gong, Z., Li, X., Cao, K., Deng, H., He, Y., & Liao, Q. (2020). The role of microenvironment in tumor angiogenesis. *Journal of Experimental & Clinical Cancer Research, 39*(1), 1–9.
120. Ferrara, N. (2004). Vascular endothelial growth factor: basic science and clinical progress. *Endocrine Reviews, 25*(4), 581–611.
121. Claesson-Welsh, L., & Welsh, M. (2013). VEGFA and tumour angiogenesis. *Journal of Internal Medicine, 273*(2), 114–127.
122. Lee, S. H., Jeong, D., Han, Y. S., & Baek, M. J. (2015). Pivotal role of vascular endothelial growth factor pathway in tumor angiogenesis. *Annals of Surgical Treatment and Research, 89*(1), 1–8.
123. Roskoski, Jr. R. (2007). Vascular endothelial growth factor (VEGF) signaling in tumor progression. *Critical Reviews in Oncology/Hematology, 62*(3), 179–213.
124. Lamalice, L., Le Boeuf, F., & Huot, J. (2007). Endothelial cell migration during angiogenesis. *Circulation Research, 100*(6), 782–794.
125. van Hinsbergh, V. W., & Koolwijk, P. (2008). Endothelial sprouting and angiogenesis: Matrix metalloproteinases in the lead. *Cardiovascular Research, 78*(2), 203–212.

126. Weis, S. M., & Cheresh, D. A. (2005). Pathophysiological consequences of VEGF-induced vascular permeability. *Nature, 437*(7058), 497–504.
127. Böckelmann, L. C., & Schumacher, U. (2019). Targeting tumor interstitial fluid pressure: Will it yield novel successful therapies for solid tumors?. *Expert Opinion on Therapeutic Targets, 23*(12), 1005–1014.
128 . Fernandes, C., Suares, D., & Yergeri, M. C. (2018). Tumor microenvironment targeted nanotherapy. *Frontiers in Pharmacology, 9*, 1230.
129. Hofer, E., & Schweighofer, B. (2007). Signal transduction induced in endothelial cells by growth factor receptors involved in angiogenesis. *Thrombosis and Haemostasis, 97*(3), 355–363.
130. Autiero, M. (2003). Role of PlGF in the intra- and intermolecular cross talk between the VEGF receptors Flt1 and Flk1. *Nature Medicine, 9*(7), 936–943.
131. Schomber, T. (2007). Placental growth factor-1 attenuates vascular endothelial growth factor-A-dependent tumor angiogenesis during beta cell carcinogenesis. *Cancer Research, 67*(22), 10840–10848.
132. Fischer, C. (2007). Anti-PlGF inhibits growth of VEGF(R)- inhibitor-resistant tumors without afecting healthy vessels. *Cell, 131*(3), 463–475.
133. Bais, C. (2010). PlGF blockade does not inhibit angiogenesis during primary tumor growth. *Cell, 141*(1), 166–177.
134. Quintero-Fabián, S., Arreola, R., Becerril-Villanueva, E., Torres-Romero, J. C., Arana-Argáez, V., Lara-Riegos, J., Ramírez-Camacho, M. A., & Alvarez-Sánchez, M. E. (2019). Role of matrix metalloproteinases in angiogenesis and cancer. *Frontiers in Oncology, 9*, 1370.
135. Ornitz, D. M., & Itoh, N. (2015). The fbroblast growth factor signaling pathway. *Wiley Interdisciplinary Reviews: Developmental Biology, 4*(3), 215–266.
136. Presta, M. (2005). Fibroblast growth factor/fbroblast growth factor receptor system in angiogenesis. *Cytokine Growth Factor Review, 16*(2), 159–178.
137. Compagni, A. (2000). Fibroblast growth factors are required for efcient tumor angiogenesis. *Cancer Research, 60*(24), 7163–7169.
138. Yu, P. (2017). FGF-dependent metabolic control of vascular development. *Nature, 545*(7653), 224–228.
139. Incio, J. (2018). Obesity promotes resistance to anti-VEGF therapy in breast cancer by up-regulating IL-6 and potentially FGF-2. *Science Translational Medicine, 10*(432), eaag0945.
140. Alvarez, R. H., Kantarjian, H. M., & Cortes, J. E. (2006). Biology of platelet-derived growth factor and its involvement in disease. *Mayo Clinic Proceedings, 9*, 1241–1257.
141. Franco, M. (2011). Pericytes promote endothelial cell survival through induction of autocrine VEGF-A signaling and Bcl-w expression. *Blood, 118*(10), 2906–2917.
142. Betsholtz, C. (2004). Insight into the physiological functions of PDGF through genetic studies in mice. *Cytokine Growth Factor Review, 15*(4), 215–228.
143. Guo, P. (2003). Platelet-derived growth factor-B enhances glioma angiogenesis by stimulating vascular endothelial growth factor expression in tumor endothelia and by promoting pericyte recruitment. *American Journal of Pathology, 162*(4), 1083–1093.
144. Davis, S. (1996). Isolation of angiopoietin-1, a ligand for the TIE2 receptor, by secretion-trap expression cloning. *Cell, 87*(7), 1161–1169.

145. Bhardwaj, V., Zhang, X., Pandey, V., & Garg, M. (2023). Neo-vascularization-based therapeutic perspectives in advanced ovarian cancer. *Biochimica et Biophysica Acta (BBA)-Reviews on Cancer, 29*, 188888.
146. Kiss, E. A., & Saharinen, P. (2018). Anti-angiogenic targets: Angiopoietin and angiopoietin-receptors. In D. Marmé (Ed.), *Tumor angiogenesis: A key target for cancer therapy* (pp. 1–24). Springer.
147. Lugano, R., Ramachandran, M., & Dimberg, A. (2020). Tumor angiogenesis: Causes, consequences, challenges and opportunities. *Cellular and Molecular Life Sciences, 77*, 1745–1770.
148. Fiedler, U. (2006). Angiopoietin-2 sensitizes endothelial cells to TNF-alpha and has a crucial role in the induction of infammation. *Nature Medicine, 12*(2), 235–239.
149. Chae, S. S. (2010). Angiopoietin-2 interferes with antiVEGFR2-induced vessel normalization and survival beneft in mice bearing gliomas. *Clinical Cancer Research, 16*(14), 3618–3627.
150. Peterson, T. E. (2016). Dual inhibition of Ang-2 and VEGF receptors normalizes tumor vasculature and prolongs survival in glioblastoma by altering macrophages. *Proceedings of the National Academy of Sciences of the United States of America, 113*(16), 4470–4475.
151. Kloepper, J. (2016). Ang- 2/VEGF bispecifc antibody reprograms macrophages and resident microglia to anti-tumor phenotype and prolongs glioblastoma survival. *Proceedings of the National Academy of Sciences of the United States of America, 113*(16), 4476–4481.
152. Wu, F. T. (2016). Efficacy of cotargeting angiopoietin-2 and the VEGF pathway in the adjuvant postsurgical setting for early breast, colorectal, and renal cancers. *Cancer Research, 76*(23), 6988–7000.
153. Kullander, K., & Klein, R. (2002). Mechanisms and functions of Eph and ephrin signalling. *Nature Reviews Molecular Cell Biology, 3*(7), 475–486.
154. Zhang, J., & Hughes, S. E. (2006). Role of the ephrin and Eph receptor tyrosine kinase families in angiogenesis and development of the cardiovascular system. *The Journal of Pathology: A Journal of the Pathological Society of Great Britain and Ireland, 208*(4), 453–461.
155. Cheng, N., Brantley, D. M., & Chen, J. (2002). The ephrins and Eph receptors in angiogenesis. *Cytokine & Growth Factor Reviews, 13*(1), 75–85.
156. Papadakos, S. P., Petrogiannopoulos, L., Pergaris, A., & Theocharis, S. (2022). The EPH/ephrin system in colorectal cancer. *International Journal of Molecular Sciences, 23*(5), 2761.
157. Surawska, H., Ma, P. C., & Salgia, R. (2004). The role of ephrins and Eph receptors in cancer. *Cytokine & Growth Factor Reviews, 15*(6), 419–433.
158. Dong, Y. (2009). Downregulation of EphA1 in colorectal carcinomas correlates with invasion and metastasis. *Modern Pathology, 22*(1), 151–160.
159. Hafner, C. (2003). Loss of EphB6 expression in metastatic melanoma. *International Journal of Oncology, 23*(6), 1553–1559.
160. Herath, N. I., & Boyd, A. W. (2010). The role of Eph receptors and ephrin ligands in colorectal cancer. *International Journal of Cancer, 126*(9), 2003–2011.

161. Tandon, M., Vemula, S. V., & Mittal, S. K. (2011). Emerging strategies for EphA2 receptor targeting for cancer therapeutics. *Expert Opinion on Therapeutic Targets,15*(1), 31–51.
162. Han, B., Zhang, H., Tian, R., Liu, H., Wang, Z., Wang, Z., Tian, J., Cui, Y., Ren, S., Zuo, X., & Tian, R. (2022). Exosomal EPHA2 derived from highly metastatic breast cancer cells promotes angiogenesis by activating the AMPK signaling pathway through Ephrin A1-EPHA2 forward signaling. *Theranostics, 12*(9), 4127.
163. Chen, J. (2012). Regulation of tumor initiation and metastatic progression by Eph receptor tyrosine kinases. *Advances in Cancer Research, 114*, 1–20.
164. Du, E., Li, X., He, S., Li, X., & He, S. (2020). The critical role of the interplays of EphrinB2/EphB4 and VEGF in the induction of angiogenesis. *Molecular Biology Reports, 47*, 4681–4690.
165. Djokovic, D., Trindade, A., Gigante, J., Badenes, M., Silva, L., Liu, R., Li, X., Gong, M., Krasnoperov, V., Gill, P. S., & Duarte, A. (2010). Combination of Dll4/Notch and Ephrin-B2/EphB4 targeted therapy is highly effective in disrupting tumor angiogenesis. *BMC Cancer, 10*(1), 1–2.
166. Krusche, B. (2016). EphrinB2 drives perivascular invasion and proliferation of glioblastoma stem-like cells. *Elife, 5*, e14845.
167. Wang, Y. (2010). Ephrin-B2 controls VEGF-induced angiogenesis and lymphangiogenesis. *Nature, 465*(7297), 483–486.
168. Sawamiphak, S. (2010). Ephrin-B2 regulates VEGFR2 function in developmental and tumour angiogenesis. *Nature, 465*(7297), 487–491.
169. Perjés, Á., Kilpiö, T., Ulvila, J., Magga, J., Alakoski, T., Szabó, Z., Vainio, L., Halmetoja, E., Vuolteenaho, O., Petäjä-Repo, U., & Szokodi, I. (2016). Characterization of apela, a novel endogenous ligand of apelin receptor, in the adult heart. *Basic Research in Cardiology, 111*, 1–2.
170 . Lugano, R., Ramachandran, M., & Dimberg, A. (2020). Tumor angiogenesis: Causes, consequences, challenges and opportunities. *Cellular and Molecular Life Sciences, 77*, 1745–1770.
171. Testa, U., Pelosi, E., Castelli, G. (2020). Endothelial progenitors in the tumor microenvironment. In *Tumor microenvironment: State of the science* (pp. 85–115).
172. Hu, L., Hayashi, Y., Kidoya, H., & Takakura, N. (2021). Endothelial cell-derived Apelin inhibits tumor growth by altering immune cell localization. *Scientific Reports, 11*(1), 14047.
173. Wysocka, M. B., Pietraszek-Gremplewicz, K., & Nowak, D. (2018). The role of apelin in cardiovascular diseases, obesity and cancer. *Frontiers in Physiology, 9*, 557.
174. Chen, H., Wong, C. C., Liu, D., Go, M. Y., Wu, B., Peng, S., Kuang, M., Wong, N., & Yu, J. (2019). APLN promotes hepatocellular carcinoma through activating PI3K/Akt pathway and is a druggable target. *Theranostics, 9*(18), 5246.
175. Kälin, R. E., & Glass, R. (2021). APLN/APLNR signaling controls key pathological parameters of glioblastoma. *Cancers, 13*(15), 3899.
176. Liu, L., Yi, X., Lu, C., Wang, Y., Xiao, Q., Zhang, L., Pang, Y., & Guan, X. (2021). Study progression of apelin/APJ signaling and apela in different types of cancer. *Frontiers in Oncology, 11*, 658253.
177. Uribesalgo, I., Hoffmann, D., Zhang, Y., Kavirayani, A., Lazovic, J., Berta, J., Novatchkova, M., Pai, T. P., Wimmer, R. A., László, V., & Schramek, D. (2019).

Apelin inhibition prevents resistance and metastasis associated with anti-angiogenic therapy. *EMBO Molecular Medicine, 11*(8), e9266.

178. Mastrella, G., Hou, M., Li, M., Stoecklein, V. M., Zdouc, N., Volmar, M. N., Miletic, H., Reinhard Herold-Mende, C. C., Kleber, S., & Eisenhut, K. (2019). Targeting APLN/APLNR improves antiangiogenic efficiency and blunts proinvasive side effects of VEGFA/VEGFR2 blockade in glioblastoma. *Cancer Research, 79*(9), 2298–2313.
179. Lugano, R., Ramachandran, M., & Dimberg, A. (2020). Tumor angiogenesis: Causes, consequences, challenges and opportunities. *Cellular and Molecular Life Sciences, 77*, 1745–1770.
180. Wysocka, M. B., Pietraszek-Gremplewicz, K., & Nowak, D. (2018). The role of apelin in cardiovascular diseases, obesity and cancer. *Frontiers in Physiology, 9*, 557.
181. Masoumi, J., Jafarzadeh, A., Khorramdelazad, H., Abbasloui, M., Abdolalizadeh, J., & Jamali, N. (2020). Role of Apelin/APJ axis in cancer development and progression. *Advances in Medical Sciences, 65*(1), 202–213.
182. Frisch, A., Kälin, S., Monk, R., Radke, J., Heppner, F. L., & Kälin, R. E. (2020). Apelin controls angiogenesis-dependent glioblastoma growth. *International Journal of Molecular Sciences, 21*(11), 4179.
183. Chen, J., Li, Z., Zhao, Q., & Chen, L. (2020). Roles of apelin/APJ system in cancer Biomarker, predictor, and emerging therapeutic target. *Journal of Cellular Physiology, 237*(10), 3734–3751.
184. Sorli, S. C. (2006). Therapeutic potential of interfering with apelin signalling. *Drug Discovery Today, 11*(23–24), 1100–1106.
185. Wysocka, M. B., Pietraszek-Gremplewicz, K., & Nowak, D. (2018). The role of apelin in cardiovascular diseases, obesity and cancer. *Frontiers in Physiology, 9*, 557.
186. Lugano, R., Ramachandran, M., & Dimberg, A. (2020). Tumor angiogenesis: Causes, consequences, challenges and opportunities. *Cellular and Molecular Life Sciences, 77*, 1745–1770.
187. Harford-Wright, E. (2017). Pharmacological targeting of apelin impairs glioblastoma growth. *Brain, 140*(11), 2939–2954.
188. Laing, K. J., & Secombes, C. J. (2004). Chemokines. *Developmental & Comparative Immunology, 28*(5), 443–460.
189. Strieter, R. M., Burdick, M. D., Gomperts, B. N., Belperio, J. A., & Keane, M. P. (2005). CXC chemokines in angiogenesis. *Cytokine & Growth Factor Reviews, 16*(6), 593–609.
190. Angara, K., Borin, T. F., Rashid, M. H., Lebedyeva, I., Ara, R., Lin, P. C., Iskander, A. S., Bollag, R. J., Achyut, B. R., & Arbab, A. S. (2018). CXCR2-expressing tumor cells drive vascular mimicry in antiangiogenic therapy–resistant glioblastoma. *Neoplasia, 20*(10), 1070–1082.
191. Boissière-Michot, F., Jacot, W., Fraisse, J., Gourgou, S., Timaxian, C., & Lazennec, G. (2020). Prognostic value of CXCR2 in breast cancer. *Cancers, 12*(8), 2076.
192. Ijichi, H. (2011). Inhibiting Cxcr2 disrupts tumor-stromal interactions and improves survival in a mouse model of pancreatic ductal adenocarcinoma. *Journal of Clinical Investigation, 121*(10), 4106–4117.

193. Yang, G. (2010). CXCR196 promotes ovarian cancer growth through dysregulated cell cycle, diminished apoptosis, and enhanced angiogenesis. *Clinical Cancer Research, 16*(15), 3875–3886.
194. Smith, M. L., Olson, T. S., & Ley, K. (2004). CXCR197- and E-selectininduced neutrophil arrest during infammation in vivo. *Journal of Experimental Medicine, 200*(7), 935–939.
195. Smith, D. R. (1994). Inhibition of interleukin 8 attenuates angiogenesis in bronchogenic carcinoma. *Journal of Experimental Medicine, 179*(5), 1409–1415.
196. Ha, H., Debnath, B., & Neamati, N. (2017). Role of the CXCL8- CXCR199/2 axis in cancer and infammatory diseases. *Theranostics*, *7*(6), 1543–1588.
197. Xu, J. (2017). Vascular CXCR206 expression promotes vessel sprouting and sensitivity to sorafenib treatment in hepatocellular carcinoma. *Clinical Cancer Research, 23*(15), 4482–4492.

CHAPTER 2

Cancer Treatment Through Gene Therapy: Methods, Challenges, and Current Progress

ABSTRACT

Even while gene therapy may not be as effective as chemotherapy, it might be a more effective choice for treating cancer since it is more selective and avoids causing non-targeted side effects. Numerous challenges have to be overcome before cancer therapy can be successfully implemented including non-targeted expression, ineffective delivery, and biosafety in the clinic. Reconstructing vectors and transgenes to improve their safety and efficacy is being pursued using a variety of cutting-edge genetic methods. Gene expression may now be tailored to particular tissues and organs thanks to cutting-edge delivery technology. Gene therapy has the potential to replace conventional medicine for neoplastic disorders as a result of recent advancements in the field. Preclinical and clinical implications of recent breakthroughs in gene therapy are explored in this chapter.

2.1 INTRODUCTION

Using a normal form of a damaged or missing gene, gene therapy may repair an underlying illness in an international setting. In the 1960s, researchers studying viruses found that the cells they infected absorbed the virus's genetic code, changing their genomes in malignant ways [1]. In 1966, he advocated for the possibility of using viruses in somatic cell genetic modification for therapeutic purposes. It was not until a few years after the

DNA- and m-RNA-Based Vaccines: An Immunotherapeutic Approach to Cancer.
Sonali Sundram and Rishabha Malviya (Authors)

DOI: 10.1201/9781774919613-2

initial gene therapy proof of concept was achieved, and even then, all that was needed was for the tobacco mosaic virus to be used as a vector to insert the RNA polyadenylate stretch [2–4]. Treatment of two seriously disabled young girls with hyperuricemia in the 1970s was achieved by giving the arginase gene-producing wild-type Shope papillomavirus. Despite our best efforts, we were only partially successful. In 1990, using a retrovirus (RV) vector, the ADA gene was effectively introduced into the T-cells of two infants born with severe combined immunodeficiency (SCID) [5]. Only one of the patients responded favorably, but disagreement arose because the patient had both gene therapy and enzyme replacement therapy at the same time [6]. Another investigation was done on a patient, age 18, who had ornithine transcarbamylase insufficiency, a relatively modest nitrogen metabolism issue. The practice was temporarily put on hold when a patient who had vector-related toxicity as a result of gene therapy passed away. Cancer, congenital X-linked severe combined immunodeficiency (SCID-X1), thalassemia major, Leber's congenital amaurosis, and many more debilitating diseases affect far too many people and -thalassemia minor and others have been demonstrated to respond favorably to gene therapy despite the widespread public outcry after this incidence. It is also possible that a therapeutic breakthrough may be approaching because of breakthroughs in genetics, improved vectors to reduce the risk of undesired toxicity, and new techniques for controlling DNA expression and delivery in a targeted way. As a result, more than 1800 clinical studies have been done or are now underway across the globe [7–10].

Gene therapy once concentrated on treating (orphan) diseases with genetic causes [11]. From heart failure to dementia, gene therapy has been utilized to treat conditions that refuse to go away. Although 60% of ongoing gene therapy experiments are concentrating on cancer, gene therapy has a wide range of potential applications [12–15]. This chapter discusses several gene therapy approaches, as well as challenges, and issues related to cancer gene therapy, as well as a few instances of recent achievements in the field.

2.2 METHODS FOR TREATING CANCER WITH GENES

Rogers and Pfuderer [16] pioneered virus-mediated gene transfer proof-of-concept. It was demonstrated that the transfer of foreign genetic material to specific cells may be achieved via the employment of viruses [16]. Rogers carried out the first-ever human gene therapy study using this technique. Rogers utilized a wild-type Shope papilloma virus in that work to introduce the gene for arginase into two girls who were suffering from a urea cycle abnormality (also known as hyperargininemias) [17, 18]. The researcher postulated that the Shope papillomavirus would inherently possess the genetic information necessary for arginase activity and that this genetic material might be transmitted by introducing the virus to the subjects. Both the clinical course of the illness in these individuals and their arginine levels remained unchanged. The first gene therapy regimen was approved by the United States Food and Drug Administration (FDA) and subsequently implemented in 1989. In this study, tumor-infiltrating lymphocytes obtained from patients with advanced melanoma were genetically modified *ex vivo* with a marker gene, which does not have therapeutic properties. These modified cells were then cultured in a laboratory setting to increase their numbers and then reintroduced into the same patients [19].

The resistance of cancer cells to apoptosis, which may be attributed to either genetic mutations or an imbalance in the expression of pro- and antiapoptotic genes, can be elucidated by the use of genomic therapies [20]. One often-used strategy in cancer therapy is the utilization of genes that possess the ability to suppress the development of cancer. A frequently utilized approach within this context is the introduction of genes that encode inducers, mediators, or executors of apoptosis. Recent findings have shown that the apoptosis-inducing ligand known as TNF-related apoptosis-inducing ligand (TRAIL) can effectively eliminate a diverse range of cancer cell types while causing relatively little damage to normal, healthy cells [21–23]. It has been demonstrated that the apoptosis-inducer member of the interleukin *(IL)-10* gene family *IL-24* causes cell death preferentially in some malignancies while not affecting normal tissue of similar composition (mda-7) [24–26]. Caspases, which are apoptosis executioner genes, are efficient against cancer cells notwithstanding the health of the apoptosis machinery [27]. When cancer gene therapy is administered to malignant cells, its primary mechanism of action is enhancing their susceptibility to antiapoptotic gene suppression via the use of small interfering RNAs (siRNAs) and microRNAs (miRNAs). The process of sensitization is achieved by the use of pro-apoptotic pharmaceutical agents or radiation therapy [28, 29].

The *IL-24*, which belongs to the *IL-10* gene family, induces selective cell death in some cancerous cells while exhibiting no impact on normal tissue with comparable composition (mda-7). Regardless of the optimal functionality of the apoptosis mechanism, cancer cells may be efficiently eradicated via the action of caspases, which are genes responsible for executing apoptosis [30, 31]. Cancer gene therapy typically seeks to sensitize malignant cells to the targeted antiapoptotic gene silencing through siRNA or microRNA by using pro-apoptotic drugs or radiation. Lung cancer that is not a tiny cell was first treated using retroviral vectors producing human p53 controlled by an actin promoter in 1996. For treating cancer, oncogenes may also have their biological activity regulated and reduced at the RNA or DNA level [32–34]. In many types of human cancer, the transcription factor MYC, which controls many cellular functions, is dysregulated. Antisense oligonucleotides against the *c-Myc* gene are effective genes that inhibit the growth of melanoma cells. A common RAS gene mutation, K-Ras, is often seen in human colon cancer (approximately 40–60%), and antisense RNA treatment of K-Ras results in animal models of apoptosis and tumor growth suppression. The discovery of oncogenic microRNAs, molecules of 20–22 nucleotides that regulate genes posttranscriptionally, has paved the way for a novel kind of gene therapy. In recent years, antisense drugs have been employed in clinical settings due to their success in targeting oncomirs in animal models, both *in vitro* and *in vivo* investigations [35–39].

The introduction of genes encoding enzymes that are capable of transforming prodrugs into their active forms is one method that has shown to be highly successful in the treatment of cancer via gene therapy. The combination of ganciclovir and herpes simplex virus (HSV)-thymidine kinase is largely regarded as the most effective strategy for treating herpes simplex virus [40, 41]. Patients diagnosed with prostate cancer and malignant glioma are now undergoing treatment in many Phase I clinical trials using this approach. The failure of several chemotherapy treatments may be attributed to the emergence of chemoresistance throughout treatment. To address this resistance, the use of gene therapy might potentially contribute to the elucidation of the genetic basis and targeted suppression of proto-oncogenes [42, 43]. These methods are well established in preclinical studies, but new techniques are required for successful clinical translation.

Understanding the obstacles and ways being utilized to overcome these obstructions, which will be explored in this chapter, will help us understand why gene therapy's promise in cancer treatment has not been fully recognized.

2.3 A FEW OF THE CHALLENGES WITH GENE THERAPY

The achievement of long-term therapeutic effects or, ideally, a cure can only be realized when there is a comprehensive understanding of the challenges to therapeutic engagement and the development of measures to overcome them [44]. Transgenic expression is challenging to achieve, which makes it difficult to silence a gene linked to cancer or deliver therapeutic doses of a cancer-treating gene to the afflicted tissue. Identifying the appropriate treatment gene(s) capable of impeding or halting the progression of the disease is equally crucial. In the following sections, an examination will be conducted on several strategies aimed at surmounting the aforementioned barriers to achieve efficacious gene therapy.

2.3.1 HIGHEST POSSIBLE TRANSGENE EXPRESSION

The regulation of therapeutic transgene expression is crucial, as it should be customized to the specific clinical requirements. Moreover, in the event of any adverse consequences, it is essential to completely suppress gene expression. Transgene expression in certain cells or tissues is regulated by two essential components, namely promoters and enhancers [45–48]. Promoters may be either constitutive or inducible. A gene's constitutive promoter ensures that it will continue to be expressed at a steady rate. For example, melanoma tyrosinase and prostate-specific antigen (PSA) are constitutive promoters, whereas others, such as hTERT and progression-elevated gene, are functional in many different types of cancer (PEG-3). An inducible promoter is characterized by its transient expression and may be activated to generate transgenes by the application of exogenous hormones or small molecules. To ensure adequate expression of effector proteins, it is crucial to possess a promoter that exhibits both specificity and potency. This objective may be achieved by using enhancers derived from many genes or a single gene. Nettelbeck et al. devised an enhancer element, which was positioned upstream of the human tyrosinase promoter, to selectively target malignant melanoma by particularly binding to pigment cells [49, 50]. The prostate-cancer-targeted adenovirus was generated by inserting an enhancer fragment into the *PSMA* gene nearer the start of the RNA polymerase II elongation phase than the E1A transcription initiation site/TATA. It is possible to use restricted expression silencers to prevent the vector from activating in healthy cells. The need to manage transgenic expression is contingent upon the characteristics of the encoded product and the requirements of the recipient cell. Adenoviruses expressing the tumor suppressor p53 have been extensively used in several clinical investigations due to their nontoxicity toward normal cells, resulting in little negative consequences [51]. When a potentially dangerous gene product needs to be delivered, however, inducible controlled systems function better than constitutive expression [52–54].

2.3.2 ADMINISTRATION OF GENE THERAPY

Two of the most crucial elements in establishing a treatment's therapeutic value are its efficacy and safety. Tissue-specific expression of therapeutic genes is a well-suited strategy for maximizing treatment effects [55]. As a consequence of this, gene therapy has prioritized individualized distribution as one of its principal objectives, owing to its shown efficacy [56]. It is possible to distribute genes via catheters, gene guns, etc., in the first method of physical targeting. This review will not go into detail on these subjects, since they have been well covered elsewhere [57, 58]. The second approach employs genetically modified elements delivered using viral or nonviral vectors, which effectively hinder their interaction with healthy cells while selectively enabling their attachment to malignant cells. This chapter will discuss ways to achieve cell-specific targeting. Several methods are now being investigated in experimental animals for research purposes, with the possibility of further clinical studies using this method shortly [59].

2.4 METHODS OF GENE TRANSFER AND VECTORS USED IN GENE THERAPY

Delivering a sufficient quantity of genetic information into target tissues or cells and sustaining gene expression for the intended length of time are challenges in gene therapy. Various techniques of delivery may be used to transfer genetic material into target cells or tissues. The categorization of these methods may be broadly classified as follows: (i) physical techniques; (ii) viral approaches; (iii) nonviral methodologies; and (iv) bacterial or yeast-based strategies (see Figure 2.1) [60]. Physical approaches such as electroporation ultrasound imaging, and gene gun delivery have been used. The use of viral vectors in gene transfer involves the employment of a biological vector, specifically a virus, to facilitate the delivery of genetic information into cells. Conversely, nonviral gene transfer techniques employ synthetic carriers such as liposomes or nanoparticles for this purpose. Other vector systems, such as lentiviruses and adeno-associated viruses (AAVs), have been demonstrated to be less inflammatory and immunogenic than Ads. If the vectors enter cells that are good at presenting antigens, like dendritic cells, the modified result could lead to a T-cell reaction [61]. Because there are tools for mass production, transgene expression is robust in diseased tissues, and genetic editing makes it simple to create safe, non-immunogenic vectors [62, 63]. Common therapeutic viral vectors include AAV, Adenovirus (Ad), RV, and lentiviruses. Factors including the vector's capacity for packing, its selectivity toward its host, its gene expression profile, and its potential to elicit an immunological response, particularly in response to repeated doses, all play a role in determining which vector to use [64–67].

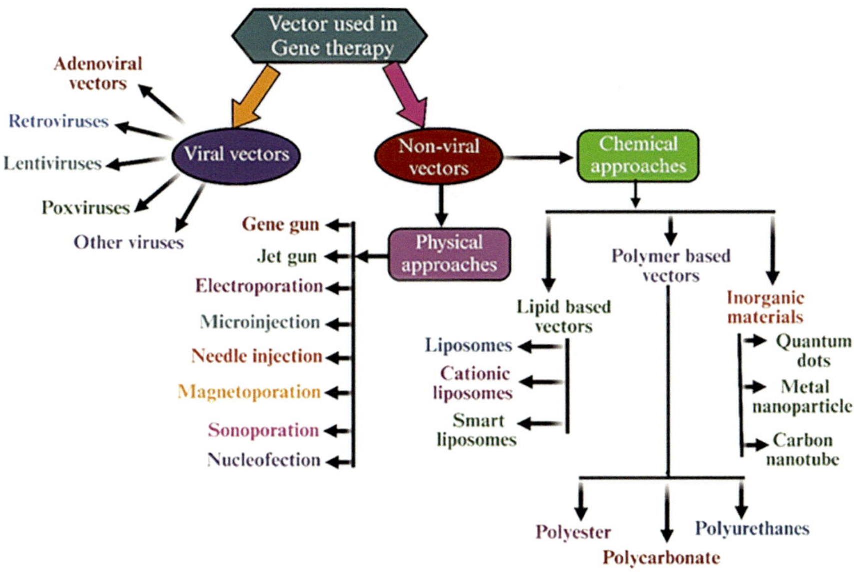

FIGURE 2.1 Classification of different types of vectors for gene therapy.

Recent developments have shown the flexibility and potential therapeutic uses of adenoviral (Ad) vectors, which have been at the forefront of gene therapy research. The improvement of Ad vector design, which includes initiatives to lower immunogenicity and increase safety, is one noteworthy advancement. Minimal viral genes or fiber alterations in modified ads are intended to reduce human immune reactions, which enables them to be administered again. Targeted gene expression is also made possible by the use of tissue-specific promoters, which reduces off-target effects. Additionally, continuing research aims to improve the Ad vectors' ability to transport particular tissues or cell types, which is critical for treating a variety of illnesses, including cancer and inherited genetic abnormalities. Ad gene therapy has shown therapeutic promise as demonstrated by recent achievements in studies treating hereditary retinal disorders and hemophilia. In the field of gene therapy, these advancements in Ad gene therapy are encouraging milestones toward realizing the full therapeutic potential of non-integrating viral vectors [68–70]. Various vectors exhibit specific features, their transduction effectiveness, and their ability to express the inserted genes. Additionally, they vary in transgenic expression length and safety profile. Various vectors can be utilized for various therapy goals, based on the needs. *In vivo*, gene transfer with virus vectors is thought to be the most successful way available right now. The ideal gene transfer vector targets a particular tissue with high transmission efficiency, maintaining consistent gene expression without side effects or immunological reactions. Regrettably, the existing gene delivery vectors do not meet all of these requirements. When a vector is injected locally, it usually has a small but accurate effect area. However, when a vector is given systemically, it might affect the whole body. Targeted delivery and improved transduction efficiencies have resulted from tweaks to vectors and vector administration [71]. Many viral vectors include intrinsic tropism toward certain cell types or tissues, making them valuable for therapeutic applications [72].

2.4.1 VIRAL VECTORS FOR GENE DELIVERY

The most popular viral vectors for gene transfer are adenoviruses, lenti- and RVs (including HIV), vaccinia viruses, AAV, and baculoviruses. These vectors vary from one another in terms of cell tropisms, expression patterns, transgenic capabilities, immunogenicity, and transgene expression duration. Furthermore, viral vectors may be categorized into two distinct types based on their ability to integrate into the host genome: integrating vectors and non-integrating vectors. Non-integrating vectors include baculoviruses and adenoviruses. They exhibit a deficiency in their capacity to integrate their genetic material, including the transgene, into the genetic material of the host organism. Lentiviruses, RVs, and AAVs are examples of vectors that possess the ability to integrate into the genome of the host organism (Figure 2.2). The transgene's expression is temporary in the case of non-integrating viral vectors, often declining within a few weeks. However, integrating vectors sometimes leads to long-term expression, lasting for months to years. The incorporation of the transgene into the genome of the host organism has elicited apprehensions over the safety of these vectors. This is because integration has been known to sometimes take place at areas that are actively expressed when using retroviral vectors (insertional mutagenesis) [73–75]. Figure 2.2 shows the mechanism of the viral vector for gene delivery. The *ex vivo* gene transfer technique may also be used for the delivery of genetic material. In this process, the genetic material is administered *ex vivo*, meaning that it is supplied to the cell outside the patient's body. This is done by isolating autologous cells, introducing the genetic material to them, and then reintroducing these modified cells back into the patient.

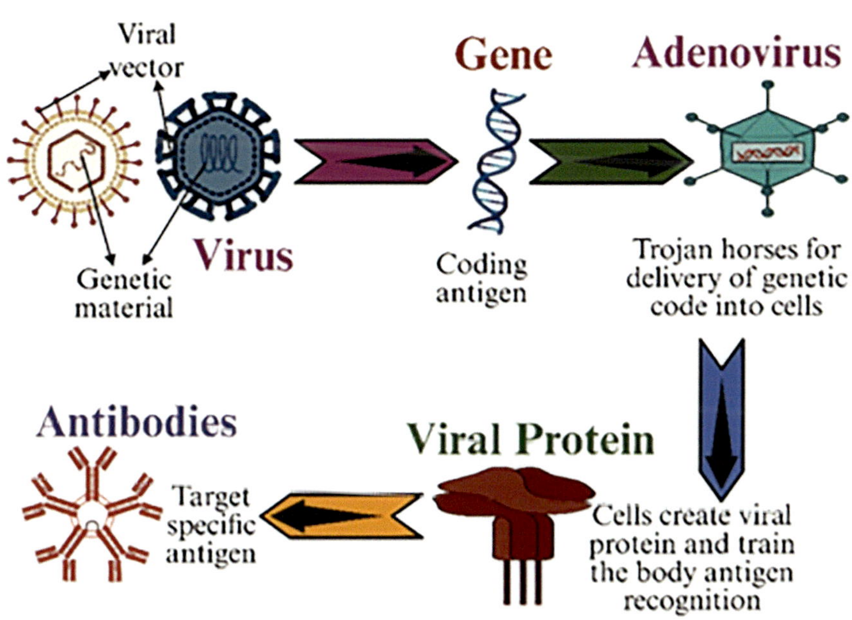

FIGURE 2.2 Mechanism of viral vector for gene delivery.

At now, adenoviruses represent the prevailing transmission of gene vectors used in the field of gene therapy. Over 50 distinct serotypes of adenoviruses have been found, and they may be further classified into six subgroups labeled A through F [76]. Among the several serotypes, serotypes 2 and 5 are frequently used in the field of gene therapy. One of the limitations associated with adenoviruses is the presence of measurable amounts of preexisting antibodies in around 97% of persons. This feature has the potential to impact the effectiveness of transmission and the medicinal result.

2.4.2 NONVIRAL VECTORS FOR GENE DELIVERY

The efficacy of viral vectors as gene transfer methods has been shown. However, the presence of some limitations, such as the fast elimination of viral vectors from the circulatory system (when administered systematically), as well as their tendency to provoke immune responses and inflammation, has necessitated the development of novel synthetic gene delivery vectors. Indeed, nonviral gene delivery technologies (Figure 2.3) are now the subject of significant study as potential substitutes for viral delivery techniques. The most basic manifestation of a nonviral mechanism is represented by the use of bare plasmid DNA. One benefit of using a naked plasmid is its little potential for toxicity or undesirable responses. Furthermore, it is simple to create and is affordable to manufacture. However, one drawback of this method is its relatively lower transfection effectiveness when compared to gene transfer facilitated by viruses [77]. To optimize transfection effectiveness, many strategies have been devised, such as the use of cationic polymers or lipid formulations. These approaches include the condensation of plasmid DNA to safeguard against DNA degradation and facilitate the absorption and transfection of plasmid. One benefit of using such formulations is that polymers or lipids may be readily engineered to achieve certain qualities. For instance, nonviral vectors may conveniently target certain tissues or cells by connecting cell- or tissue-specific targeting moieties to the carrier. In addition, the biodistribution, cellular uptake, and intracellular trafficking of micro- or nanoparticles may be modified by altering their size [78]. However, the practical use of nonviral delivery technologies in gene therapy has encountered limitations in terms of achieving success. Nonviral vectors lack the evolutionary process experience of viruses, resulting in lower transduction efficiency *in vivo*. The effectiveness of nonviral gene therapy relies on many obstacles, both extracellular and intracellular, that impact the performance of gene delivery methods. These obstacles include cellular absorption, endosomal escaping, nuclear intake, and the expression of genes [78–80].

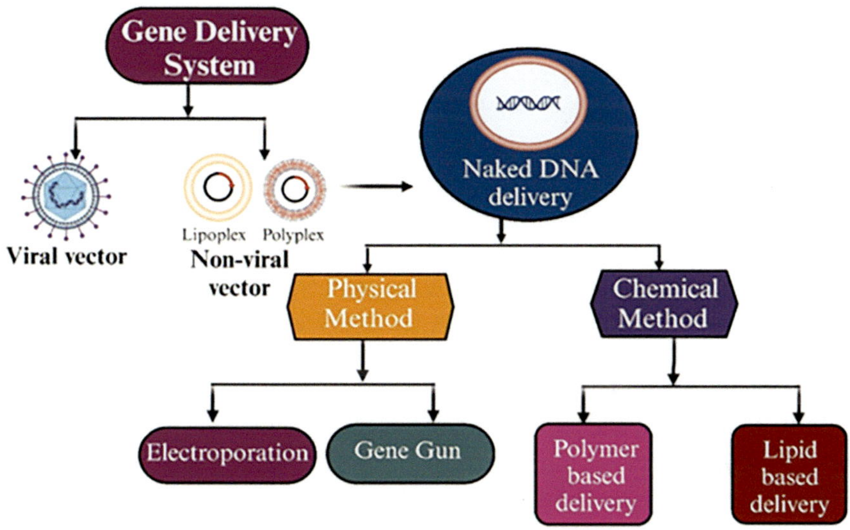

FIGURE 2.3 Describe various methods of nonviral vectors for gene delivery.

2.5 IMMUNOLOGICAL RESPONSES INDUCED BY VECTORS AS A MEAN OF AROUND INFECTION BARRIERS

Preexisting immunity in humans to certain Ad serotypes, whether from spontaneous infection or vaccination, is a significant obstacle for viral vectors, especially Ads [81]. Immunoglobulins against wild-type Ad viral vectors complicate systemic administration. It could be possible to resolve this problem using heterologous prime-boosting regimens, which deliver similar antigens via various vectors [82]. Following repeated viral vector infusions, neutralizing antibodies might potentially diminish therapeutic efficacy. Temporary immunosuppression may alleviate this issue [83]. Alternatively, Ad capsid chimeras are produced by combining fibers. Using Ad serotype 45, a less immunogenic Ad can reduce serological identification. Due to its high degree of conservation across a wide variety of Ad serotypes, the peptide H910–924 has the potential to lessen the efficacy of Ad-based treatments; most persons also show virus-specific memory immunological responses in addition to humoral responses [84–86]. The safety and immunogenicity of hexon chimeric vectors, produced by substituting immunodominant hypervariable regions (HVRs), are being studied as a breakthrough in gene therapy and vaccine development. Researchers hope to minimize the host immune response to adenoviral vectors by selectively altering these HVRs, enabling repeated delivery and better therapeutic effects [87].

Synthetic polypeptides, such as polyethylene glycol (PEG), could be inserted into the viral capsid to dampen the body's natural defenses. Ads can be rendered less effective when coated with poly [N-(2-hydroxypropyl) methacrylamide], similar to the effects of PEGylation, to minimize host–vector interactions [88]. Viral particles that activate the complement system prevent the delivery of antiviral genes. Incorporating host proteins into membranes aids in preventing complement system activation. Proteins produced by viruses, such as the complement control protein from Vaccinia (VCP), prevent complement activation via both the traditional and alternate pathways by interacting with and inactivating C4b and C3b [89–91]. Membrane-attack complex deposition may be prevented by PEG-containing shielding advertisements or genetic modifications that express soluble CD59 [92, 93].

Initial therapeutic adenoviruses were created by removing the early *E1* genes while either retaining the *E3* genes or having only a few deletions, which led to faulty viral replication. Removing all viral coding, scientists have developed the next generation of "gutless" ad vectors [94]. Sequences are specifically engineered to reduce the immunogenicity of these adenoviruses, or to render them non-immunogenic or less immunogenic. The use of an organ-specific promoter might potentially be advantageous in mitigating inflammatory responses via the downregulation of professional antigen-presenting cells (APCs) that carry the transgene [95].

Other vector systems, such as lentiviruses and AAVs, have been demonstrated to be less inflammatory and immunogenic than Ads [96]. If the vectors transduce cells with a high capacity for antigen presentation, like dendritic cells, the transgenic consequence may trigger a T-cell response. The severity of an adverse reaction can be affected by the organ being targeted, the method of administration, and the dosing schedule [97]. Multiple *in vivo* animal models have shown successful suppression of immunological responses to the transgenic product by the use of various techniques for immunosuppression, by means such as preemptive injection of an immunosuppressant medication like rapamycin combined with IL-10. The likelihood that transgenic products may trigger an immune response is reduced by the use of certain promoters, such as Ad vectors. Inhibiting transgene expression in expert APCs is most successful when a target sequence is included in several copies [98–103].

2.6 TARGETED TRANSDUCTION REDUCES THE POSSIBILITY OF TRANSMISSION TO UNINTENDED RECIPIENTS

The success of virus-mediated gene therapy relies on the high-affinity binding of viral fiber proteins to strain- or serotype-specific host receptors. Low or absent receptor expression in the infected tissue reduces the infection's effectiveness [104]. An inherent safety problem associated with the use of viruses as vectors lies in their intrinsic tendency to infect non-targeted cells. Numerous approaches in viral gene therapy include the modification of viral surface proteins to express ligands that selectively target tumor cells [105]. Although CARs (coxsackie and adenovirus) are frequently utilized in therapeutic settings, the most common serotypes used are Ad5 vectors, which target cells that are not widely expressed in human cancer cells [106, 107]. To enable CAR-independent cell entrance, ads containing a Hi loop with an integrin-binding RGD motif have been tropism-modified. In primary tumors and cell lines from ovarian cancer, the Ad increased transductional efficiency and gene delivery by a factor of two to three, indicating that it may be clinically useful [108]. Chimeric adenovirus vectors were created by splicing fiber proteins into the capsid of the CAR-nontargeting serotype Ad5 [109]. Low levels of CAR expression have been seen in many cancers, including melanoma, ovarian cancer, and renal cancer, which are resistant to Ad.5, and others, they have demonstrated exceptional transductional effectiveness. Additionally, they now more effectively induce cytopathology in primary melanoma cells. The oncoprotein c-erbB-2, which is prominently expressed in breast cancer, was the target of a ScFv. A CAR-independent method of targeting Ads has been developed using the resultant protein, which binds to the oncoprotein c-erbB-2 further limiting Ad infection to cells that express CAR. Cancers, on the other hand, are not a homogeneous group. It may not be possible to get the most out of a single-cell surface receptor. As a result, it makes sense to use numerous ligands inside a single virion in Ad-targeting techniques. Ad.5 with an RGD motif and a polylysine ligand is the first adenovirus to attach to Integrins on cell surfaces as well as heparin sulfate proteoglycan. Using this technique, by developing a viral vector for adenovirus that carried both wild-type and knob-less fibrin (6-His motif displaying) fibers, Pereboeva et al. demonstrated the transduction of genes specific to the CAR and synthetic 6-His receptors [110]. A brief antibody mimetic or target peptide with cellular specificity (like SY-GYLPLP, vascular endothelial cell-targeting peptide) may also be added into the HI loop to improve transduction in a variety of cancer cell types. Researchers employed a neutralizing anti-fiber antibody in combination with an Ad expressing an anti-EpCAM antibody to target this protein, which is produced by tumor cells (EpCAM). Two-specificity antibodies were effective in transferring genes to human colon cancer cells [111].

To address the issue of nonspecific absorption of viral vectors, particularly in the liver and spleen, a promising approach involves the modification of the adenoviral vector's hexon protein. The Ad5 hexon protein, known for its affinity for factor X and its role in liver sequestration, might potentially be substituted by hexon proteins derived from other adenoviral serotypes, such as Ad serotype 48 hexon, which have a comparatively lower affinity for factor X. The objective of this change is to decrease the uptake of viral vectors by the liver, hence reducing their susceptibility to being captured by Kupffer cells in the liver. The evasion of capture by modified adenoviral vectors holds promise for achieving more systemic availability, hence boosting their therapeutic effectiveness. This is of particular significance within the fields of gene therapy and oncolytic virotherapy. The aforementioned technique demonstrates a potentially advantageous advancement in enhancing the efficiency of administering and disseminating viral vectors, hence leading to enhanced therapeutic results [112].

2.7 TARGETING TRANSCRIPTS FOR TUMOR EXPRESSION

When employing viral vectors to deliver transgenes, the most crucial aspect is to achieve tumor-specific expression [110]. Oncolytic viruses need rigorous regulation of this characteristic. A variety of different approaches are now being tested to reach this goal. It is presently being investigated *in vitro* and *in vivo* utilizing promoters that are tumor- or cancer-selective and restrict expression to particular cell types Symbol. A crucial step in this method is to identify a promoter that is tumor-selective or tumor-specific [113, 114]. Recent developments in molecular biology and bioinformatics, such as database searching and sequence analysis tools, have allowed for the identification of these promoters [115].

Several promoters are utilized to sustain viral replication or to sustain viral-mediated gene expression in a tumor-specific manner. For instance, a virus with a high selectivity for the prostate was generated by adding a PSA promoter/enhancement element upstream of E1A [116–118]. The observed elevated levels of hTERT expression and promoter activity in many cancer cell types provide substantial evidence for the potential use of this promoter in the development of replicative recombinant viruses [119–121].

Target tumor cells are effectively lysed by these viruses, which demonstrates limited replication in telomerase-positive tumor cells. Many cancer cells have been shown to employ hTERT as a method of selective gene suppression [122]. The disadvantage of this technique is that it cannot identify the promoter-transduction influence in tumors lacking hTERT expression. Various promoters have been used to activate genes in malignancies that replicate viruses. Examples include the surviviN promoter, the tyrosinase promoter for melanoma, and the catenin-sensitive promoter [123, 124] for colorectal and liver cancer. Oncolytic viruses have been used to specifically target cancer cells in the pancreas, ovaries, and cervix, using the assistance of the cyclooxygenase-2 promoter.

One potential approach to enhance the tumor selectivity of oncolytic viruses involves modifying gene expressions that are specific to healthy cells, but not present in malignant cells, to facilitate viral replication [124]. The *E1B-55kd* gene in the wild-type adenovirus is responsible for carrying out the functions of attaching to *p53* and subsequently inactivating it. The advertisement was developed in the absence of *E1B-55kd* to enhance the proliferation of viral particles inside tumor cells that had a nonfunctional *p53* gene (referred to as *dl1520*). Recent investigations have shown that the inhibition of *E1B-55kd*-mediated late viral RNA export has a more significant role in the regulation of viral replication in normal cells compared to the inhibition of p53 inactivation [125, 126].

While studies have demonstrated that tissue-specific oncolytic viruses can be successful, combining therapy with a virus-derived substance has shown significant clinical benefits. In a colon xenograft model, Ad.TKRC, an *E1B-55k* deleted Ad with HSV-TK, had better survival when combined with ganciclovir than when used alone [127–129]. Numerous structural modifications and synergistic interactions with various pharmaceutical agents have shown efficacy in preclinical studies. The use of this approach has been shown in the advancement of a virus known as cancer terminator viruses (CTV), which exhibits the capability to induce apoptosis in cancerous cells. A specific kind of chimeric antigen receptor T-cell therapy (CTV) involves the use of the *media-7/IL-24* therapeutic cytokine gene, which is controlled by the promoter known as progressively elevated *gene-3* (PEG-Prom). The administration of CTV has shown potential in the therapeutic management of several malignancies, including breast cancer, prostate cancer, and melanoma. This statement presents a case supporting the diverse range of prospective uses of this treatment in the context of addressing human tumors [130].

2.8 SAFE AND EFFECTIVE VECTOR DELIVERY

When viruses are injected systemically, nonspecific absorption by other organs like the liver or spleen can still cause unpleasant side effects or a loss of efficacy despite significant advancements in retargeting vectors to boost their activity in tumor cells [131]. One of the primary obstacles in the field of tumor detection is the ability of tumor cells to evade detection, which may be attributed to many factors such as the presence of endothelial–matrix barriers, vector neutralization, nonspecific adhesion, and sequestration. These factors significantly contribute to the failure of vectors to accurately identify tumor cells, hence leading to suboptimal clinical results. These challenges underscore the need to establish dependable delivery methods to guarantee the delivery of sufficient dosage to the targeted region. The presence of organs that are inaccessible to targeted catheter-based therapies or surgical bed injections is a unique problem [132]. A systems administration approach is the only viable method of delivering services to a specific target location.

Ultrasound contrast agents known as microbubbles (MBs) transfer therapeutic agents such as therapeutic proteins, inhibitory siRNA/shRNA, transgenes, viral vectors, and transfection to safely and effectively target cells. Perfluorocarbon or sulfur hexafluoride are common heavy-molecular-weight gases used to fill MBs, which reduces their solubility and increases their lifespan while also enabling them to travel by the use of microcirculation [133]. The low metabolic rate of MBs results in the absence of an immunological response in the host, enabling the stealthy systemic delivery of treatments such as viral vectors, transgenes, or medications. The use of ultrasonic technology leads to the generation of micro- or microscopic streams, resulting in an augmentation of cellular permeability and an improvement in the effectiveness of transfection and/ or transduction processes. MBs, employing an Ad vector expressing a GFP marker gene, have been used for site-specific gene delivery *in vivo*, as reported by Howard et al. [134]. This technique has shown potential in the delivery of therapeutic viruses in xenograft and spontaneous tumor models, underscoring the need for further investigation [135].

A combination of MB size and ultrasonography amplitude is crucial for understanding their behavior. Enlarged microbeads (MBs) of 2.5–4 nm in diameter are ideal for encasing viral vectors, which prevents them from being trapped in the pulmonary capillary bed. To maximize transmission efficiency while minimizing tissue harm, the frequencies used must be tailored to the target organ [152]. Membrane-bound beads (MBs) targeting tissues or organs have been produced for a brief duration by linking an antibody chemically or via a biotin-streptavidin spacer. Single-chain VEGF molecules on MB may target tumor vasculature that overexpresses VEGFR2. Targeted imaging with VCAM-1 is also employed in mouse tumor models. It is being examined if this ornamented MB may transmit therapeutic viruses [136].

2.9 IDENTIFYING GENES FOR TREATMENT

To make gene therapy work, the right beneficial gene must be picked so that it works best while also being safe. A lot of beneficial gene groups are now being used in clinical studies. As a result, scientists are now trying to find new genes that seem to change the way cancerous cells behave [137]. There are several advantages of using cancer genomic data to identify molecular alterations in cancer cells. Comprehensive molecular profiling of tumors, which makes it easier to identify target genes, may help researchers discover new treatment targets in these situations. Indeed, this strategy often encounters difficulties in the areas of large-scale genomic characterization and adequate data analysis. Improved high-throughput methods including gene expression array profiling and genome sequencing, on the other hand, are leading to better-quality data that can be interpreted thanks to the addition of new computational tools [138]. Researchers may find novel genes and treatments for cancer with the help of the Gene Expression Omnibus (GEO), a useful resource. It provides access to an extensive collection of high-throughput data on the levels of gene expression seen in a broad variety of cancer types. Researchers may use this data to find genes whose expression is altered in cancer cells compared to healthy ones, and therefore possibly new therapeutic targets for cancer treatment. Gene expression patterns, genetic variations, and molecular signatures associated with different cancer subtypes can be explored by scientists thanks to the comprehensive datasets provided by GEO. This paves the way for the development of treatment strategies that are more targeted and effective in the fight against cancer, which is a disease that is both complex and heterogeneous [139].

2.10 SAFETY OF GENE THERAPY

Although Jesse Gelsinger died from gene therapy utilizing adenoviral vectors, safety data from several human gene therapy experiments has been consistently positive. As viral vectors employed in gene therapy are often human infections, preexisting antibodies against them may cause an undesirable immune response. For example, adenoviral vector injections trigger a nonspecific immune response, releasing various cytokines, followed by a targeted antibody and cell-mediated reaction against transduced cells. However, adenovirus responses vary by serotype. Thoma et al. [140], for example, established that the initial cytokine response of macrophages upon viral stimulation varies across adenovirus serotypes and is therefore serotype-specific. In a long-term study, Ad11 showed no/mild toxicity whereas Ad5 caused moderate/severe toxicity when injected intraperitoneally [140]. In general, the availability of long-term safety data about the use of viral vectors in human subjects remains limited. However, multiple meta-analyses have shown that adenoviruses are safe for human usage [141]. The tolerance of adenoviral vectors has been satisfactory, and the side effects have been largely minor, with no significant adverse events associated with gene therapy.

Various methods have been used to improve gene therapy safety. One potential method involves the development of targeting techniques to optimize the delivery of gene transfer vectors, hence enhancing the length and effectiveness of gene expression. One of the primary limitations associated with gene therapy is the fundamental lack of selectivity toward target cells and the relatively poor effectiveness of transduction. Enhancing the specificity and/or transduction effectiveness would eventually lead to an improved safety profile as well. The enhancement of gene transfer vectors' transduction effectiveness has been achieved by advancements in vector technology, such as the modification of viral vectors through epitope insertion, chemical alteration, and the evolution of molecules [142]. Kim et al. [143] showed this principle in action by modifying the RGD fiber knob of adenoviruses, hence increasing viral infectivity of cancer cells, in a phase I clinical study. The investigation of the innate immune response and the subsequent activation of T and B cells in reaction to the vector and its transgenic product is now a subject of significant academic study. The assessment of the potential impacts of gene transfer vectors and/or the proteins they produce on nearby lymph nodes is an area that requires more investigation.

There are already neutralizing antibodies in the body, for example against different types of viral or AAVs. This has been known for a while, and it has been demonstrated that these neutralizing antibodies can make transmission much less effective [144]. To enhance selectivity and transduction effectiveness, viral surface proteins have been altered, deleted, or replaced. For instance, lentiviral vectors may be made by fusing a ligand or antibody that targets a certain cell type to the viral envelope (i.e., pseudotyping) [145]. The focused incorporation of transgenes into specific genomic regions has emerged as an important field of study in contemporary vector advancement. DNA double-strand break-enhanced homologous recombination (HR) is considered to be one of the most effective approaches for achieving tailored integration into human cells [146]. Moreover, lentivirus/transposon hybrids have been created to mitigate the risk of insertional mutagenesis [147]. The Sleeping Beauty transposon system is a promising method for stable transgene integration into the target cell genome [148, 149]. The Sleeping Beauty transposon system is useful because it does not happen to insert itself into active genes, and the reversed repeats do not have much promoter or enhancer activity left over. One of the primary concerns raised about human gene therapy is the potential for it to produce genotoxicity or mutagenesis. Traditional cancer treatments (such as radiation and chemotherapy) may also result in genetic changes, although this is generally overlooked. Multiple chemotherapeutic medications, in addition to radiation treatment, have been shown to increase the risk of genetic changes and oncogenesis in patients [150–152].

2.11 THE CLINICAL EFFECTIVENESS OF GENE THERAPY

For cancer gene treatment, many gene therapy techniques involving various gene transfer vectors have been investigated. The various strategies encompassed in this field encompass the induction of apoptosis, oncolytic virotherapy, immune modulation, antiangiogenic gene therapies, gene deficiencies modification, preventing tumor invasion, gene therapy for enhancing chemo- and radiotherapy, cytoprotective gene treatment, strategies involving antisense and RNA interference (RNAi), as well as prodrug activation/suicide gene therapy. Regrettably, only a small number of these approaches have been implemented in clinical settings. Utilizing a mutation that is naturally occurring in the p53 protein is one approach that has been used often in the field of gene therapy for cancer. Lang et al. [153] conducted a phase I clinical trial to evaluate the efficacy of an adenoviral vector carrying the tumor suppressor gene *TP53* in the management of patients with frequent malignancy. The study involved 15 patients who received an intratumoral stereotactic injection of the adenoviral vector through an implanted catheter. Subsequently, the tumor was surgically removed as a whole, and the post-resection cavity was treated [153]. The assessment of tumor response was not possible due to the trial's methodology; nevertheless, the study showed low toxicity. In this trial, there was no evidence of systemic viral spread, and the maximum tolerable dosage was not achieved. Moreover, examination of tumor tissues revealed limited transgenic expression in proximity to the site of injection. Another study, similar to the viral agent used by Lang et al. [153], is Gendicine™. Gendicine™ is an adenovirus that cannot replicate and has the *TP53* gene instead of the viral *E1* gene. It is used as a therapeutic intervention for a range of cancer types.

A significant feature of Gendicine™ is its distinction as the first gene therapy medication to have received approval for clinical use [154]. In a clinical study of phase I, including a cohort of 12 patients diagnosed with laryngeal cancer, the therapeutic potential of Gendicine™ was seen. Particularly, none of the patients who received therapy with Gendicine™ had tumor recurrence throughout the 5 years of posttreatment follow-up [155]. Furthermore, Gendicine™ had a favorable safety profile, as shown by a clinical study including 132 patients with head and neck squamous cell carcinoma in phase II/III studies. In this study, it was shown that 32% of participants had fever as the only adverse effect of the medication [156]. When Gendicine™ was administered in conjunction with radiotherapy, a significant proportion of patients (64%) exhibited a complete regression, while 29% experienced a partial regression. In comparison, when radiotherapy was administered alone, only 19% of patients achieved a complete regression, with 60% experiencing a partial regression. These outcomes indicate a synergistic effect resulting from the combined treatment [156].

Another gene therapy medicine approved by the Chinese SFDA is Oncorine™, created by Shanghai Sunway Biotech. Oncorine™ is a conditionally replicative adenovirus created by deleting the *E1B 55K* gene. Eliminating this gene inhibits the virus from binding and inactivating the wild-type p53 protein, a crucial host defense mechanism against viral infection [157]. Removing E1B 55K activity prevents normal cell replication, enabling only p53-deficient cells to replicate. Malignant cells undergo viral growth, resulting in oncolysis, a cancer treatment for solid tumors. One intriguing aspect of this medicine is that ONYX-015, created by Onyx Pharmaceuticals, was never approved for the market. ONYX-015 did not show a therapeutic effect in clinical settings compared to Oncorine™. In a phase I dose-escalation experiment by Chiocca et al. [158], 24 patients with recurrent malignant glioma received 10 injections of the oncolytic virus into 10 areas of the tumor cavity.

The research found that ONYX-015 was safe and no significant side effects were reported; however, all patients suffered tumor growth. A patient with anaplastic astrocytoma had stable disease, whereas two patients who received a second resection showed lymphocyte and plasmacytoid cell infiltration at the injection site. Based on extensive safety data, Oncorine™ and ONYX-015 have shown acceptable safety profiles for glioma, pancreatic, and ovarian malignancies [20]. Typical side effects include fever, injection site soreness, nausea, hair loss, leucopenia, and flu-like symptoms [159].

2.12 IMPROVED DELIVERY AND EXPRESSION METHODS THAT ARE SPECIFIC TO CANCER

Even though the nonviral majority of patients have responded positively to MDA-7/IL-24 treatment investigations connected to this compound have used Adenovirus serotype 5 (Ad.5). Due to its reliance on surface-expressed CARs for viral absorption, Ad.5 serotype's clinical value is restricted since CARs are frequently not numerous in tumors. To circumvent this limitation, broaden its host range, and increase its infectious potential, Chimeric adenoviruses harboring mda-7/IL-24 (Ad.5 modified with an Ad.3 fiber, Ad.5/3). Both a spontaneous Hi-my prostate cancer animal model and tumor xenografts derived from poor CAR human prostate cancer cells showed improved mda-7/IL-24 transduction efficiency after exposure to this modified virus. In later research evaluations, Ad.5/3.mda-7 demonstrated greater efficacy than Ad.5.mda-7 against glioblastoma multiforme, renal carcinoma, colorectal carcinoma, and breast cancer [160]. Several low CAR human cancer xenografts were found to benefit from a lower multiplicity of infection when treated with either adolescent adenovirus five composite type V (Ad.5-CTV) or tropism-modified adenovirus composite type V (Ad.5/3) both of which demonstrated superior transduction efficiency.

Inducing apoptosis in many human malignancies by Mda-7/IL-24-mediated adenoviral tropism has to be seen; it is clear that this therapeutic virus has limited practical application. When administered systemically, the improved effectiveness and infectivity of the Ad.5/3-CTV are restricted due to nonspecific liver trapping, immune clearance, and a dearth of choices for properly delivering internal organs such as the prostate, pancreas, kidney, and others have been affected by the virus. This virus is not the only one with challenges when it comes to systemically administering the Ad.5/3-CTV, since these same issues plague many other viral-based treatment techniques as well. A method known as ultrasonic-targeted microbubble destruction (UTMD) uses MBs and ultrasound to get around these issues [161]. This technique reduces the chance of viruses becoming caught in the liver by discharging viruses into the tumor microenvironment, straight into internal organs, and malignant tissues. In immunocompetent Hi-Myc mice, a spontaneous prostate cancer transgenic mouse model that develops localized adenocarcinoma at the age of 6 months, a therapeutic virus (Ad.5/3.mda-7) was administered selectively to the prostate gland using UTMD. For a total of 4 weeks, Ad.5/3.mda-7 with MB was given intravenously three times each week. According to data from immunohistochemistry, the MDA-7/IL-24 protein was delivered directly to tumors. Additionally, combining *mda-7/IL-24* gene therapy with chemotherapy was investigated (Sabutoclax). Azab et al. [9] modeled their work after Dash et al. [27] who successfully used Ad.5/3-mda-7 (a nonreplicating adenovirus expressing mda-7/IL-24). They used the UTMD approach to deliver Ad.5/3-CTV to Hi-Myc mice. This strategy has the potential to be exploited for the effective and targeted delivery of cytokines to internal organs, as in the case of MDA-7/IL-24.

2.13 SUICIDE GENE TREATMENT

The technique of suicide gene therapy involves the introduction of genes derived from viruses or bacteria into cancerous cells. These genes facilitate the conversion of a nontoxic prodrug into a toxic chemical inside the targeted cells. Multiple suicide gene systems have been reported, such as the HSV-thymidine kinase (TK) gene in combination with ganciclovir (GCV), as well as the cytosine deaminase gene (CD) in conjunction with 5-fluorocytosine (5-FC) [162]. Gene-mediated cytotoxic immunotherapy is a therapeutic approach involving the use of an adenoviral vector containing the *herpes virus thymidine kinase* gene (*AdV-TK*). This vector is administered directly to the tumor site, leading to the localized expression of the *HSV-TK* gene. Consequently, viral thymidine kinase is synthesized, which facilitates the conversion of GCV to GCV monophosphate. The subsequent stage involves the injection of GCV, which serves as a substrate for *HSV-TK* and undergoes phosphorylation to generate GCV monophosphate. Subsequently, intracellular kinases facilitate the metabolic conversion of guanosine-5'-monophosphate (GVC-monophosphate) into guanosine-5'-triphosphate (GVC-triphosphate). GCV triphosphate is an analog of deoxyguanosine triphosphate that is integrated into the DNA chain, resulting in the termination of the chain and subsequent demise of tumor cells [163].

The TK/GCV system demonstrated a favorable antitumor impact in animal models, indicating potential therapeutic efficacy. The study examines the treatment of individuals with hormone-refractory prostate cancer using HSV-TK given via adenovirus, followed by GCV administration. The findings indicated that the response seen was at the surrogate marker level and demonstrated safety. Numerous investigations are now undergoing Phase III clinical trials [164]. The enzyme CD is present in fungi and bacteria, but not in human cells. Its function is to convert cytosine into uracil. The enzyme CD facilitates the metabolic conversion of the nontoxic prodrug 5-FC into 5-fluorouracil (5-FU). Subsequently, cellular enzymes further metabolize 5-FU into 5-fluoro-2'-deoxyuridine monophosphate (5-FdUMP), 5-fluoro-2'-deoxyuridine triphosphate (5-FdUTP), and 5-fluorouridine triphosphate (5-FUTP). The CD/5-FC suicide mechanism induces cell death via the inhibition of thymidylate synthase and the subsequent synthesis of (5-FU) DNA and RNA.

The use of 5-FU in the treatment of cancer necessitates the administration of a substantial dosage. The use of this suicide system leads to the administration of tumor-targeted chemotherapy with minimal adverse effects. The CD/5-FC system was enhanced by the incorporation of the *uracil phosphoribosyltransferase* (*UPRT*) gene, which facilitates the phosphorylation of 5-FU into 5-fluorouridine mono-phosphate. This enzymatic reaction represents the first stage in the process of activating 5-FU [165]. The combination of CD/5-FC had a more pronounced antitumor impact in animal models, indicating improved effectiveness. A clinical investigation was conducted on individuals with refractory cancer, whereby the intratumoral delivery of TAPET-CD attenuated Salmonella bacteria was used. This bacterium was engineered to encode the *E. coli CD* gene. The study included three patients. The research findings demonstrated a substantial impact and absence of adverse reactions. In a phase I clinical trial, individuals diagnosed with prostate cancer were treated with an oncolytic adenovirus that included a *CD/HSV-1 TK* gene. The findings indicated that the transgene responsible for sustained presence in the prostate was seen for 3 weeks after injection. Developing gene transfer vector manufacturing, including cell lines, techniques, and purification stages, may enhance their safety profile. For example, gutless adenoviral vectors replace all genes save those necessary for virus generation with the desired gene driven by an appropriate promoter. Gutless adenoviruses have good transduction efficiency and comparable properties to earlier vectors but are less immunogenic than first-generation vectors. Gutless vectors lack viral genes, necessitating coinfection with a helper adenovirus for genome replication, packing, and capsid formation. Since helper and gutless vectors share a viral capsid, separating them before purification is tedious and challenging.

2.14 CONCLUSION

Although cancer gene therapy has been more effective in treating monogenetic illnesses, progress in this area is still slow. Gene therapy is a new strategy that offers a promising option for the treatment of illnesses that now lack effective remedies. In the last three decades, significant advancements have been made in the field of gene therapy for the treatment of cancer. While a limited number of medications have received approval, many more are now undergoing clinical trials. Gene therapy has been shown to have superior effectiveness and safety in comparison to chemotherapy in the management of cancer. Genome integration raises valid concerns about current cancer treatments, particularly the risk of transmitting genetic mutations to offspring. Each agent used in gene therapy is considered an orphan drug since it only helps a limited subset of patients with a specific type of cancer. Another problem with cancer gene therapy is that it has not been able to zero in on the cells responsible for metastasis, the leading cause of death from the disease. The difficulties of detecting metastases and overcoming resistance are two of the key reasons why metastasis-specific gene treatments have not been more effective. Gene therapy can be used to treat both primary and secondary cancers, with only little side effects on healthy cells. The use of gene products that either engage the immune system to stop distant invasion or boost their translation in a way that is particular to cancer cells could be a solution. Combining gene therapy with chemotherapy, small molecule inhibitor therapy, radiation therapy, and/or immunotherapy has been shown to significantly increase the success rate of gene therapy for several forms of human cancer.

KEYWORDS

- **clinical trial**
- **DNA**
- **gene therapy**
- **oncolytic virus**
- **siRNAs**

REFERENCES

1. Conti, C. J. (2020). The mouse skin as a model for chemical carcinogenesis. In *Handbook of mouse mutations with skin and hair abnormalities* (Vol. 26, pp. 39–46).
2. Ahmad, M. Z., Akhter, S., Rahman, Z., Akhter, S., Anwar, M., Mallik, N., & Ahmad, F. J. (2013). Nanometric gold in cancer nanotechnology: Current status and prospect. *Journal of Pharmacy and Pharmacology, 65*, 634–651.

3. Ahrendt, S. A., Hu, Y., Buta, M., McDermott, M. P., Benoit, N., Yang, S. C., Wu, L., & Sidransky, D. (2003). P53 mutations and survival in stage I non-small-cell lung cancer: Results of a prospective study. *Journal of National Cancer Institute, 95*, 961–970.
4. Tholomier, C., Martini, A., Mokkapati, S., & Dinney, C. P. (2023). The current status of gene therapy in bladder cancer. *Expert Review of Anticancer Therapy, 23*(5), 531–543.
5. Thomas, A., Samykutty, A., Gomez-Gutierrez, J. G., Yin, W., Egger, M. E., McNally, M., Chuong, P., MacCuaig, W. M., Albeituni, S., Zeiderman, M., & Li, M. (2020). Actively targeted nano delivery of echinomycin induces autophagy-mediated death in chemoresistant pancreatic cancer in vivo. *Cancers, 12*, 2279.
6. Alba, R., Bosch, A., & Chillon, M. (2005). Gutless adenovirus: Last-generation adenovirus for gene therapy. *Gene Therapy, 12*, S18–S27.
7. Odiba, A. S., Okoro, N. O., Durojaye, O. A., & Wu, Y. (2021). Gene therapy in PIDs, hemoglobin, ocular, neurodegenerative, and hemophilia B disorders. *Open Life Sciences, 16*(1), 431–441.
8. Crenshaw, B. J., Jones, L. B., Bell, C. R., Kumar, S., & Matthews, Q. L. (2019). Perspective on adenoviruses: Epidemiology, pathogenicity, and gene therapy. *Biomedicines, 7*(3), 61.
9. Azab, B., Dash, R., Das, S. K., Bhutia, S. K., Shen, X.-N., Quinn, B. A., Sarkar, S., Wang, X.-Y., Hedvat, M., Dmitriev, I. P., Curiel, D. T., Grant, S., Dent, P., Reed, J. C., Pellecchia, M., Sarkar, D., & Fisher, P. B. (2012). Enhanced delivery of mda-7/IL-24 using a serotype chimeric adenovirus (Ad.5/3) in combination with the Apogossypol derivative BI-97C1 (Sabutoclax) improves therapeutic efficacy in low CAR colorectal cancer cells. *Journal of Cell Physiology, 227*, 2145–2153.
10. Gonzalez-Pastor, R., Goedegebuure, P. S., & Curiel, D. T. (2021). Understanding and addressing barriers to successful adenovirus-based virotherapy for ovarian cancer. *Cancer Gene Therapy, 28*(5), 375–389.
11. Zhao, W., Hou, X., Vick, O. G., & Dong, Y. (2019). RNA delivery biomaterials for the treatment of genetic and rare diseases. *Biomaterials, 217*, 119291.
12. Bhoopathi, P., Pradhan, A. K., Kumar, A., Maji, S., Mannangatti, P., Deng, X., Bandyopadhyay, D., Sarkar, D., Wang, X. Y., Landry, J. W., & Das, S. K. (2022). Conversion of a non-cancer-selective promoter into a cancer-selective promoter. *Cancers, 14*(6), 1497.
13. Bhatia, S., Menezes, M. E., Das, S. K., Emdad, L., Dasgupta, S., Wang, X. Y., Sarkar, D., & Fisher, P. B. (2013). Innovative approaches for enhancing cancer gene therapy. *Discovery Medicine, 15*, 309–317.
14. Mantwill, K., Klein, F. G., Wang, D., Hindupur, S. V., Ehrenfeld, M., Holm, P. S., & Nawroth, R. (2021). Concepts in oncolytic adenovirus therapy. *International Journal of Molecular Sciences, 22*(19), 10522.
15. Debela, D. T., Muzazu, S. G., Heraro, K. D., Ndalama, M. T., Mesele, B. W., Haile, D. C., Kitui, S. K., & Manyazewal, T. (2021). New approaches and procedures for cancer treatment: Current perspectives. *SAGE Open Medicine, 9*, 20503121211034366.
16. Rogers, S., & Pfuderer, P. (1968). Use of viruses as carriers of added genetic information. *Nature, 219*, 749–751.

17. Zhao, L., & Yang, X. (2022). Development of cationic lipid-assisted PEG-b-PLA nanoparticle for nucleic acid therapeutics. *Gene Delivery, 29*, 543–554.
18. Terheggen, H. G., Lowenthal, A., Lavinha, F., Colombo, J. P., & Rogers, S. (1975). Unsuccessful trial of gene replacement in arginase deficiency. *Zeitschrift für Kinderheilkunde, 119*, 1–3.
19. Rosenberg, S. A., Aebersold, P., Cornetta, K., Kasid, A., Morgan, R. A., Moen, R., Karson, E. M., Lotze, M. T., Yang, J. C., & Topalian, S. L. (1990). Gene transfer into humans—Immunotherapy of patients with advanced melanoma, using tumor-infiltrating lymphocytes modified by retroviral gene transduction. *New England Journal of Medicine, 323*, 570–578.
20. Plati, J., Bucur, O., & Khosravi-Far, R. (2008). Dysregulation of apoptotic signaling in cancer: Molecular mechanisms and therapeutic opportunities. *Journal of Cellular Biochemistry*, *104*(4), 1124–1149.
21. Sayers, T. J., & Murphy, W. J. (2006). Combining proteasome inhibition with TNF-related apoptosis-inducing ligand (Apo2L/TRAIL) for cancer therapy. *Cancer Immunology, Immunotherapy*, *55*, 76–84.
22. Holoch, P. A., & Griffith, T. S. (2009). TNF-related apoptosis-inducing ligand (TRAIL): A new path to anti-cancer therapies. *European Journal of Pharmacology*, *625*(1–3), 63–72.
23. Pistritto, G., Trisciuoglio, D., Ceci, C., Garufi, A., & D'Orazi, G. (2016). Apoptosis as an anticancer mechanism: Function and dysfunction of its modulators and targeted therapeutic strategies. *Aging*, *8*(4), 603.
24. Curiel, D. T., & Fisher, P. B. (2012). Applications of viruses for cancer therapy. *Advances in Cancer Research*, *115*, 1–334.
25. Das, S. K., Sarkar, S., Dash, R., Dent, P., Wang, X.-Y., Sarkar, D., & Fisher, P. B. (2012). Cancer terminator viruses and approaches for enhancing therapeutic outcomes. *Advances in Cancer Research*, *115*, 1–38.
26. Dash, R., Azab, B., Quinn, B. A., Shen, X. N., Wang, X.-Y., Das, S. K., Rahmani, M., Wei, J., Hedvat, M., Dent, P., Dmitriev, I. P., Curiel, D. T., Grant, S., Wu, B. N., Stebbins, J. L., Pellecchia, M., Reed, J. C., Sarkar, D., & Fisher, P. B. (2011a). Apogossypol derivative BI-97C1 (Sabutoclax) targeting Mcl-1 sensitizes prostate cancer cells to mda-7/IL-24-mediated toxicity. *Proceedings of the National Academy of Science of the United States of America*, *108*, 8785–8790.
27. Dash, R., Azab, B., Shen, X.-N., Sokhi, U. K., Sarkar, S., Su, Z. Z., Wang, X. Y., Claudio, P. P., Dent, P., Dmitriev, I. P., Curiel, D. T., Grant, S., Sarkar, D., & Fisher, P. B. (2011b). Developing an effective gene therapy for prostate cancer: New technologies with potential to translate from the laboratory into the clinic. *Discovery Medicine*, *11*, 46–56.
28. El Sayed, S. R., Cristante, J., Guyon, L., Denis, J., Chabre, O., & Cherradi, N. (2021). MicroRNA therapeutics in cancer: Current advances and challenges. *Cancers*, *13*(11), 2680.
29. Du, L., & Pertsemlidis, A. (2012). MicroRNA regulation of cell viability and drug sensitivity in lung cancer. *Expert Opinion on Biological Therapy*, *12*(9), 1221–1239.
30. Pestka, S., Krause, C. D., Sarkar, D., Walter, M. R., Shi, Y., & Fisher, P. B. (2004). Interleukin-10 and related cytokines and receptors. *Annual Review of Immunology*, *22*, 929–979.

31. Jain, K. K., & Jain, K. K. (2014). Gene Therapy of Cancer. In *Applications of Biotechnology in oncology* (pp. 509–547).
32. Dmitriev, I., Krasnykh, V., Miller, C. R., Wang, M., Kashentseva, E., Mikheeva, G., Belousova, N., & Curiel, D. T. (1998). An adenovirus vector with genetically modified fibers demonstrates expanded tropism via the utilization of a coxsackievirus and adenovirus receptor-independent cell entry mechanism. *Journal of Virology*, *72*, 9706–9713.
33. Ellegala, D. B., Leong-Poi, H., Carpenter, J. E., Klibanov, A. L., Kaul, S., Shaffrey, M. E., Sklenar, J., & Lindner, J. R. (2003). Imaging tumor angiogenesis with contrast ultrasound and microbubbles targeted to alpha(v) beta3. *Circulation*, *108*, 336–341.
34. Emdad, L., Lebedeva, I. V., Su, Z. Z., Gupta, P., Sarkar, D., Settleman, J., & Fisher, P. B. (2007). Combinatorial treatment of non-small-cell lung cancers with gefitinib and Ad.*mda-7* enhances apoptosis-induction and reverses resistance to a single therapy. *Journal of Cell Physiology*, *210*(2), 549–559.
35. Emdad, L., Lebedeva, I. V., Su, Z. Z., Gupta, P., Sauane, M., Dash, R., Grant, S., Dent, P., Curiel, D. T., Sarkar, D., & Fisher, P. B. (2009). Historical perspective and recent insights into our understanding of the molecular and biochemical basis of the antitumor properties of *mda-7*/IL-24. *Cancer Biology & Therapy*, *8*, 391–400.
36. Esquela-Kerscher, A., & Slack, F. J. (2006). Oncomirs - microRNAs with a role in cancer. *Nature Reviews Cancer*, *6*, 259–269.
37. Eulitt, P. J., Park, M. A., Hamed, H. A., Cruikshank, N., Yang, C., Dmitriev, I. P., Yacoub, A., Curiel, D. T., Fisher, P. B., & Dent, P. (2010). Enhancing *mda 7*/ IL-24 therapy in renal carcinoma cells by inhibiting multiple protective signaling pathways using sorafenib and by Ad.5/3 gene delivery. *Cancer Biology Therapy*, *10*, 1290–1305.
38. Farma, J. M., Puhlmann, M., Soriano, P. A., Cox, D., Paciotti, G. F., Tamarkin, L., & Alexander, H. R. (2007). Direct evidence for rapid and selective induction of tumor neovascular permeability by tumor necrosis factor and a novel derivative, colloidal gold bound tumor necrosis factor. *International Journl of Cancer*, *120*, 2474–2480.
39. Fisher, P. B. (2005). Is mda-7/IL-24 a "magic bullet" for cancer? *Cancer Research, 65*, 10128–10138.
40. Fillat, C., Carrio, M., Cascante, A., & Sangro, B. (2003). Suicide gene therapy mediated by the Herpes Simplex virus thymidine kinase gene/Ganciclovir system: fifteen years of application. *Current Gene Therapy*, *3*(1), 13–26.
41. Van der Eb, M. M., Cramer, S. J., Vergouwe, Y., Schagen, F. H., Van Krieken, J. H., Van der Eb, A. J., Rinkes, I. H., Van de Velde, C. J., & Hoeben, R. C. (1998). Severe hepatic dysfunction after adenovirus-mediated transfer of the herpes simplex virus thymidine kinase gene and ganciclovir administration. *Gene Therapy*, *5*(4), 451–458.
42. McAuliffe, S. M., Morgan, S. L., Wyant, G. A., Tran, L. T., Muto, K. W., Chen, Y. S., Chin, K. T., Partridge, J. C., Poole, B. B., Cheng, K. H., & Daggett, Jr. J. (2012). Targeting Notch, a key pathway for ovarian cancer stem cells, sensitizes tumors to platinum therapy. *Proceedings of the National Academy of Sciences*, *109*(43), E2939–E2948.
43. Kicielinski, K. P., Chiocca, E. A., John, S. Y., Gill, G. M., Coffey, M., & Markert, J. M. (2014). Phase 1 clinical trial of intratumoral reovirus infusion for the treatment of recurrent malignant gliomas in adults. *Molecular Therapy*, *22*(5), 1056–1062.

44. World Health Organization. (2003). Adherence to long-term therapies: Evidence for action. *World Health Organization*, 216.
45. Fournillier, A., Frelin, L., Jacquier, E., Ahlen, G., Brass, A., Gerossier, E., Holmstrom, F., Broderick, K. E., Sardesai, N. Y., Bonnefoy, J. Y., Inchauspe, G., & Sallberg, M. (2013). A heterologous prime/boost vaccination strategy enhances the immunogenicity of therapeutic vaccines for hepatitis C virus. *Journal of Infectious Diseases*, *208*, 1008–1019.
46. Freeman, S. M., Abboud, C. N., Whartenby, K. A., Packman, C. H., Koeplin, D. S., Moolten, F. L., & Abraham, G. N. (1993). The bystander effect-tumor-regression when a fraction of the tumor mass is genetically-modified. *Cancer Research*, *53*, 5274–5283.
47. Friedmann, T. (1992). A brief history of gene therapy. *Nature Genetics*, *2*, 93–98.
48. Fuerer, C., & Iggo, R. (2002). Adenoviruses with Tcf binding sites in multiple early promoters show enhanced selectivity for tumour cells with constitutive activation of the wnt signalling pathway. *Gene Therapy*, *9*, 270–281.
49. Fujiwara, T., Shirakawa. Y., & Kagawa, S. (2011). Telomerase-specific oncolytic virotherapy for human gastrointestinal cancer. *Expert Review of Anticancer Therapy*, *11*, 525–532.
50. Nettelbeck, D. M. (2008). Cellular genetic tools to control oncolytic adenoviruses for virotherapy of cancer. *Journal of Molecular Medicine*, *86*, 363–377.
51. Hall, P. A. (1998). p53: The challenge of linking basic science and patient management. *The Oncologist*, *3*(4), 218–224.
52. Gabrilovich, D. I. (2006). INGN 201 (Advexin): Adenoviral p53 gene therapy for cancer. *Expert Opinion on Biological Therapy*, *6*, 823–832.
53. Gao, P., Sun, X., Chen, X., Wang, Y., Foster, B. A., Subjeck, J., Fisher, P. B., & Wang, X.-Y. (2008). Secretable chaperone Grp170 enhances therapeutic activity of a novel tumor suppressor, *mda-7*/IL-24. *Cancer Research*, *68*, 3890–3898.
54. Goel, R., Shah, N., Visaria, R., Paciotti, G. F., & Bischof, J. C. (2009). Biodistribution of TNF-alpha-coated gold nanoparticles in an in vivo model system. *Nanomedicine (London)*, *4*, 401–410.
55. Gotoh, A., Ko, S. C., Shirakawa, T., Cheon, J., Kao, C., Miyamoto, T., Gardner, T. A., Ho, L. J., Cleutjens, C. B., Trapman, J., Graham, F. L., & Chung, L. W. (1998). Development of prostate-specific antigen promoter-based gene therapy for androgen-independent human prostate cancer. *Journal of Urology*, *160*, 220–229.
56. Lee, C. S., Bishop, E. S., Zhang, R., Yu, X., Farina, E. M., Yan, S., Zhao, C., Zeng, Z., Shu, Y., Wu, X., & Lei, J. (2017). Adenovirus-mediated gene delivery: Potential applications for gene and cell-based therapies in the new era of personalized medicine. *Genes & Diseases*, *4*(2), 43–63.
57. Greco, A., Di Benedetto, A., Howard, C. M., Kelly, S., Nande, R., Dementieva, Y., Miranda, M., Brunetti, A., Salvatore, M., Claudio, L., Sarkar, D., Dent, P., Curiel, D. T., Fisher, P. B., & Claudio, P. P. (2010). Eradication of therapy-resistant human prostate tumors using an ultrasound-guided site-specific cancer terminator virus delivery approach. *Molecular Theraphy*, *18*, 295–306.
58. Griffith, T. S., Stokes, B., Kucaba, T. A., Earel, J. K. Jr., VanOosten, R. L., Brincks, E. L., Norian, L. A. (2009). TRAIL gene therapy: From preclinical development to clinical application. *Current Gene Theraphy*, *9*, 9–19.

59. Dogbey, D. M., Torres, V. E., Fajemisin, E., Mpondo, L., Ngwenya, T., Akinrinmade, O. A., Perriman, A. W., & Barth, S. (2023). Technological advances in the use of viral and non-viral vectors for delivering genetic and non-genetic cargos for cancer therapy. *Drug Delivery and Translational Research*, *13*(11), 1–20.
60. Wirth, T., & Ylä-Herttuala, S. (2014). Gene therapy used in cancer treatment. *Biomedicines*, *2*(2), 149–162.
61. Gamvrellis, A., Leong, D., Hanley, J. C., Xiang, S. D., Mottram, P., & Plebanski, M. (2004). Vaccines that facilitate antigen entry into dendritic cells. *Immunology and Cell Biology*, *82*(5), 506–516.
62. Huang, T. G., Savontaus, M. J., Shinozaki, K., Sauter, B. V., & Woo, S. L. (2003). Telomerase-dependent oncolytic adenovirus for cancer treatment. *Gene Therapy*, *10*, 1241–1247.
63. Irving, J., Wang, Z., Powell, S., O'Sullivan, C., Mok, M., Murphy, B., Cardoza, L., Lebkowski, J. S., & Majumdar, A. S. (2004). Conditionally replicative adenovirus driven by the human telomerase promoter provides broad-spectrum antitumor activity without liver toxicity. *Cancer Gene Therapy*, *11*, 174–185.
64. Jain, K. (2009). *Pharmacology-VolII-Gene therapy* (pp. 331–359).
65. Jain, S., Hirst, D. G., O'Sullivan, J. M. (2012). Gold nanoparticles as novel agents for cancer therapy. *British Journal of Radiology*, *85*, 101–113.
66. Jia, L. T., Chen, S. Y., & Yang, A. G. (2012). Cancer gene therapy targeting cellular apoptosis machinery. *Cancer Treatment Review*, *38*, 868–876.
67. Jiang, H., & Fisher, P. B. (1993). Use of a sensitive and efficient subtraction hybridization protocol for the identification of genes differentially regulated during the induction of differentiation in human melanoma cells. *Molecular Cell Different*, *1*, 285–299.
68. Jiang, H., Lin, J. J., Su, Z. Z., Goldstein, N. I., & Fisher, P. B. (1995). Subtraction hybridization identifies a novel melanoma differentiation associated gene, *mda-7*, modulated during human melanoma differentiation, growth and progression. *Oncogene*, *11*, 2477–2486.
69. Jiang, H., Su, Z. Z., Lin, J. J., Goldstein, N. I., Young, C. S., & Fisher, P. B. (1996). The melanoma differentiation associated gene mda-7 suppresses cancer cell growth. *Proceedings of the Natuaral Academy of Science of the United States of America*, *93*, 9160–9165.
70. Kanerva, A., Mikheeva, G. V., Krasnykh, V., Coolidge, C. J., Lam, J. T., Mahasreshti, P. J., Barker, S. D., Straughn, M., Barnes, M. N., Alvarez, R. D., Hemminki, A., & Curiel, D. T. (2002). Targeting adenovirus to the serotype 3 receptor increases gene transfer efficiency to ovarian cancer cells. *Clinical Cancer Research*, *8*, 275–280.
71. Raty, J. K., Lesch, H. P., Wirth, T., & Yla-Herttuala, S. (2008). Improving safety of gene therapy. *Current Drug Safety*, *3*, 46–53.
72. Coughlan, L., Alba, R., Parker, A. L., Bradshaw, A. C., McNeish, I. A., Nicklin, S. A., & Baker, A. H. (2010). Tropism-modification strategies for targeted gene delivery using adenoviral vectors. *Viruses*, *2*, 2290–2355.
73. Montini, E. (2011). Quest for safety at AAValon. *Blood*, *117*, 3249–3250.
74. Biffi, A., Bartolomae, C. C., Cesana, D., Cartier, N., Aubourg, P., Ranzani, M., Cesani, M., Benedicenti, F., Plati, T., Rubagotti, E., & et al. (2011). Lentiviral vector

common integration sites in preclinical models and a clinical trial reflect a benign integration bias and not oncogenic selection. *Blood*, *117*, 5332–5339.

75. Matrai, J., Chuah, M. K., & VandenDriessche, T. (2010). Recent advances in lentiviral vector development and applications. *Molecuar Therapy*, *18*, 477–490.
76. Sharma, A., Li, X., Bangari, D. S., & Mittal, S. K. (2009). Adenovirus receptors and their implications in gene delivery. *Virus Research*, *143*, 184–194.
77. Heyde, M., Partridge, K. A., Oreffo, R. O., Howdle, S. M., Shakesheff, K. M., & Garnett, M. C. (2007). Gene therapy used for tissue engineering applications. *Journal of Pharmacy and Pharmacology*, *59*, 329–350.
78. Pathak, A., Patnaik, S., & Gupta, K. C. (2009). Recent trends in non-viral vector-mediated gene delivery. *Biotechnology Journal*, *4*, 1559–1572.
79. Mudhakir, D., & Harashima, H. (2009). Learning from the viral journey: How to enter cells and how to overcome intracellular barriers to reach the nucleus. *AAPS Journal*, *11*, 65–77.Biomedicines 2014, *2* 160.
80. Escoffre, J. M., Teissie, J., & Rols, M. P. (2010). Gene transfer: How can the biological barriers be overcome? *Journal of Membrane Biology*, *236*, 61–74.
81. Kashentseva, E. A., Seki, T., Curiel, D. T., & Dmitriev, I. P. (2002). Adenovirus targeting to c-erbB-2 oncoprotein by single-chain antibody fused to trimeric form of adenovirus receptor ectodomain. *Cancer Research*, *62*, 609–616.
82. Fausther-Bovendo, H., & Kobinger, G. P. (2014). Pre-existing immunity against Ad vectors: Humoral, cellular, and innate response, what's important?. *Human Vaccines & Immunotherapeutics*, *10*(10), 2875–2884.
83. Kawabe, S., Nishikawa, T., Munshi, A., Roth, J. A., Chada, S., & Meyn, R. E. (2002). Adenovirus-mediated *mda-7* gene expression radiosensitizes non-small cell lung cancer cells via TP53-independent mechanisms. *Molecular Theraphy*, *6*, 637–644.
84. Kawakami, Y., Li, H., Lam, J. T., Krasnykh, V., Curiel, D. T., & Blackwell, J. L. (2003). Substitution of the adenovirus serotype 5 knob with a serotype 3 knob enhances multiple steps in virus replication. *Cancer Research*, *63*, 1262–1269.
85. Kim, E., Kim, J.H., Shin, H. Y., Lee, H., Yang, J. M., Kim, J., Sohn, J. H., Kim, H., & Yun, C. (2003). O. Ad-mTERT-delta19, a conditional replication-competent adenovirus driven by the human telomerase promoter, selectively replicates in and elicits cytopathic effect in a cancer cell-specific manner. *Human Gene Therapy*, *14*, 1415–1428.
86. Kircher, M., & Kelso, J. (2010). High-throughput DNA sequencing–concepts and limitations. *Bioessays*, *32*, 524–536.
87. Singh, S., Kumar, R., & Agrawal, B. (2019). Adenoviral vector-based vaccines and gene therapies: Current status and prospects. *Adenoviruses*, *4*, 53–91.
88. Krens, L. L., Baas, J. M., Gelderblom, H., & Guchelaar, H. J. (2010). Therapeutic modulation of k-ras signaling in colorectal cancer. *Drug Discovery Today*, *15*, 502–516.
89. Lai, T. C., Kataoka, K., & Kwon, G. S. (2012). Bioreducible polyether-based pDNA ternary polyplexes: Balancing particle stability and transfection efficiency. *Colloids Surfuce B Biointerfaces*, *99*, 27–37. [PMC free article] [PubMed] [Google Scholar]
90. Lanson, N. A. Jr., Friedlander, P. L., Schwarzenberger, P., Kolls, J. K., & Wang, G. (2003). Replication of an adenoviral vector controlled by the human telomerase

reverse transcriptase promoter causes tumor-selective tumor lysis. *Cancer Research*, *63*, 7936–7941.
91. Larina, I. V., Evers, B. M., Ashitkov, T. V., Bartels, C., Larin, K. V., & Esenaliev, R. O. (2005). Enhancement of drug delivery in tumors by using interaction of nanoparticles with ultrasound radiation. *Technology in Cancer Research and Treatment*, *4*, 217–226.
92. Larocca, C., & Schlom, J. (2011). Viral vector-based therapeutic cancer vaccines. *Cancer Journal*, *17*, 359–371.
93. Lawrie, A., Brisken, A. F., Francis, S. E., Cumberland, D. C., Crossman, D. C., & Newman, C. M. (2000). Microbubble-enhanced ultrasound for vascular gene delivery. *Gene Therapy*, *7*, 2023–2027.
94. Lebedeva, I. V., Emdad, L., Su, Z. Z., Gupta, P., Sauane, M., Sarkar, D., Staudt, M. R., Liu, S. J., Taher, M. M., Xiao, R., Barral, P., Lee, S. G., Wang, D., Vozhilla, N., Park, E. S., Chatman, L., Boukerche, H., Ramesh, R., Inoue, S., Chada, S., Li, R., De Pass, A. L., Mahasreshti, P. J., Dmitriev, I. P., Curiel, D. T., Yacoub, A., Grant, S., Dent, P., Senzer, N., Nemunaitis, J. J., Fisher, P. B. (2007). Mda-7/IL-24, novel anticancer cytokine: Focus on bystander antitumor, radiosensitization and antiangiogenic properties and overview of the phase I clinical experience (Review). *International Journal of Oncology*, *31*, 985–1007.
95. Alba, R., & Bosch, A., & Chillon, M. (2005). Gutless adenovirus: last-generation adenovirus for gene therapy. *Gene Therapy*, *12*(1), S18–S27.
96. Lebedeva, I. V., Su, Z. Z., Sarkar, D., & Fisher, P. B. (2003). Restoring apoptosis as a strategy for cancer gene therapy: Focus on p53 and mda-7. *Seminars in Cancer Biology*, *13*, 169–178.
97. Lebedeva, I. V., Su, Z. Z., Vozhilla, N., Chatman, L., Sarkar, D., Dent, P., Athar, M., Fisher, P. B. (2008a). Chemoprevention by perillyl alcohol coupled with viral gene therapy reduces pancreatic cancer pathogenesis. *Molecular Cancer Therapy*, *7*, 2042–2050.
98. Lebedeva, I. V., Su, Z. Z., Vozhilla, N., Chatman, L., Sarkar, D., Dent, P., Athar, M., & Fisher, P. B. (2008b). Mechanism of in vitro pancreatic cancer cell growth inhibition by melanoma differentiation-associated gene-7/interleukin-24 and perillyl alcohol. *Cancer Resarch*, *68*, 7439–7447.
99. Lee, S. J., Kim, H. S., Yu, R., Lee, K., Gardner, T. A., Jung, C., Jeng, M. H., Yeung, F., Cheng, L., & Kao, C. (2002). Novel prostate-specific promoter derived from PSA and PSMA enhancers. *Molecular Therapy*, *6*, 415–421.
100. Leszczyniecka, M., Roberts, T., Dent, P., Grant, S., & Fisher, P. B. (2001). Differentiation therapy of cancer: Basic science and clinical applications. *Pharmacology & Therapeutics*, *90*, 105–156.
101. Li, Y. H. G., Diakur, J., & Wiebe, L. I. (2008). Targeted delivery of macromolecular drugs: Asialoglycoprotein receptor (ASGPR) expression by selected hepatoma cell lines used in antiviral drug development. *Current Drug Delivery*, *5*, 4–10.
102. Li, X., Zhang, Y. P., Kim, H. S., Bae, K. H., Stantz, K. M., Lee, S. J., Jung, C., Jimenez, J. A., Gardner, T. A., Jeng, M. H., & Kao, C. (2005). Gene therapy for prostate cancer by controlling adenovirus E1a and E4 gene expression with PSES enhancer. *Cancer Research*, *65*, 1941–1951.
103. Liu, G., Wong-Staal, F., Li. Q. X. (2007). Development of new RNAi therapeutics. *Histology and Histopathology*, *22*, 211–217.

104. Philipson, L., & Pettersson, R. F. (2004). The coxsackie-adenovirus receptor—A new receptor in the immunoglobulin family involved in cell adhesion. *Current Topics in Microbiology and Immunology*, *273*, 87–111.
105. Buchholz, C. J., Friedel, T., & Büning, H. (2015). Surface-engineered viral vectors for selective and cell type-specific gene delivery. *Trends in Biotechnology*, *33*(12), 777–790.
106. Putney, S. D., Brown, J., Cucco, C., Lee, R., Skorski, T., Leonetti, C., Geiser, T., Calabretta, B., Zupi, G., & Zon, G. (1999). Enhanced anti-tumor effects with microencapsulated c-myc antisense oligonucleotide. *Antisense Nucl Acid Drug Devlopment*, *9*, 451–458.
107. Ramesh, R., Ito, I., Saito, Y., Wu, Z., Mhashikar, A. M., Wilson, D. R., Branch, C. D., Roth, J. A., & Chada, S. (2004). Local and systemic inhibition of lung tumor growth after nanoparticle-mediated mda-7/IL-24 gene delivery. *DNA Cell Biology*, *23*, 850–857.
108. Ramesh, R., Mhashilkar, A. M., Tanaka, F., Saito, Y., Branch, C. D., Sieger, K., Mumm, J. B., Stewart, A. L., Boquoi, A., Dumoutier, L., Grimm, E. A, Renauld, J. C., Kotenko, S., & Chada, S. (2003). Melanoma differentiation-associated gene 7/interleukin (IL)-24 is a novel ligand that regulates angiogenesis via the IL-22 receptor. *Cancer Research*, *63*, 5105–5113.
109. Raty, J. K., Pikkarainen, J. T., Wirth, T., & Yla-Herttuala, S. (2008). Gene therapy: The first approved gene-based medicines, molecular mechanisms and clinical indications. *Current Molecular Pharmacology*, *1*, 13–23.
110. Reid, T., Warren, R., & Kirn, D. (2002). Intravascular adenoviral agents in cancer patients: Lessons from clinical trials. *Cancer Gene Therapy*, *9*, 979–986.
111. Rein, D. T., Breidenbach, M., Kirby, T. O., Han, T., Siegal, G. P., Bauerschmitz, G. J., Wang, M., Nettelbeck, D. M., Tsuruta, Y., Yamamoto, M., Dall, P., Hemminki, A., & Curiel, D. T. (2005). A fiber-modified, secretory leukoprotease inhibitor promoter-based conditionally replicating adenovirus for treatment of ovarian cancer. *Clin Cancer Research*, *11*, 1327–1335.
112. Rivera, A. A., Davydova, J., Schierer, S., Wang, M., Krasnykh, V., Yamamoto, M., Curiel, D. T., & Nettelbeck, D. M. (2004). Combining high selectivity of replication with fiber chimerism for effective adenoviral oncolysis of CAR-negative melanoma cells. *Gene Therapy*, *11*, 1694–1702.
113. Rodriguez, R., Schuur, E. R., Lim, H. Y., Henderson, G. A., Simons, J. W., & Henderson, D. R. (1997). Prostate attenuated replication competent adenovirus (ARCA) CN706: A selective cytotoxic for prostate-specific antigen- positive prostate cancer cells. *Cancer Research*, *57*, 2559–2563.
114. Rogers, S., Lowentha, A., Terhegge, H. G., & Columbo, J. P. (1973). Induction of arginase activity with shope papilloma virus in tissue-culture cells from an argininemic patient. *Journal of Experimental Medicine*, *137*, 1091–1096.
115. Rogers, S., & Pfuderer, P. (1968). Use of viruses as carriers of added genetic information. *Nature*, *219*, 749–756.
116. Rosenberg, S. A., Aebersold, P., Cornetta, K., Kasid, A., Morgan, R. A., Moen, R., Karson, E. M., Lotze, M. T., Yang, J. C., Topalian, S. L., & et al. (1990). Gene transfer into humans—Immunotherapy of patients with advanced melanoma, using

tumor-infiltrating lymphocytes modified by retroviral gene transduction. *New England Journal of Medicine*, *323*, 570–578.

117. Roth, J. A., Nguyen, D., Lawrence, D. D., Kemp, B. L., Carrasco, C. H., Ferson, D. Z., Hong, W. K., Komaki, R., Lee, J. J., Nesbitt, J. C., Pisters, K. M., Putnam, J. B., Schea, R., Shin, D. M., Walsh, G. L., Dolormente, M. M., Han, C. I., Martin, F. D., Yen, N., Xu, K., Stephens, L. C., McDonnell, T. J., Mukhopadhyay, T., & Cai, D. (1996). Retrovirus-mediated wild-type p53 gene transfer to tumors of patients with lung cancer. *Nature Medicine*, *2*, 985–991.
118. Sarkar, D., Lebedeva, I. V., Gupta, P., Emdad, L., Sauane, M., Dent, P., Curiel, D. T., & Fisher, P. B. (2007a). Melanoma differentiation associated gene-7 (*mda-7*)/ IL-24: A 'magic bullet' for cancer therapy. *Expert Opinion on Biological Therapy*, *7*, 577–586.
119. Sarkar, D., Lebedeva, I. V., Su, Z. Z., Park, E. S., Chatman, L., Vozhilla, N., Dent, P., Curiel, D. T., & Fisher, P. B. (2007b). Eradication of therapy-resistant human prostate tumors using a cancer terminator virus. *Cancer Research, 67*, 5434–5442.
120. Sarkar, S., Quinn, A. B., Shen, B. A., Dent, X., Klibanov, P., Emdad, A. L., Das, L., Sarkar, S. K., & Fisher, D. (2013). Chemoprevention gene therapy (CGT) of pancreatic cancer using perillyl alcohol and a novel chimeric serotype Cancer Terminator Virus. *Current Molecular Medicone*, *14*, 125–140.
121. Sarkar, D., Su, Z. Z., & Fisher, P. B. (2006). Unique conditionally replication competent bipartite adenoviruses-cancer terminator viruses (CTV): Efficacious reagents for cancer gene therapy. *Cell Cycle*, *5*, 1531–1536.
122. Sarkar, D., Su, Z. Z., Vozhilla, N., Park, E. S., Gupta, P., & Fisher, P. B. (2005a). Dual cancer-specific targeting strategy cures primary and distant breast carcinomas in nude mice. *Proceedings of the National Academy of Science of the United States of America*, *102*, 14034–14039.
123. Sarkar, D., Su, Z. Z., Vozhilla, N., Park, E. S., Randolph, A., Valerie, K., & Fisher, P. B. (2005b). Targeted virus replication plus immunotherapy eradicates primary and distant pancreatic tumors in nude mice. *Cancer Research*, *65*, 9056–9063.
124. Sauane, M., Gopalkrishnan, R. V., Sarkar, D., Su, Z.-Z., Lebedeva, I. V., Dent, P., Pestka, S., & Fisher, P. B. (2003). Mda-7/IL-24: Novel cancer growth suppressing and apoptosis inducing cytokine. *Cytokine Growth Factor Reviews*,*14*, 35–51.
125. Sauane, M., Gupta, P., Lebedeva, I. V., Su, Z. Z., Sarkar, D., Randolph, A., Valerie, K., Gopalkrishnan, R. V, & Fisher, P. B. (2006). N-glycosylation of MDA-7/ IL-24 is dispensable for tumor cell-specific apoptosis and "bystander" antitumor activity. *Cancer Research*, *66*, 11869–11877.
126. Sauane, M., Su, Z. Z., Gupta, P., Lebedeva, I. V., Dent, P., Sarkar, D., & Fisher, P. B. (2008). Autocrine regulation of mda-7/IL-24 mediates cancer-specific apoptosis. *Proceedings of the National Academy of Sciences of the United States of America*, *105*, 9763–9768.
127. Stolberg, S. G. (1999). The biotech death of Jesse Gelsinger. *NY Times Magazine*, *136–140*, 149–150.
128. Studeny, M., Champlin, M.F., Zompetta, R. E., & Fidler, C. (2002). Bone marrow-derived mesenchymal stem cells as vehicles for interferon-β delivery into tumors. *Cancer Research*, *62*, 3603–3608.

129. Su, Z. Z., Emdad, L., Sauane, M., Lebedeva, I. V., Sarkar, D., Gupta, P., James, C. D., Randolph, A., Valerie, K., Walter, M. R., Dent, P., & Fisher, P. B. (2005a). Unique aspects of *mda-7*/IL-24 antitumor bystander activity: establishing a role for secretion of MDA-7/IL-24 protein by normal cells. *Oncogene*, *24*, 7552–7566.
130. Su, Z., Lebedeva, I. V., Gopalkrishnan, R. V., Goldstein, N. I., Stein, C. A., Reed, J. C., Dent, P., & Fisher, P. B. (2001). A combinatorial approach for selectively inducing programmed cell death in human pancreatic cancer cells. *Proceedings of the National Academy of Sciences of the United States of America*, *98*, 10332–10337.
131. Su, Z., Lebedeva, I. V., Gopalkrishnan, R. V., Goldstein, N. I., Stein, C. A., Reed, J. C., Dent, P., & Fisher, P. B. (2001). A combinatorial approach for selectively inducing programmed cell death in human pancreatic cancer cells. *Proceedings of the National of Academy of Sciences of the United States of the America*, *98*, 10332–10337.
132. Das, S. K., Menezes, M. E., Bhatia, S., Wang, X. Y., Emdad, L., Sarkar, D., & Fisher, P. B. (2015). Gene therapies for cancer: Strategies, challenges and successes. *Journal of Cellular Physiology*, *230*(2), 259–271.
133. Terheggen, H. G., Lowenthal, A., Lavinha, F., Colombo, J. P., & Rogers, S. (1975). Unsuccessful trial of gene replacement in arginase deficiency. *Zeitschrift für Kinderheilkunde*, *119*, 1–3.
134. Howard, C. M., Forsberg, F., Minimo, C., Liu, J. B., Merton, D. A., & Claudio, P. P. (2006). Ultrasound guided site specific gene delivery system using adenoviral vectors and commercial ultrasound contrast agents. *Journal of Cell Physiology*, *209*, 413–421.
135. Santiago-Ortiz, J. L., & Schaffer, D. V. (2016). Adeno-associated virus (AAV) vectors in cancer gene therapy. *Journal of Controlled Release*, *240*, 287–301.
136. Danhier, F., Feron, O., & Préat, V. (2010). To exploit the tumor microenvironment: passive and active tumor targeting of nanocarriers for anti-cancer drug delivery. *Journal of Controlled Release*, *148*(2), 135–146.
137. Marshall, E. (1995). Gene therapy's growing pains: With more than 100 clinical trials started and hundreds of millions of dollars at stake the field is struggling to meet expectations. *Science*, *269*(5227), 1050–1055.
138. Vita, M., & Henriksson, M. (2006). The Myc oncoprotein as a therapeutic target for human cancer. *Seminars in Cancer Biology*, *16*, 318–330.
139. Li, K., Du, Y., Li, L., & Wei, D. Q. (2020). Bioinformatics approaches for anti-cancer drug discovery. *Current Drug Targets*, *21*(1), 3–17.
140. Thoma, C., Bachy, V., Seaton, P., Green, N. K., Greaves, D. R., Klavinskis, L., Seymour, L. W., & Morrison, J. (2013). Adenovirus serotype 11 causes less long-term intraperitoneal inflammation than serotype 5: Implications for ovarian cancer therapy. *Virology*, *447*, 74–83.
141. Wirth, T., Hedman, M., Makinen, K., Manninen, H., Immonen, A., Vapalahti, M., & Yla-Herttuala, S. (2006). Safety profile of plasmid/liposomes and virus vectors in clinical gene therapy. *Current Drug Safety*, *1*, 253–257. Biomedicines 2014, 2 162.
142. Wang, J., Faust, S. M., & Rabinowitz, J. E. (2011). The next step in gene delivery: Molecular engineering of adeno-associated virus serotypes. *Journal of Molecular and Cellular Cardiology*, *50*, 793–802.
143. Kim, K. H., Ryan, M. J., Estep, J. E., Miniard, B. M., Rudge, T. L., Peggins, J. O., Broadt, T. L., Wang, M., Preuss, M. A., Siegal, G. P., & et al. (2011). A new generation

of serotype chimeric infectivity-enhanced conditionally replicative adenovirals: The safety profile of ad5/3-Delta24 in advance of a phase I clinical trial in ovarian cancer patients. *Human Gene Theraphy*, *22*, 821–828.
144. Wang, L., Calcedo, R., Bell, P., Lin, J., Grant, R. L., Siegel, D. L., & Wilson, J. M. (2011). Impact of pre-existing immunity on gene transfer to nonhuman primate liver with adeno-associated virus 8 vectors. *Human Gene Theraphy*, *22*, 1389–1401.
145. Barnett, B. G., Crews, C. J., & Douglas, J. T. (2002). Targeted adenoviral vectors. *Biochimica et Biophysica Acta*, *1575*, 1–14.
146. Urnov, F. D., Rebar, E. J., Holmes, M. C., Zhang, H. S., & Gregory, P. D. (2010). Genome editing with engineered zinc finger nucleases. *Nature Reviews Genetics*, *11*, 636–646.
147. Staunstrup, N. H., Moldt, B., Mates, L., Villesen, P., Jakobsen, M., Ivics, Z., Izsvak, Z., & Mikkelsen, J. G. (2009). Hybrid lentivirus-transposon vectors with a random integration profile in human cells. *Molecular Theraphy*, *17*, 1205–1214.
148. Mates, L., Chuah, M. K., Belay, E., Jerchow, B., Manoj, N., Acosta-Sanchez, A., Grzela, D. P., Schmitt, A., Becker, K., Matrai, J., & et al. (2009). Molecular evolution of a novel hyperactive sleeping beauty transposase enables robust stable gene transfer in vertebrates. *Nature Genetics*, *41*, 753–761.
149. VandenDriessche, T., Ivics, Z., Izsvak, Z., & Chuah, M. K. (2009). Emerging potential of transposons for gene therapy and generation of induced pluripotent stem cells. *Blood*, *114*, 1461–1468.
150. Patel, S. R. (2000). Radiation-induced sarcoma. *Current Treatment Options in Oncology*, *1*, 258–261.
151. Harris, C. C. (1976). The carcinogenicity of anticancer drugs: A hazard in man. *Cancer*, *37*, 1014–1023.
152. Boffetta, P., & Kaldor, J. M. (1994). Secondary malignancies following cancer chemotherapy. *Acta Oncology*, *33*, 591–598.
153. Lang, F. F., Bruner, J. M., Fuller, G. N., Aldape, K., Prados, M. D., Chang, S., Berger, M. S., McDermott, M. W., Kunwar, S. M., Junck, L. R., & et al. (2003). Phase I trial of adenovirus-mediated p53 gene therapy for recurrent glioma: Biological and clinical results. *Journal of Clinical Oncology*, *21*, 2508–2518.
154. Raty, J. K., Pikkarainen, J. T., Wirth, T., & Yla-Herttuala, S. (2008) Gene therapy: The first approved gene-based medicines, molecular mechanisms, and clinical indications. *Current Molecular Pharmacology*, *1*, 13–23.
155. Han, D. M., Huang, Z. G., Zhang, W., Yu, Z. K., Wang, Q., Ni, X., Chen, X. H., Pan, J. H., & Wang, H. (2003). Effectiveness of recombinant adenovirus p53 injection on laryngeal cancer: Phase I clinical trial and follow up. *Zhonghua Yi Xue Za Zhi*, *83*, 2029–2032.
156. Peng, Z. (2005). Current status of gendicine in China: Recombinant human Ad-p53 agent for treatment of cancers. *Human Gene Therapy*, *16*, 1016–1027.
157. Bischoff, J. R., Kirn, D. H., Williams, A., Heise, C., Horn, S., Muna, M., Ng, L., Nye, J. A., Sampson-Johannes, A., Fattaey, A., & et al. (1996). An adenovirus mutant that replicates selectively in p53-deficient human tumor cells. *Science*, *274*, 373–376.
158. Chiocca, E. A., Abbed, K. M., Tatter, S., Louis, D. N., Hochberg, F. H., Barker, F., Kracher, J., Grossman, S. A., Fisher, J. D., Carson, K., & et al. (2004). A phase I open-label, dose-escalation, multi-institutional trial of injection with an E1B-Attenuated

adenovirus, ONYX-015, into the peritumoral region of recurrent malignant gliomas, in the adjuvant setting. *Molecular Therapy*, *10*, 958–966.

159. Yu, W., & Fang H. (2007). Clinical trials with oncolytic adenovirus in China. *Current Cancer Drug Targets*, *7*, 141–148.
160. Wiman, K. G. (1993). The retinoblastoma gene: Role in cell cycle control and cell differentiation. *FASEB Journal, 7*, 841–845.
161. Wirth, T., Parker, N., & Yla-Herttuala, S. (2013). History of gene therapy. *Gene, 525*, 162–169.
162. Düzgüneş, N. (2019). Origins of suicide gene therapy. In *Suicide gene therapy* (pp. 1–9). Humana Press
163. Dey, D., Evans, G. R. (2011). Suicide gene therapy by herpes simplex virus-1 thymidine kinase (HSV-TK). In *Targets gene therapy* (Vol. 65).
164. Sonabend, A. M., Ulasov, I. V., & Lesniak, M. S. (2007). Gene therapy trials for the treatment of high-grade gliomas. *Gene Therapy and Molecular Biology*, *11*(A), 79.
165. Aučynaitė, A., Rutkienė, R., Tauraitė, D., Meškys, R., & Urbonavičius, J. (2018). Discovery of bacterial deaminases that convert 5-fluoroisocytosine into 5-fluorouracil. *Front Microbiology*, *9*, 2375. DOI: 10.3389/ fmicb.2018.02375
166. Zarogoulidis, P., Darwiche, K., Sakkas, A., & et al. (2013). Suicide gene therapy for cancer–current strategies. *Journal of Genetic Syndromes and Gene Therapy, 4*, 16849.

CHAPTER 3

Current Status and Prospects for Cancer Gene Therapy

ABSTRACT

Novel discoveries in human genomics have shown the critical function of somatic abnormalities in the host genome as cancer mediators, generating great excitement among specialists in the field. In an effort to accelerate the regression of cancer and find a cure, they have adopted therapeutic genetic mutation treatments. At the forefront of these efforts is gene therapy, which introduces genetic information into host cells via bacterial, viral, or non-viral vectors. Important components include controlling the tumor microenvironment and adjusting the tumor cells or the immune system of the host to produce significant advancements with few adverse effects. The likelihood of retrovirus integration into the host genome has been greatly decreased by a new generation of vectors, allaying worries about mutagenesis, recurrent cancers, resistance to treatment, and disease recurrence. A number of vaccines targeting cancer and genetically modified immune cells have made it to market, but many more are in clinical studies and show great promise for future development. When combined with traditional therapies, such as surgery, radiation, and chemotherapy, gene therapy has the potential to completely transform the area of cancer treatment. Individualized treatment regimens that consider genetics, immunological status of the host, cancer-specific characteristics, and genomic profiles will be created to determine which gene therapy technique and type is best for each patient. Which could be a paradigm shift in the way cancer is treated in the future.

DNA- and m-RNA-Based Vaccines: An Immunotherapeutic Approach to Cancer.

Sonali Sundram and Rishabha Malviya (Authors)

DOI: 10.1201/9781774919613-3

3.1 INTRODUCTION

Gene therapy allows researchers to alter the genetic composition and properties of cancerous or immunological cells. Tumor microenvironment, the environment a cancer develops around itself to promote development and inhibit the immune system is being studied by researchers to help understand how different types of cancer start and what distinguishes cancer cells from healthy tissue. These cellular variations typically show up as changed, added, or removed genes that foster the development of cancer. Gene therapy uses therapeutic agents that have been developed to target these alterations, such as CAR-T cells. With an emphasis on the function of genes in cancer, the Alliance for Cancer Gene Therapy is trying to pinpoint the particular genetic changes connected to certain tumors. Genes are short segments of DNA that provide instructions on how to make proteins that control different parts of life. Gene alterations or mutations can throw off the body's delicate equilibrium and cause issues with cell division and overproduction. The project aims to create efficient gene-targeting cancer medications [1]. As with any revolutionary method of therapy, there are serious safety risks. The early excitement around gene therapy as a therapeutic method was dashed in 1999 after a patient died in a dose-escalation trial [2]. For many human diseases, somatic gene therapy is presently a safe therapeutic option. Gene therapy is an effective treatment for many ailments, thanks to advancements in gene delivery technology and a better understanding of disease etiology [3]. Among the various applications of gene therapy are gene replacement and knockdown for genetic disorders including cancer, hemophilia, hypercholesterolemia, and neurodegenerative diseases, as well as immunization; each of these uses calls for a unique method of gene delivery [4]. Gene delivery systems consist of a plasmid-based gene encoding system that regulates gene activity in the target organ, a gene that generates essential therapeutic peptides, and a gene delivery system that regulates the distribution of the encoding gene to host tissue [5]. A significant quantity of data has been produced by recent research on cancer gene treatments to evaluate the effectiveness of genes and vectors. The only way to eradicate cancer cells is through gene therapy, which involves precisely expressing a set of known genes in the right amounts and locations. To overcome the limitations of gene delivery, approaches such as inducing a bystander effect, developing gene therapies for immunogenes and antiangiogenesis, and combining adjuvants with conventional cancer treatments are being researched. A comprehensive understanding of the disease and its clinical environment is necessary to maximize therapeutic effect and optimize the potential of cancer gene therapy [6–14]. Generally speaking, pharmaceuticals fall into two categories: biological macromolecular drugs and chemical small-molecule drugs. The focus of cell medicines has moved from research and development to application with the advancement of science and technology. Furthermore, it is anticipated that artificial organ cloning would become feasible in the future. Drug creation has grown more difficult as medications' structures and functions have gotten more complicated [15]. The goal of the chapter is to give a thorough review of cancer gene therapy, taking into account the field's difficulties and ethical issues as well as its historical background, contemporary methods, and potential future applications.

3.1.1 IMPORTANCE AND RELEVANCE OF THE TOPIC

The issue is relevant and important because it has the potential to completely change how cancer is treated. Targeting the genetic causes of cancer through novel approaches is possible with cancer gene therapy, which may lead to more individualized and efficient treatment plans. Gaining knowledge in and improving the area can have a big influence on patient outcomes and lessen the worldwide cancer burden.

3.1.2 OBJECTIVES OF THE CHAPTER

The chapter's goals are to provide readers with a thorough grasp of cancer gene therapy, including its background, present methods, and potential applications, while also discussing the difficulties and moral dilemmas that the area presents.

3.2 CURRENT APPROACHES IN CANCER GENE THERAPY

3.2.1 GENE DELIVERY METHODS

Since the advent of recombinant DNA technology, the primary challenge in gene therapy has been how to distribute gene products safely and effectively. A vector is a tool used to transfer the desired gene. An optimal vector is one that is safe, non-immunogenic, can provide a gene to the target tissue, can accommodate a foreign gene of sufficient size, and can achieve transgenic expression at a level and duration necessary to fix the defective gene [16]. The delivery of gene products can be achieved using bactofection, viral vectors, or non-viral vectors (physical/chemical) as presented in the Figure 3.1 [17].

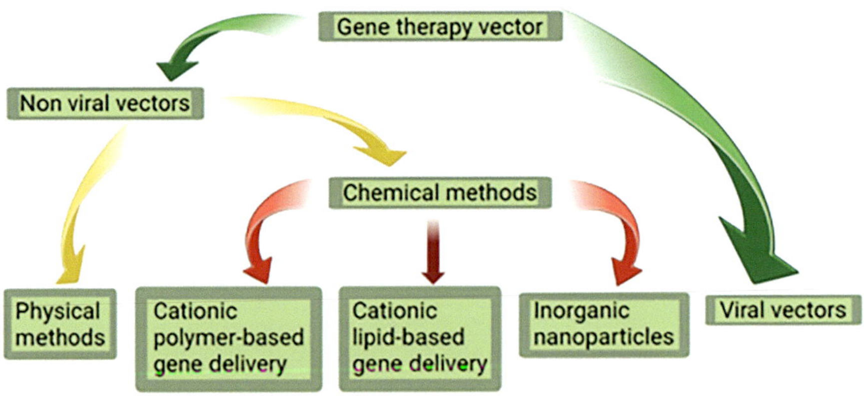

FIGURE 3.1 An overview of the gene therapy delivery methods.

3.2.1.1 *VIRAL VECTORS*

First and most popular vectors for delivering genes to the intended tissue were viruses. Nearly, all cells can become infected because of the viral vectors, which do not compromise cell viability. Because of their unique characteristics, viruses can be used to deliver genes in therapeutic settings. Endocytosis is triggered by the interaction of viral surface proteins with host receptors. Viruses release their genome into the nucleus as soon as they enter the cell to enable gene expression. Lentivovirus (LV), adenovirus (Ad), adeno-associated virus (AAV), and herpes simplex virus (HSV) are among the most important viral vectors [18–21].

3.2.1.1.1 Retrovirus

Retroviruses' capacity to incorporate into dividing cells makes them popular candidates for use in gene-transfer techniques for cancer applications.

They are the best vector for integrating foreign DNA into target cells because of their high transduction efficiency. Nevertheless, they have a number of drawbacks, such as a low attainable titer, a restricted capacity of around 8 kilobases, probable inactivation by serum complement, and challenges with large-scale synthesis. Packaging cell lines have been created to divide packaging signals across two plasmids in order to solve these problems. Additionally, certain retroviruses could have a limited host range. Nevertheless, pseudotyping techniques can get around this constraint by encasing cell lines with envelop proteins that have the right host range. For example, a packaging cell line that distributes a Sendai virus surface-F glycoprotein was able to circumvent the limitations of the amphotropic Moloney leukemia virus, hence granting infectivity to hepatocytes [22–28].

3.2.1.1.2 Adenovirus

For gene therapy to be successful, more adaptable vectors are required due to the shortcomings of recombinant retroviral vectors. The Ad5 viral vector, a double-stranded DNA virus, has gained interest due to its ability to transduce several cell types without relying on the cell's mitotic state. First-generation recombinant adenoviruses are created by homologous recombination into the E1 or E3 regions of the viral genome using the embryonic kidney cell line 293 as a helper cell. With minimal modification, the vector can provide greater viral titers than retrovirus. Studies have shown that relatively low doses of the virus may induce high-level transduction of cells with functional gene expression in most tissues, with the exception of hematopoietic cells. Recently, emphasis has shifted to cancer applications, wherein the vector is used to carry genes that are resistant to drugs or suppressor genes [29–33]. Because of its promise, gene therapy has been used extensively to adenovirus. On the other hand, reduced gene expression brought on by intact viral genes might result in cellular toxicity and cell death. Second-generation recombinant adenoviruses have been developed with the goals of reducing late gene expression, inhibiting the host immune response, and extending the duration of therapeutic gene expression. IL-12 can reduce the amount of immunoglobulin. Humoral immune responses can be strengthened, but they can also be weakened by immunosuppressive medications like cyclosporin. It is possible to get around the neutralizing antibody reaction by progressively administering different viral serotypes [34–41].

3.2.1.2 BACTERIAL-MEDIATED GENE TRANSFER (BACTOFECTION)

Some bacteria specifically target tumor cells, blocking RNA functions including protein synthesis and leading to gene silencing and RNA interference (RNAi). Numerous studies, both *in vivo* and *in vitro*, have shown how intracellular bacteria may be used to deliver plasmids harboring deadly chemicals and pro-drug converting enzymes into target cells. *Salmonella* species, *Listeria* monocytogenes, *Shigella flexneri*, *Bifidobacterium longum*, *Escherichia coli*, and *Yersinia enterocolitica* are among these microorganisms. A phase I clinical trial is using gene therapy for *Listeria*, *Bifidobacterium*, *Salmonella*, *Shigella*, and *Clostridium* to treat cancer. The anti-colitis effects of *Lactococcus* synthesizing interleukin 10 are now being studied in phase II clinical trials [42–44].

3.2.1.3 NON-VIRAL VECTORS

Unlike viral vectors, non-viral vectors are synthetic vectors mostly based on liposomes or polymers. Complexes are created when the positive charge provided by cationic liposomes or polymers engages and binds to DNA due to the presence of negative charges associated with the phosphate group. DNA is compacted to a tiny size by the electrostatic interaction of cationic non-viral vectors with DNA [45–47].

3.2.1.3.1 Lipoplexes

Lipoplexes are intricate structures that are created when positively charged liposomes and negatively charged DNA interact. They improve the stability and effectiveness of transfection. Lipids, which can be neutral, cationic, or anionic, are essential to the process. In order to increase transfection stability and efficiency, researchers have used techniques like PEGylation, which decreases aggregation and lengthens circulation duration. Transfection results have been enhanced by PEGylated lipoplexes that contain a cholesterol domain. Helper lipids such as DOPE facilitate endosomal egress, hence augmenting lipoplex efficacy. Novel cationic lipids with good transfection effectiveness and little cytotoxicity, gene material stability and protection have been improved by the development of substances like Gemini cationic lipids (GCL). High transfection efficiency and DNA protection have also been successfully attained by encasing DNA in lipid envelopes such as protamine and DOTAP [48–52].

3.2.1.3.2 Polyplexes

Because of their excellent stability and effective compaction of genetic information, polyplexes—which are created when positively charged cationic polymers combine with negatively charged DNA—are a preferred option for gene delivery. Because of its high transfection effectiveness, polyethylenimine (PEI) is a commonly used material; yet, it has significant toxicity and non-biodegradability concerns. In order to get over these limitations, researchers have developed techniques such as grafting branched PEI with O-carboxymethyl chitosan-grafted branching polyethylenimine (OCMPEI) for high transfection efficiency and low toxicity and enhancing biodegradability and transfection levels. Studies employing polycationic cyclodextrins and PLPEI have shown improved transfection efficiency in both *in vitro* and *in vivo* settings. While certain polyplexes have shown little endosome-lytic activity, scientists have created polycationic clusters based on β-CD-scaffolds that facilitate endosomal escape and DNA release, resulting in strong expression of genes even when serum is present [53–57].

3.3 TARGETING STRATEGIES

Many researchers think that by comprehending the molecular basis of cancer and using efficient medications that target aberrant molecules that control tumor development and metastasis, significant advancements in cancer treatment may be made which is known as targeted treatment, because it has minimal adverse effects while killing cancer cells on a selective basis. The selection of appropriate targets and the safe and efficient delivery of those targets into the tumor mass are key components of an effective targeted treatment. Over the last few decades, numerous significant tumor targets have been utilized [58].

3.3.1 TARGETING TUMORS BY DYSFUNCTIONAL PATHWAYS

Receptor overexpression combined with aberrant intracellular kinase mutation activation leads to downstream signaling pathway enhancement, which in turn causes cell transformation, proliferation, resistance to apoptosis, and ultimately cancer. As a result, the signaling system has emerged as a possible cancer treatment target.

3.3.1.1 TARGETING THE EGFR SIGNALING PATHWAY

Numerous critical physiological functions in both healthy and malignant cells are mediated by the EGFR pathway. Owing to the EGFR pathway's role, several therapeutic drugs that target EGFR have been discovered. Thus far, the FDA has approved five EGFR-targeting drugs for use in the treatment of cancer patients. The combination of erlotinib (OSI-774, Tarceva) and gemcitabine has been approved for the treatment of pancreatic cancer and metastatic non-small cell lung cancer (NSCLC). Another small-molecule EGFR kinase inhibitor used for locally advanced and metastatic NSCLC is gefitinib (ZD1839, Iressa) (Lo). A small-molecule inhibitor called lapatinib (GW572016, Tykerb/Tyverb) targets both EGFR and HER2. When a patient has HER2-positive advanced or metastatic breast cancer that has not responded to prior treatment, it is used in combination with other drugs to treat them [59].

3.3.1.2 TARGETING THE NF-KB PATHWAY

Many cancer cells have abnormal or constitutive NF-κB activity, which makes them more resistant to chemotherapy and radiation. Because of its pivotal role in the growth of tumors, the NF-κB signaling pathway has become a viable target for pharmaceutical intervention. Both an upstream and an NF-κB targeted technique can be used to inhibit NF-κB. The goal of the NF-κB targeting technique is to prevent the NF-κB signaling pathway from being activated. One such method is the use of glucocorticoids, which impede NF-κB transactivation. (b) Decoy oligodeoxynucleotides (ODNs) that prevent NF-κB from binding to DNA. Conversely, the upstream approach consists of the following: (a) PS-341 and MG132, proteasome inhibitors; (b) NSAIDs, sulfasalazine, arsenic trioxide, curcumin, and thalidomide; (c) overexpression of the *IκBα* gene by recombinant adenovirus; (d) The cell-permeable peptide SN-50; (e) The antioxidants glutathione and disulfiram [60–63].

3.3.1.3 TARGETING THE PTEN/PI3K/AKT SIGNALING PATHWAY

The PTEN/PI3K/AKT pathway, which controls cell division, survival, apoptosis, and metabolism, is implicated in the development of cancer. In the procedure, Akt inhibitors are essential because they block PI3K signaling and stop tumor development. The selective mTOR inhibitor rapamycin has been studied for possible medical use. Other inhibitors with better qualities and less toxicity include TGX115 and LY294002. Perifosine and other Akt inhibitors have demonstrated effectiveness in preventing the development of cells in solid tumors. These inhibitors have shown promise in the treatment of lung cancer, breast cancer, prostate cancer, and multiple myeloma [64–71].

3.3.1.4 TARGETING THE MAPK SIGNALING PATHWAY

Human tumors usually have an overexpression of the RAS-mitogen-activated protein kinase (MAPK) pathway, which is well-known for its function in cell survival and proliferation. Clinical trials on the first attempts to use farnesyltransferase inhibitors (FTIs) to target the route were unsuccessful. Then, clinical studies were conducted on small-molecule RAF inhibitors, such as BAY 43-9006, which had some promise but lacked selectivity, particularly in Phase III trials. Within the field of MEK inhibition, Phase I studies of CI-1040 showed anticancer effectiveness, while Phase II trials were not as successful. The discovery of PD0325901, a structurally comparable MEK inhibitor with enhanced efficacy and bioavailability, presents a more encouraging strategy for treating cancer by targeting the RAS-MAPK axis [72–73].

3.3.2 TARGETING TUMOR VASCULATURE

To change from benign to malignant, tumor cells must undergo angiogenesis in order to build blood vessels and adjust to the growing oxygen and nutritional needs of cancer cells that have undergone mutations. Hypoxia induces the synthesis of cellular hypoxia-inducible factor (HIF), which in turn causes proangiogenic proteins including PDGF, vascular endothelial growth factor, and TNF-α (tumor necrosis factor-α) to be overexpressed (VEGF). Due to their ability to obstruct intravenous chemotherapy treatments through *in vivo* barriers like the vascular endothelium, endothelial cells are crucial targets in disease processes like cancer. Nanoparticles can break through cell membranes and release the chemotherapeutic payload from the DDS by attaching to these cell surface markers. Targeting the endothelium is beneficial since it is more accessible than circulating bodies such as tumor cells [74–80]. One of the major challenges in tumor vascular-focused treatments is the potential for substantial adverse effects associated with standard intravenous chemotherapy treatment. Bevacizumab and other encapsulated medications that target angiogenesis have been studied for their efficacy and less harmful characteristics. Medication resistance and poor patient compliance may result from the free medication form, though. Drugs like bevacizumab are more attractive when they are encapsulated in nanoparticle form since they allow for prolonged gradual delivery and longer intervals between doses. Combining bevacizumab with camptothecin in the form of nanoparticles (CRXL101) has demonstrated encouraging synergistic effects in preclinical animals, leading to longer medication exposure and better tumor reduction [81–87]. By blocking VEGF receptors and targeting αvβ3 integrin, RGD nanoparticles have demonstrated potential in targeting cancer cells via the vascular system. By controlling cell adhesion, motility, and dissemination, these integrins inhibit apoptosis and encourage angiogenesis. Drug distribution into tumor cells can be improved by conjugating RGD-based sequences to the surfaces of nanoparticles. Research has demonstrated that RGD-peptides can enhance intracellular environment acidity and integrin receptor-mediated endocytosis to enhance cellular uptake and drug release. The combination of photodynamic therapy (PDT) with tumor-targeting has been shown to increase anticancer medication therapeutic effectiveness. RGD nanoparticles have been shown to be beneficial in treating cancer cells and preventing cell death in both *in vitro* and *in vivo* experiments [88–97].

3.4 APPROVED GENE THERAPY FOR CANCER

The U.S. Food and Drug Administration has approved Adstiladrin (nadofaragene firadenovec-vncg), a non-replicating adenoviral vector gene therapy (FDA). The medication is intended for adult patients with high-risk non-muscle-invasive bladder cancer (NMIBC) who do not respond to treatment with Bacillus Calmette-Guérin (BCG). One common kind of cancer is bladder cancer. Treatment for high-risk NMIBC, such as carcinoma *in situ* (CIS), can be challenging, and BCG treatment is often required in addition to tumor removal. Patients who do not react to BCG therapy now have a new therapeutic alternative in the form of adsteladrin. In a clinical research that evaluated the safety and efficacy of Adstiladrin, 51% of patients experienced a full response, with a median response duration of 9.7 months. Hematuria, exhaustion, urinary problems, and bladder discharge are typical adverse effects. Adstiladrin is injected straight into the bladder, and immunocompromised people should not use it. The approval is important in the battle against bladder cancer since it fills a gap in the treatment of high-risk NMIBC [98].

3.5 PROBLEMS WITH GENE THERAPY

Common negative reactions to gene therapy include transient grade 3 hypersensitivity upon intravenous infusion response symptoms including fever and flu-like symptoms, which can be addressed with standard supportive care. White blood cell redistribution to tumors, such as lymphopenia, may be the cause of leukocytopenia and lymphopenia. There have also been reports of mild transitory anemia [99]. Concerns about viral vector therapy's potential for toxicity, mutagenicity, and immunogenicity have been raised [100].

The integration of retroviruses into the host genome during lentiviral gene therapy, for instance, has been linked to mutagenesis events and secondary malignancies [101]. Five out of 30 patients with severe combined immunodeficiency who received the murine leukemia retrovirus vector developed leukemia, but Gene therapy for cancer has not yet been associated with any secondary malignancies. A virus's ability to cause mutations is site-specific. The FDA has required that all clinical research using viral vectors with genomic integration track and assess viral vector insertion sites. Recent years have seen the development of high-throughput DNA sequencing techniques using the linear amplification-mediated polymerase chain reaction (LAMP) [102–104]. It' is common for clinical studies to be stopped when they reveal signs of greater mutagenicity. In establishing novel and safer treatment options, the findings of these trials are critical [105].

Resistance to treatment is a problem with gene therapy for cancer, which results in tumor recurrences and shorter life spans. One putative mechanism, for instance, is the dysregulation and release of Bcl-2 or Bcl-XL proteins, which may allow tumor cells to withstand therapy-induced cell death (apoptosis) [106]. Some pharmaceutical companies have recently developed compounds that suppress the Bcl-2 protein, which lengthens remission during gene therapy, prevents or delays tumor resistance, and promotes cell death (apoptosis) and tumor regression, include Novartis-LBH589, cIAP1, and cIAP2. There are presently active clinical trials for these medicines [107].

3.6 CONCLUSION

Within the cancer field one potential avenue in the fight against cancer is gene therapy. Experts are excited by the recent discoveries in human genomics that shed light on the critical role somatic genetic alterations play as cancer drivers. Gene therapy is one of the therapeutic genetic mutation treatments that is leading attempts to accelerate cancer regression and maybe find a cure. The mainstay of these efforts is gene therapy, which introduces genetic material into host cells via bacterial, viral, or non-viral vectors. Restructuring the tumor microenvironment and using the immune system are important goals that will result in notable progress with little side effects. The creation of sophisticated vectors has allayed worries about mutagenesis and resistance resulting from retrovirus integration into the host DNA. While a number of genetically engineered immune cells and vaccines that target cancer have already been commercialized, many more are still in clinical studies and show tremendous potential for future advancements. Gene therapy has the potential to completely transform the treatment of cancer by providing individualized regimens based on genetics, immunological condition, cancer-specific traits, and genomic profiles when paired with conventional cancer therapies. While concerns regarding safety and resistance must be thoroughly addressed to ensure gene therapy's efficacy and safety in the battle against cancer, the technique might herald a dramatic shift in the way cancer is treated by providing patients with more individualized and potent treatments.

KEYWORDS

- **genomic aberrations**
- **gene therapy**
- **cancer treatment**
- **somatic mutations**
- **therapeutic strategies**
- **tumor microenvironment**
- **genetic mutation**

REFERENCES

1. https://acgtfoundation.org/news/gene-therapy-for-cancer/#:~:text=Types%20of%20gene%20therapy%20for%20cancer&text=Gene%20therapy%20aims%20to%20control,is%20called%20somatic%20gene%20therapy (accessed November 1, 2023).
2. Raper, S. E., Chirmule, N., Lee, F. S., Wivel, N. A., Bagg, A., Gao, G. P., Wilson, J. M., & Batshaw, M. L. (2003). Fatal systemic inflammatory response syndrome in a ornithine transcarbamylase deficient patient following adenoviral gene transfer. *Molecular Genetics and Metabolism, 80*(1–2), 148–158.
3. Reis, R. L. (2019). *Encyclopedia of tissue engineering and regenerative medicine*. Academic Press.
4. Ginn, S. L., Amaya, A. K., Alexander, I. E., Edelstein, M., & Abedi, M. R. (2018). Gene therapy clinical trials worldwide to 2017: An update. *The Journal of Gene Medicine, 20*(5), e3015.
5. Sung, Y. K., & Kim, S. W. (2018). The practical application of gene vectors in cancer therapy. *Integrative Cancer Science and Therapeutics, 5*, 1–5.
6. Verma, I. M., & Somia, N. (1997). Gene therapy-promises, problems and prospects. *Nature, 389*(6648), 239–242.
7. Roth, J. A., Nguyen, D., Lawrence, D. D., Kemp, B. L., Carrasco, C. H., Ferson, D. Z., Hong, W. K., Komaki, R., Lee, J. J., Nesbitt, J. C., & Pisters, K. M. W. (1996). Retrovirus–mediated wild–type P53 gene transfer to tumors of patients with lung cancer. *Nature Medicine, 2*(9), 985–991.
8. Ram, Z., Culver, K. W., Oshiro, E. M., Viola, J. J., DeVroom, H. L., Otto E., Long, Z., Chiang, Y., McGarrity, G. J., Muul, L. M., Katz, D., Blaese, R. M., & Oldfield, E. H. (1997). Therapy of malignant brain tumors by intratumoral implantation of retroviral vector-producing cells. *Nature Medicine, 3*(12), 1354–1361.
9. Soiffer, R., Lynch, T., Mihm, M., Jung, K., Rhuda, C., Schmollinger, J. C., Hodi, F. S., Liebster, L., Lam, P., Mentzer, S., Singer, S., Tanabe, K. K., Cosimi, A. B., Duda, R., Sober, A., Bhan, A., Daley, J., Neuberg, D., Parry, G., Rokovich, J., Richards, L., Drayer, J., Berns, A., Clift, S., Cohen, L. K., Mulligan, R. C., & Dranoff, G. (1998).

Vaccination with irradiated autologous melanoma cells engineered to secrete human granulocyte-macrophage colony-stimulating factor generates potent antitumor immunity in patients with metastatic melanoma. *Proceedings of the National Academy of Sciences, 95*(22), 13141–13146.

10. Palu, G., Cavaggioni, A., Calvi, P., Franchin, E., Pizzato, M., Boschetto, R., Parolin, C., Chilosi, M., Ferrini, S., Zanusso, A., & Colombo, F. (1999). Gene therapy of glioblastoma multiforme via combined expression of suicide and cytokine genes: a pilot study in humans. *Gene Therapy, 6*(3), 330–337.
11. Peng, K.-W., & Vile R. (1999). Vector development for cancer gene therapy. *Tumor Targeting, 4*(3–11), 1999.
12. Ramesh, R., Saeki, T., Templeton, N. S., Ji, L., Stephens, L. C., Ito, I., Wilson, D. R., Wu, Z., Branch, C. D., Minna, J. D., & Roth, J. A. (2001). Successful treatment of primary and disseminated human lung cancers by systemic delivery of tumor suppressor genes using an improved liposome vector. *Molecular Therapy, 3*(3), 337–350.
13. Plautz, G. E., Yang, Z. Y., Wu, B. Y., Gao, X., Huang, L., & Nabel, G. J. (1993). Immunotherapy of malignancy by in vivo gene transfer into tumors. *Proceedings of the National Academy of Sciences, 90*(10), 4645–4649.
14. Heise, C., Sampson-Johannes, A., Williams, A., Mccormick, F., Von Hoff, D. D., & Kirn, D. H. (1997). ONYX-015, an E1B gene-attenuated adenovirus, causes tumor-specific cytolysis and antitumoral efficacy that can be augmented by standard chemotherapeutic agents. *Nature Medicine, 3*(6), 639–645.
15. Wang, L., Liu, G., Zheng, L., Long, H., & Liu, Y. (2023). A new era of gene and cell therapy for cancer: A narrative review. *Annals of Translational Medicine, 11*(9), 321.
16. Belete, T. M. (2021). The current status of gene therapy for the treatment of cancer. *Biologics: Targets and Therapy,* 67–77.
17. Mali, S. (2013). Delivery systems for gene therapy. *Indian journal of human Genetics, 19*(1), 3. doi:10.4103/0971-6866.112870.
18. Sung, Y. K., & Kim, S. W. (2019). Recent advances in the development of gene delivery systems. *Biomaterials Research, 23*(1), 8. doi:10.1186/s40824-019-0156-z.
19. Humphreys, I. R., & Sebastian, S. (2018). Novel viral vectors in infectious diseases. *Immunology, 153*(1), 1–9. doi:10.1111/imm.12829
20. Bouard, D., Alazard-Dany, N., & Cosset, F. L. (2009). Viral vectors: from virology to transgene expression. *British Journal of Pharmacology, 157*(2), 153–165. doi:10.1038/bjp.2008.349
21. Goswami, R., Subramanian, G., Silayeva, L., Newkirk, I., Doctor, D., Chawla, K., Chattopadhyay, S., Chandra, D., Chilukuri, N., & Betapudi, V. (2019). Gene therapy leaves a vicious cycle. *Frontiers in Oncology, 9*, p.297.
22. Herrmann, F. (1995). Cancer gene therapy: principles, problems, and perspectives. *Journal of Molecular Medicine, 73*(4), 157–163.
23. Hodgson, C. P. (1995). The vector void in gene therapy. *Bio/Technology, 13*(3), 222–225.
24. Habib, N. A., Ding, S. F., El-Masry, R., Dalla Serra, G., Mikhail, N. E., & Izzi, G. (1995). Contrasting effects of direct p53 DNA injection in primary and secondary liver tumors. *Tumor Targeting, 1*, 295–298.

25. Markowitz, D., Goff, S., & Bank, A. (1988). Construction and use of a safe and efficient amphotropic packaging cell line. *Virology, 167*(2), 400–406.
26. Heinrich, M., Keebel, W. W., Grompe, M., Bagby Jr, G. C., & Hoatlin, M. E. (1995). A gibbon ape leukemia virus (GALV) pseudotyped retroviral vector for gene therapy of Fanconi Anemia complementation group C (FACC). In *Cancer biotechnology weekly.* (pp. 22–23).
27. Yam, P., Chow, W., Zaia, J. A., & Yee, J. K. (1995). Comparison of pseudo-type and aphotropic retro viral mediated gene transfer into human hematopoietic progenitors and cell line. *Cancer Gene Therapy, 2*, 323.
28. Spiegel, M., Gregor, M., & Lauer, U. (1995). Generation of recombinant hepatotropic retro-viral pseudotypes for usage in liver-restricted in vivo gene therapy. *Gut, 37*, A133.
29. Li, Q., Kay, M. A., Finegold, M., Stratford-Perricaudet, L. D., & Woo, S. L. (1993). Assessment of recombinant adenoviral vectors for hepatic gene therapy. *Human Gene Therapy, 4*(4), 403–409.
30. Mittal, S. K., Bett, A. J., Prevec, L., & Graham, F. L. (1995). Foreign gene expression by human adenovirus type 5-based vectors studied using firefly luciferase and bacterial β-galactosidase genes as reporters. *Virology, 210*(1), 226–230.
31. Kremer, E. J., & Perricaudet, M. (1995). Adenovirus and adeno-associated virus mediated gene transfer. *British Medical Bulletin, 51*(1), 31–44.
32. Engelhardt, J. F., Simon, R. H., Yang, Y., Zepeda, M., Weber-Pendleton, S., Doranz, B., Grossman, M., & Wilson, J. M. (1993). Adenovirus-mediated transfer of the CFTR gene to lung of nonhuman primates: biological efficacy study. *Human Gene Therapy, 4*(6), 759–769.
33. Sobol, R., & Scanlon, K. J. (1995). Clinical protocols list. *Cancer Gene Therapy, 2*, 225–234.
34. Engelhardt, J. F., Ye, X., Doranz, B., & Wilson, J. M. (1994). Ablation of E2A in recombinant adenoviruses improves transgene persistence and decreases inflammatory response in mouse liver. *Proceedings of the National Academy of Sciences, 91*(13), 6196–6200.
35. Yang, Y., Nunes, F. A., Berencsi, K., Furth, E. E., Gönczöl, E., & Wilson, J. M. (1994). Cellular immunity to viral antigens limits E1-deleted adenoviruses for gene therapy. *Proceedings of the National Academy of Sciences, 91*(10), 4407–4411.
36. Engelhardt, J. F., Litzky, L., & Wilson, J. M. (1994). Prolonged transgene expression in cotton rat lung with recombinant adenoviruses defective in E2a. *Human Gene Therapy, 5*(10), 1217–1229.
37. Fisher, K. J., Choi, H., Burda, J., CHEN, S. J., & Wilson, J. M. (1996). Recombinant adenovirus deleted of all viral genes for gene therapy of cystic fibrosis. *Virology, 217*(1), 11–22.
38. Yang, Y., Trinchieri, G., & Wilson, J. M. (1995). Recombinant IL–12 prevents formation of blocking IgA antibodies to recombinant adenovirus and allows repeated gene therapy to mouse lung. *Nature Medicine, 1*(9), 890–893.
39. Dai, Y., Schwarz, E. M., Gu, D., Zhang, W. W., Sarvetnick, N., & Verma, I. M. (1995). Cellular and humoral immune responses to adenoviral vectors containing factor IX gene: tolerization of factor IX and vector antigens allows for long-term expression. *Proceedings of the National Academy of Sciences, 92*(5), 1401–1405.

40. Fang, B., Eisensmith, R. C., Wang, H., Kay, M. A., Cross, R. E., Landen, C. N., Gordon, G., Bellinger, D. A., Read, M. S., Hu, P. C., & Woo, S. L. C. (1995). Gene therapy for hemophilia B: host immunosuppression prolongs the therapeutic effect of adenovirus-mediated factor IX expression. *Human Gene Therapy, 6*(8), 1039–1044.
41. Roth, J. A. (1996). Modification of tumor suppressor gene expression in non-small cell lung cancer (NSCLC) with a retroviral vector expressing wildtype (normal) p53. University of Texas MD Anderson Cancer Center, Houston, Texas. *Human Gene Therapy, 7*(7), 861–874.
42. Pilgrim, S., Stritzker, J., Schoen, C., Kolb-Mäurer, A., Geginat, G., Loessner, M. J., Gentschev, I., & Goebel, W. (2003). Bactofection of mammalian cells by Listeria monocytogenes: improvement and mechanism of DNA delivery. *Gene Therapy, 10*(24), 2036–2045. doi:10.1038/sj.gt.3302105
43. Johnson, S. A., Ormsby, M. J., McIntosh, A., Tait, S. W., Blyth, K., & Wall, D. M. (2019). Increasing the bactofection capacity of a mammalian expression vector by removal of the f1 ori. *Cancer Gene Therapy, 26*(7), 183–194. doi:10.1038/s41417-018-0039-9
44. Celec, P., & Gardlik, R. (2017). Gene therapy using bacterial vectors. *Front Bioscience, 22*, 81–95. doi:10.2741/4473
45. Al-Dosari, M. S., & Gao, X. (2009). Nonviral gene delivery: principle, limitations, and recent progress. *The AAPS Journal, 11*, 671–681. doi: 10.1208/s12248-009-9143-y
46. Kaneda, Y., & Tabata, Y. (2006). Non-viral vectors for cancer therapy. *Cancer Science, 97*(5), 348–354. doi: 10.1111/j.1349-7006.2006.00189.x
47. Sung, Y. K., & Kim, S. W. (2019). Recent advances in the development of gene delivery systems. *Biomaterials Research, 23*(1), 8. doi: 10.1186/s40824-019-0156-z
48. Felgner, Philip L., Thomas R. Gadek, Marilyn Holm, Richard Roman, Hardy W. Chan, Michael Wenz, Jeffrey P. Northrop, Gordon M. Ringold, & Mark Danielsen (1987). "Lipofection: a highly efficient, lipid-mediated DNA-transfection procedure." *Proceedings of the National Academy of Sciences, 84*, 7413–7417. doi: 10.1073/pnas.84.21.7413
49. Harvie, P., Wong, F. M., & Bally, M. B. (2000). Use of poly (ethylene glycol)–lipid conjugates to regulate the surface attributes and transfection activity of lipid–DNA particles. *Journal of Pharmaceutical Sciences, 89*(5), 652–663. doi: 10.1002/(SICI)1520-6017(200005)89:5<652::AID-JPS11>3.0.CO;2-H
50. Xu, L., Wempe, M. F., & Anchordoquy, T. J. (2011). The effect of cholesterol domains on PEGylated liposomal gene delivery in vitro. *Therapeutic Delivery, 2*(4), 451–460, 10.4155/tde.11.13
51. Martínez-Negro, M., Guerrero-Martinez, A., García-Río, L., Domènech, O., Aicart, E., Tros de Ilarduya, C., & Junquera, E. (2018). Multidisciplinary approach to the transfection of plasmid DNA by a nonviral nanocarrier based on a gemini–bolaamphiphilic hybrid lipid. *ACS Omega, 3*(1), 208–217, 10.1021/acsomega.7b01657
52. Martínez-Negro, M., Sánchez-Arribas, N., Guerrero-Martínez, A., Moyá, M. L., Tros de Ilarduya, C., Mendicuti, F., Aicart, E., & Junquera, E. (2019). A non-viral plasmid DNA delivery system consisting on a lysine-derived cationic lipid mixed with a fusogenic lipid. *Pharmaceutics, 11*(12), 632., 10.3390/pharmaceutics11120632

53. Gallego-Yerga, L., Blanco-Fernández, L., Urbiola, K., Carmona, T., Marcelo, G., Benito, J. M., Mendicuti, F., Tros de Ilarduya, C., Ortiz Mellet, C., & Garcia Fernandez, J. M. (2015). Host–Guest-Mediated DNA Templation of Polycationic Supramolecules for Hierarchical Nanocondensation and the Delivery of Gene Material. *Chemistry–A European Journal, 21*(34), 12093–12104, 10.1002/chem.201501678
54. Cho, Y. W., Kim, J. D., & Park, K. (2003). Polycation gene delivery systems: escape from endosomes to cytosol. *Journal of Pharmacy and Pharmacology, 55*(6), 721–734. doi:10.1211/0022357021311
55. ACarbajo-Gordillo, A. I., Rodríguez-Lavado, J., Blanco, J. L. J., Benito, J. M., Di Giorgio, C., Vélaz, I., de Ilarduya, C. T., Mellet, C. O., & Fernández, J. M. G. (2019). Trehalose-based Siamese twin amphiphiles with tunable self-assembling, DNA nanocomplexing and gene delivery properties. *Chemical Communications, 55*(57), 8227–8230, 10.1039/c9cc04489b
56. Elouahabi, A., & Ruysschaert, J. M. (2005). Formation and intracellular trafficking of lipoplexes and polyplexes. *Molecular Therapy, 11*(3), 336–347. 10.1016/j.ymthe.2004.12.006
57. Arnaiz, E., Doucede, L. I., Garcia-Gallego, S., Urbiola, K., Gomez, R., Tros de Ilarduya, C., & de la Mata, F. J. (2012). Synthesis of cationic carbosilane dendrimers via click chemistry and their use as effective carriers for DNA transfection into cancerous cells. *Molecular Pharmaceutics, 9*(3), 433–447, 10.1021/mp200542j
58. Ku, G. Y., & Ilson, D. H. (2010). Esophagogastric cancer: targeted agents. *Cancer Treatment Reviews, 36*(3), 235–248.
59. Moy, B., Kirkpatrick, P., Kar, S., & Goss, P. (2007). Lapatinib. *Nature Reviews Drug Discovery, 6*, 431–432.
60. D'Acquisto, F., Sautebin, L., Iuvone, T., Di Rosa, M., & Carnuccio, R. (1998). Prostaglandins prevent inducible nitric oxide synthase protein expression by inhibiting nuclear factor-κB activation in J774 macrophages. *FEBS Letters, 440*(1–2), 76–80.
61. Karin, M., Yamamoto, Y., & Wang, Q. M. (2004). The IKK NF-κB system: a treasure trove for drug development. *Nature Reviews Drug Discovery, 3*(1), 17–26.
62. Chen, L. F., Mu, Y., & Greene, W. C. (2002). Acetylation of RelA at discrete sites regulates distinct nuclear functions of NF-κB. *The EMBO Journal, 21*, 6539–6548.
63. Tomita, N., Ogihara, T., & Morishita, R. (2003). Transcription factors as molecular targets: molecular mechanisms of decoy ODN and their design. *Current Drug Targets, 4*(8), 603–608.
64. Guertin, D. A., & Sabatini, D. M. (2007). Defining the role of mTOR in cancer. *Cancer Cell, 12*(1), 9–22.
65. Granville, C. A., Memmott, R. M., Gills, J. J., & Dennis, P. A. (2006). Handicapping the race to develop inhibitors of the phosphoinositide 3-kinase/Akt/mammalian target of rapamycin pathway. *Clinical Cancer Research, 12*(3), 679–689.
66. Jiang, B. H., & Liu, L. Z. (2008). PI3K/PTEN signaling in tumorigenesis and angiogenesis. *Biochimica et Biophysica Acta (BBA)-Proteins and Proteomics, 1784*(1), 150–158.
67. Hennessy, B. T., Smith, D. L., Ram, P. T., Lu, Y., & Mills, G. B. (2005). Exploiting the PI3K/AKT pathway for cancer drug discovery. *Nature Reviews Drug Discovery, 4*(12), 988–1004.

68. Martelli, A. M., Tazzari, P. L., Tabellini, G., Bortul, R., Billi, A. M., Manzoli, L., Ruggeri, A., Conte, R., & Cocco, L. (2003). A new selective AKT pharmacological inhibitor reduces resistance to chemotherapeutic drugs, TRAIL, all-trans-retinoic acid, and ionizing radiation of human leukemia cells. *Leukemia, 17*(9), 1794.
69. Han, E. K., Leverson, J. D., McGonigal, T., Shah, O. J., Woods, K. W., Hunter, T., Giranda, V. L., & Luo, Y. (2007). Akt inhibitor A-443654 induces rapid Akt Ser-473 phosphorylation independent of mTORC1 inhibition. *Oncogene, 26*(38), 5655–5661.
70. Jin, X., Gossett, D. R., Wang, S., Yang, D., Cao, Y., Chen, J., Guo, R., Reynolds, R. K., & Lin, J. (2004). Inhibition of AKT survival pathway by a small molecule inhibitor in human endometrial cancer cells. *British Journal of Cancer, 91*(10), 1808–1812.
71. Tang, H. J., Jin, X., Wang, S., Yang, D., Cao, Y., Chen, J., Gossett, D. R., & Lin, J. (2006). A small molecule compound inhibits AKT pathway in ovarian cancer cell lines. *Gynecologic Oncology, 100*(2), 308–317.
72. Sebolt-Leopold, J. S., & Herrera, R. (2004). Targeting the mitogen-activated protein kinase cascade to treat cancer. *Nature Reviews Cancer, 4*(12), 937–947.
73. Sebolt-Leopold, J. S., Dudley, D. T., Herrera, R., Becelaere, K. V., Wiland, A., Gowan, R. C., Tecle, H., Barrett, S. D., Bridges, A., Przybranowski, S., & Leopold, W. R. (1999). Blockade of the MAP kinase pathway suppresses growth of colon tumors in vivo. *Nature Medicine, 5*(7), 810–816.
74. Huang, S., Shao, K., Liu, Y., Kuang, Y., Li, J., An, S., Guo, Y., Ma, H., & Jiang, C. (2013). Tumor-targeting and microenvironment-responsive smart nanoparticles for combination therapy of antiangiogenesis and apoptosis. *ACS Nano, 7*(3), 2860–2871.
75. Liu, Z., Yu, L., Wang, X., Zhang, X., Liu, M., & Zeng, W. (2016). Integrin (αvβ3) targeted RGD peptide based probe for cancer optical imaging. *Current Protein and Peptide Science, 17*(6), 570–581.
76. Guyot, M., Hilmi, C., Ambrosetti, D., Merlano, M., Lo Nigro, C., Durivault, J., Grepin, R., & Pages, G. (2017). Targeting the pro-angiogenic forms of VEGF or inhibiting their expression as anti-cancer strategies. *Oncotarget, 8*, 9174–9188.
77. Chen, Y., Wang, X., Liu, T., Zhang, D. S. Z., Wang, Y., Gu, H., & Di, W. (2015). Highly effective antiangiogenesis via magnetic mesoporous silica-based siRNA vehicle targeting the VEGF gene for orthotopic ovarian cancer therapy. *International Journal of Nanomedicine,* 2579–2594.
78. Danhier, F., Le Breton, A., & Préat, V. (2012). RGD-based strategies to target alpha (v) beta (3) integrin in cancer therapy and diagnosis. *Molecular Pharmaceutics, 9*(11), 2961–2973.
79. Howard, M., Zern, B. J., Anselmo, A. C., Shuvaev, V. V., Mitragotri, S., & Muzykantov, V. (2014). Vascular targeting of nanocarriers: perplexing aspects of the seemingly straightforward paradigm. *ACS Nano, 8*(5), 4100–4132.
80. Pedroso, J. D., Gutierrez, M. M., Volker, K. W., & Howard, D. L. (2017). Thermal Effect of J-Plasma® Energy in a Porcine Tissue Model: Implications for Minimally Invasive Surgery. *Surgical Technology International, 30*, 19–24.
81. Gad, A., Kydd, J., Piel, B., & Rai, P. (2016). Targeting cancer using polymeric nanoparticle mediated combination chemotherapy. *International journal of nanomedicine and nanosurgery, 2*(3), 3264.
82. Jadia, R., Scandore, C., & Rai, P. (2016). Nanoparticles for effective combination therapy of cancer. *International Journal of Nanotechnology and Nanomedicine, 1*(1).

83. Zhang, Y., Yang, C., Wang, W., Liu, J., Liu, Q., Huang, F., Chu, L., Gao, H., Li, C., Kong, D., & Liu, Q. (2016). Co-delivery of doxorubicin and curcumin by pH-sensitive prodrug nanoparticle for combination therapy of cancer. *Scientific Reports, 6*(1), 21225.
84. Somani, R. R., & Bhanushali, U. V. (2013). Targeting angiogenesis for treatment of human cancer. *Indian Journal of Pharmaceutical Sciences, 75*(1), 3.
85. Sousa, F., Cruz, A., Fonte, P., Pinto, I. M., Neves-Petersen, M. T., & Sarmento, B. (2017). A new paradigm for antiangiogenic therapy through controlled release of bevacizumab from PLGA nanoparticles. *Scientific Reports, 7*(1), 3736.
86. Pham, E., Yin, M., Peters, C. G., Lee, C. R., Brown, D., Xu, P., Man, S., Jayaraman, L., Rohde, E., Chow, A., & Lazarus, D. (2016). Preclinical efficacy of bevacizumab with CRLX101, an investigational nanoparticle–drug conjugate, in treatment of metastatic triple-negative breast cancer. *Cancer Research, 76*(15), 4493–4503.
87. Keefe, S. M., Hoffman-Censits, J., Cohen, R. B., Mamtani, R., Heitjan, D., Eliasof, S., Nixon, A., Turnbull, B., Garmey, E. G., Gunnarsson, O., & Waliki, M. (2016). Efficacy of the nanoparticle–drug conjugate CRLX101 in combination with bevacizumab in metastatic renal cell carcinoma: results of an investigator-initiated phase I–IIa clinical trial. *Annals of Oncology, 27*(8), 1579–1585.
88. Murugan, C., Rayappan, K., Thangam, R., Bhanumathi, R., Shanthi, K., Vivek, R., Thirumurugan, R., Bhattacharyya, A., Sivasubramanian, S., Gunasekaran, P., & Kannan, S. (2016). Combinatorial nanocarrier based drug delivery approach for amalgamation of anti-tumor agents in breast cancer cells: An improved nanomedicine strategy. *Scientific Reports, 6*(1), 1–22.
89. Zhu, J., Fu, F., Xiong, Z., Shen, M., & Shi, X. (2015). Dendrimer-entrapped gold nanoparticles modified with RGD peptide and alpha-tocopheryl succinate enable targeted theranostics of cancer cells. *Colloids and Surfaces B: Biointerfaces, 133*, 36–42.
90. He, X., Alves, C. S., Oliveira, N., Rodrigues, J., Zhu, J., Bányai, I., Tomás, H., & Shi, X. (2015). RGD peptide-modified multifunctional dendrimer platform for drug encapsulation and targeted inhibition of cancer cells. *Colloids and Surfaces B: Biointerfaces, 125*, 82–89.
91. Dickreuter, E., & Cordes, N. (2017). The cancer cell adhesion resistome: mechanisms, targeting and translational approaches. *Biological Chemistry, 398*(7), 721–735.
92. Lee, C., Kim, B., Lee, S., Kim, T. H., Kim, J. O., Lee, E. S., Oh, K. T., Choi, H. G., Yoo, S. D., & Youn, Y. S. (2017). Doxorubicin and paclitaxel co-bound lactosylated albumin nanoparticles having targetability to hepatocellular carcinoma. *Colloids and Surfaces B: Biointerfaces, 152*, 183–191.
93. Hu, Z., Rao, B., Chen, S., & Duanmu, J. (2011). Selective and effective killing of angiogenic vascular endothelial cells and cancer cells by targeting tissue factor using a factor VII-targeted photodynamic therapy for breast cancer. *Breast Cancer Research and Treatment, 126*, 589–600.
94. Chen, Q., Chen, J., Liang, C., Feng, L., Dong, Z., Song, X., Song, G., & Liu, Z. (2017). Drug-induced co-assembly of albumin/catalase as smart nano-theranostics for deep intra-tumoral penetration, hypoxia relieve, and synergistic combination therapy. *Journal of Controlled Release, 263*, 79–89.
95. Wu, L., Chen, M., Mao, H., Wang, N., Zhang, B., Zhao, X., Qian, J., & Xing, C. (2017). Albumin-based nanoparticles as methylprednisolone carriers for targeted

delivery towards the neonatal Fc receptor in glomerular podocytes. *International Journal of Molecular Medicine, 39*(4), 851–860.

96. Zuo, H., Chen, W., Cooper, H. M., & Xu, Z. P. (2017). A facile way of modifying layered double hydroxide nanoparticles with targeting ligand-conjugated albumin for enhanced delivery to brain tumour cells. *ACS Applied Materials & Interfaces, 9*(24), 20444–20453.
97. Chen, Q., Wang, X., Wang, C., Feng, L., Li, Y., & Liu, Z. (2015). Drug-induced self-assembly of modified albumins as nano-theranostics for tumor-targeted combination therapy. *ACS Nano, 9*(5), 5223–5233.
98. https://www.fda.gov/news-events/press-announcements/fda-approves-first-gene-therapy-treatment-high-risk-non-muscle-invasive-bladder-cancer (accessed November 8, 2023)
99. Seiradake, E., Henaff, D., Wodrich, H., Billet, O., Perreau, M., Hippert, C., Mennechet, F., Schoehn, G., Lortat-Jacob, H., Dreja, H., & Ibanes, S. (2009). The cell adhesion molecule "CAR" and sialic acid on human erythrocytes influence adenovirus in vivo biodistribution. *PLoS Pathogens, 5*(1), e1000277. doi: 10.1371/journal.ppat.1000277
100. Hemminki, O., & Hemminki, A. (2013). Oncolytic adenoviruses in the treatment of cancer in humans. In E. C. Lattime, S. L. Gerson (Eds.), *Gene Therapy of Cancer.* (pp. 153–170). Elsevier.
101. Howe, S. J., Mansour, M. R., Schwarzwaelder, K., Bartholomae, C., Hubank, M., Kempski, H., Brugman, M. H., Pike-Overzet, K., Chatters, S. J., De Ridder, D., & Gilmour, K. C. (2008). Insertional mutagenesis combined with acquired somatic mutations causes leukemogenesis following gene therapy of SCID-X1 patients. *The Journal of Clinical Investigation, 118*(9). doi: 10.1172/JCI35798.
102. Schmidt, M., Zickler, P., Hoffmann, G., Haas, S., Wissler, M., Muessig, A., Tisdale, J. F., Kuramoto, K., Andrews, R. G., Wu, T., & Kiem, H. P. (2002). Polyclonal long-term repopulating stem cell clones in a primate model. *Blood the Journal of the American Society of Hematology, 100*(8), 2737–2743. doi: 10.1182/blood-2002-02-0407.
103. Bartholomae, C. C., Glimm, H., Von Kalle, C., & Schmidt, M. (2012). Insertion site pattern: global approach by linear amplification-mediated PCR and mass sequencing. In *Mobile Genetic Elements: Protocols and Genomic Applications.* (pp. 255–265). doi: 10.1007/978-1-61779-603-6_15
104. Gillet, N. A., Malani, N., Melamed, A., Gormley, N., Carter, R., Bentley, D., Berry, C., Bushman, F. D., Taylor, G. P., & Bangham, C. R. (2011). The host genomic environment of the provirus determines the abundance of HTLV-1–infected T-cell clones. *Blood the Journal of the American Society of Hematology, 117*(11), 3113–3122. doi: 10.1182/blood-2010-10-312926.
105. Fung, H., & Gersson, S. (2013). Viral insertion site detection and analysis in cancer gene therapy. In E. C. Lattime & S. L. Gerson (Eds.), *Gene Therapy of Cancer*. (pp. 35–46). Elsevier.
106. Yuan, Z., Pastoriza, J., Quinn, T., Libutti, S. (2013). Targeting tumor vasculature using adeno-associated virus page vector coding tumor necrosis factor-a. In E. C. Lattime & S. L. Gerson (Eds.), *Gene Therapy of Cancer*. (pp. 19–33). Elsevier.
107. Novartis (2014). Investigational New Drug Development Program.

CHAPTER 4

Therapeutic Interventions and Non-Coding RNA-Mediated Mechanisms of Cancer Resistance

ABSTRACT

Non-coding RNAs (ncRNAs) represent a distinct category of RNA molecules that play a pivotal role in regulating various physiological and pathological mechanisms, encompassing cancer-related processes. ncRNA dysregulation is associated with several diseases. CircRNA expression is very high in cells that are either terminally differentiated or proliferation-stable, and they are critical to the initiation, spread, and stemness of cancer. In the fight against cancer, ncRNAs hold great promise as therapeutic targets. When ncRNAs are targeted or delivered, cancer intervention can be improved, particularly for patients who have not responded well to chemotherapy. Delivering ncRNAs that increase or lessen cellular resistance to endocrine therapies is one possible therapeutic strategy. To ensure their safety, ncRNA-based medicines must be properly developed and administered, and extensive *in vitro* and animal research is needed. Notwithstanding these difficulties, RNA-based therapeutics have demonstrated promise in the therapy of cancer; nevertheless, more study is required to create customized treatment regimens for cancer patients and to completely comprehend the mechanisms underlying pharmaceutical resistance. The significance of ncRNAs in biological processes, which contributes to the onset and spread of cancer, is discussed in this chapter along with potential treatment modalities that could enhance cancer intervention.

DNA- and m-RNA-Based Vaccines: An Immunotherapeutic Approach to Cancer.
Sonali Sundram and Rishabha Malviya (Authors)

DOI: 10.1201/9781774919613-4

4.1 INTRODUCTION

Cancer has become more common over the past few years in an unconventional, low-risk group of patients. The majority of these cases are linked to a significant rise in dangerous neck and head sarcoma cell carcinoma (HNSCC) associated with human papillomavirus (hrHPV). Nevertheless, a subset of low-risk patients still has an unidentified etiology. The latter category is particularly common in instances of oral cavity cancer [1–4]. The latter category is particularly prominent in instances of oral cavity cancer. To fully comprehend the genetic variables that separate young, low-risk patients from older, more common counterparts and contribute to the growth of cancer, more research is required. Nevertheless, the available data indicates that clinical outcomes specific to disease survival rates are comparable and unfavorable in both cohorts of patients [5–7]. In contemporary times, notable advancements have been made in the detection of over 40 single-nucleotide polymorphisms, linked to risks. This advancement has led to enhanced predictive capabilities in assessing genetic susceptibility to risks. It is currently known that several genes, including *TP53*, *PTEN/MMAC1*, *BRCA1*, and *BRCA2*, are susceptible to breast cancer. In contrast to a subset of women within the general population, certain women possessing a genetic mutation in either the *BRCA1* or *BRCA2* genes are prone to developing breast cancer during their lifetime. Females harboring genetic variations in both *BRCA1* and *BRCA2* genes are predisposed to an increased susceptibility to ovarian cancer. Therefore, assessing these genetic susceptibility prediction models has become essential for clinical decision-making to assist doctors and patients in deciding whether or not a genetic test is necessary.

The categorization of DNA damage repair pathways is primarily based on the type and severity of genetic damage. These pathways can be classified into three main categories: base excision repair, nucleotide excision repair, and double-strand break repair. Aberrant cell function, unchecked replication, and genomic instability are all caused by disruptions in cell DNA repair pathways, and these conditions can all aid in the development of tumors [8]. Nevertheless, the utilization of chemotherapy agents in clinical settings is considerably constrained as a result of the sudden onset of drug resistance, which ultimately results in treatment inefficacy and patient fatality. Cancer treatment now faces significant challenges due to drug resistance. The fundamental processes that give rise to drug resistance are extremely intricate and remain to be fully understood. Hence, acquiring a deeper comprehension of the mechanisms underlying the emergence of resistance to drugs in cancer holds the potential to unveil innovative strategies for tailoring therapeutic interventions to individual patients [9]. Non-coding RNAs, including microRNAs, long ncRNAs, and circular RNAs, form a heterogeneous collection of transcripts that lack the ability to encode proteins [10]. They play a crucial role in regulating a wide range of physiological and pathological processes. A multitude of diseases, particularly cancer, exhibit a close association with the dysregulation of non-coding RNA (ncRNA) [11]. It is noteworthy that the dysregulation of the ncRNA plays a substantial role in facilitating drug resistance in tumors through diverse mechanisms. The mechanisms encompassed in this context involve the initiation of autophagy, augmentation of the epithelial to mesenchymal transition, and inhibition of apoptosis [12]. The dysregulation of ncRNAs plays a crucial role in the development and progression of various diseases, such as cancer. These ncRNAs have significant involvement in both normal physiological processes and pathological conditions. Indeed, it has been noted that cancerous tissues and cell lines exhibit aberrant expression of ncRNAs. Through their roles as tumor suppressors or oncogenes, proteins regulate the rate at which cancer spreads [13]. The regulatory functions of gene expression encompass various post-transcriptional stages, including transcription, transmission of signals, chromatin remodeling, and the involvement of ncRNAs [14]. The ncRNAs, despite lacking the capacity to encode proteins, play a significant role in a wide range of biological processes, primarily focusing on the regulation of genes. Extensive research on genes and mechanisms of illness has demonstrated that mutations in ncRNAs can impact the beginning and course of numerous complex diseases, including cancer. Because ncRNAs affect cell growth, differentiation, and apoptosis, it is believed that they serve as tumor inhibitors or oncogene drivers in a range of cancers [15, 16]. It is challenging to pinpoint the specific roles played by ncRNAs; numerous ncRNAs exhibit intricate interactions during cancer and control the growth cycle and characteristics of cells. A complex network comprising a multitude of ncRNAs facilitates the transmission of diverse signals between various biological structures. The interactions among ncRNAs are associated with distinct structural characteristics and contribute to the formation of network motifs [17].

Numerous RNA-based treatments have been created, and the FDA has approved some of them. Notably, each of these treatments works by targeting particular mRNAs to diminish the manifestation of linked genes. Despite being the subject of recent research, none of the lncRNAs have been studied in clinical settings as potential therapeutic targets. Phase 2 and 3 clinical studies have increased the usefulness of treatments based on miRNA. The development of therapeutic modalities targeting ncRNAs typically follows one of two paths: either overexpress a tumor suppressor ncRNA or block the specific ncRNA component if it is overexpressed [18]. ncRNA inhibitors comprise a diverse array of methodologies, including CRISPR/Cas9-mediated gene editing, antisense anti-oligonucleotides, small-molecular inhibitors targeting non-coding RNA, antagomirs, siRNAs, and short hairpin RNAs, and miRNAs sponges. *In vitro* as well as *in vivo* research commonly employ ASOs and antagomirs as miRNA-targeting inhibitors. ASOs are RNA molecules with one strand that attach themselves to complementary sequences of RNA by base pairing that matches to prevent and hinder the function of the target sequences and cause RNAse-H-mediated cleavage [19]. The second way to target ncRNAs is to restore their normal function, which is diminished when therapy resistance arises. MiRNA mimic agents, an efficient substitute that is frequently used in *in vivo* research, are examples of synthetic ncRNA-like molecules that can be used to replace or substitute the lost ncRNA to restore function [20]. Despite significant progress made in the area, the domain of ncRNA-based therapeutics still encounters various challenges. Among these challenges, the concern of off-target effects causing undesirable side effects stands out as particularly prominent [18]. A total of five patients encountered significant adverse events resulting from the administration of the widely recognized miR-34 mimic MRX34. Among these patients, one individual exhibited symptoms of cytokine release syndrome. Consequently, the phase 1 clinical trial of cancer therapy was halted [21]. The occurrence of unintended effects on healthy tissue, which do not affect tumor tissue, poses an additional challenge for RNA-based therapeutics, particularly when administered systemically.

4.2 CANCER'S LONG NON-CODING RNA

Moreover, lncRNAs function as suppressors or oncogenes to control the initiation and spread of tumors. *HOXA* gene-derived HOTTIP is extremely prevalent in a variety of canines. In recent studies, it has been shown by researchers that the oncogenic HOTTIP exhibits involvement in the pathogenesis of acute myeloid leukemia (AML) [22]. An additional long non-coding RNA, or lncRNA, originating from the TCF genome locus is commonly denoted as lncTCF7. Certain researchers have reported that ncTCF7 plays a significant and clearly visible role in the ability of cancers of the liver cell stem cells or CSCs to self-renew [23]. It has been discovered that a number of long non-coding RNAs function as suppressors, preventing cancer cells from proliferating and spreading. The inhibitory effects on cancer of lung proliferation are exerted by Pvt1b, which is a variant of lncRNA, or long non-coding RNA, that is controlled by the p53 protein. This inhibition occurs through the reduction of *c-Myc* genes. A correlation exists between decreased expression of DIRC3 and reduced survival rates, as observed in melanoma cases. Additional examination indicates that DIRC3 enhances the transcription of the tumor suppressor IGFBP5, thereby impeding the proliferation of melanoma cells. Noticeable enhancements in cellular invasion, migration, or proliferation are observed following the suppression of SATB-AS1 [24–26].

LncRNAs' function is studied through their interactions with cellular macromolecules. Long ncRNAs, also referred to as l, possess the ability to influence gene expression by means of two distinct mechanisms. Firstly, they can induce alterations in the chromatin structure within close proximity. Secondly, they can attract molecules that are responsible for regulating specific genomic regions. The modulation of protein-protein interactions and the subsequent formation of protein complexes can be influenced by the relationships between lncRNAs, or long ncRNAs, and diverse proteins. The stability, translation, and isolation of mRNAs can all be impacted by interactions with lncRNAs as shown in Figure 4.1. Even more recently, research has shown that lncRNAs can function as a precursor for circRNA or miRNA [27]. Long non-coding RNAs (non-coding RNA) have been recognized as significant contributors to diverse mechanisms associated with chemoresistance. These mechanisms include mutation of drug targets, induction of apoptosis, modification of drug efflux, and interference with DNA damage repair [28]. In the modern cancer treatment arsenal, radiation therapy is a vital tool. However, due to the presence of biological heterogeneities and intricate complexities, coupled with the existence of stem cells in cancer [29,30]. The biogenesis processes of mRNAs and lncRNAs are similar because they are both poly-adenylated, capped, and spliced. The transcripts of this complex 3D structure, which is capable of multiple functions and changes quickly, account for their complexity. LncRNAs can perform trans (done far from the transcription site) and cis (done close to the transcription site) functions. Chromosomal looping, chromatin modifications, and DNA transcription are examples of typical cis activities. Precisely delineated trans functions encompass intercellular communication with other ncRNAs, association with proteins to modulate their functionality, interaction with messenger RNAs to modify their stability, and facilitation of paraspeckle formation during cellular development [31–35].

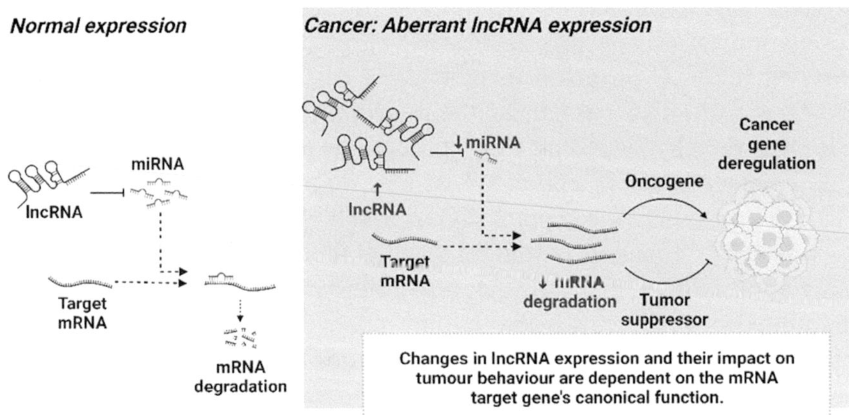

FIGURE 4.1 lncRNA—miRNA gene expression regulation in cancer.

The dysregulation of a lengthy non-coding RNA (lncRNA) has the potential to impact multiple tumor processes simultaneously, encompassing the facilitation of tumor cell proliferation, invasiveness, and metastasis. The significance of this finding is underscored by the involvement of specific lncRNAs, or long ncRNAs in the initiation and progression of colorectal cancer (CRC). The significance of long non-coding RNAs (lncRNAs) in the activation of signaling pathways associated with tumor proliferation is well-established. These pathways encompass various molecular components such as EGFR/insulin-like expansion factors 1 receptor (IGF-1R), p53, epithelial-mesenchymal transition (EMT) signaling mechanisms, KRAS, phosphatidylinositol-3-kinase (PI3K), and transforming growth factor-beta (TGF-β) [36]. A growing body of scholarly literature posits that the long non-coding RNA regulation of reprogramming (lnc-ROR), present in lung, colon, breast, and hepatocellular carcinoma, exerts a facilitative influence on the proliferation, invasiveness, migratory capacity, and drug resistance of cancer cells, thereby exerting regulatory control over the progression of diverse forms of cancer [37]. In addition, a novel prognostic marker that has been recently identified for individuals afflicted with colorectal cancer is a long non-coding RNA known as MALAT1, which stands for metastasis-associated adenocarcinoma on lung transcription. The long non-coding RNA MALAT1 has been identified as a biomarker of prognosis for metastasis in patients diagnosed with small cell non-small lung cancer [38, 39]. According to recent research, lncRNAs are crucial for the emergence and progression of all cancer types. For example, by triggering the PI3K-AKT pathway, the lncRNA HOXB-AS3 may encourage lung cancer cells to proliferate and migrate. In a different study, it was found that the long non-coding RNA GAS5 controls the expression of microRNA-216b, which affects the invasion of cancerous breast cells and the EMT. According to the research conducted by several scholars, it has been proposed that long non-coding RNA (lncRNA) OCC-1 exhibits the capability to initiate the ubiquitination process and also afterward lead to degradation of HuR protein. If this mechanism was to be implemented, it has the potential to significantly hinder the spread of cells with colorectal cancer. An increasing amount of empirical evidence suggests that lncRNAs or long ncRNAs play a role in the development of chemoresistance in cancer of the gastric (GC) through diverse mechanisms. The mechanisms encompassed in this context involve the suppression of programmed cell death, the stimulation of cellular self-digestion, the facilitation of cellular transformation from epithelial to mesenchymal state, the modification of drug levels, and the control of interconnected signaling pathways [40–43]. Both transcriptome and genomic methodologies have been utilized to evaluate the role of lncRNAs, or long ncRNAs in the development of pancreatic cancer. The research findings have unveiled atypical expression patterns of numerous long ncRNAs or lncRNAs in the context of cancer of the pancreas, particularly when comparing non-cancerous tissues and cells to pancreatic cancer tissue and cell lines. LncRNAs can control pancreatic cell migration, proliferation, apoptosis, and cell cycle transition. A lncRNA called IRAIN causes pancreatic cancer cells to undergo cell cycle arrest and increases apoptosis [44]. Drug resistance is also impacted by dysregulation of apoptosis, since most chemotherapeutic drugs work by encouraging apoptosis to stop cancer cells from proliferating. The upregulation of multiple survival factors, including the nuclear factors κB (NF-κB), Bcl-2 family molecules of protein, and the nuclear factor inhibitions of apoptotic proteins, facilitates inhibition of apoptotic death of cells. The phenomenon of reduced apoptosis in cisplatin-resistant cancer cells following treatment with cisplatin has been observed by researchers, who have attributed this effect to the overexpression of PVT1. The regulation of p53 and Bcl-XL expression in cisplatin-resistant lung cancer cells was influenced by the mitochondrial apoptotic pathways. The implementation of this regulation led to a reduction in the levels of the lncRNA, or long non-coding RNA, MEG3 expression, as well as an enhancement in the cells' responsiveness to cisplatin therapy [45–47]. The long non-coding RNA (lncRNA) H19 plays a role in promoting the acquisition of resistance to cisplatin in adenocarcinoma of the lungs by inhibiting the synthesis of proapoptotic proteins, including BAX, BAK, and FAS [48].

LncRNAs use a variety of mechanisms to carry out their roles in controlling cell fate, such as RNA interaction, protein association, DNA binding, and small peptide synthesis. First of all, lncRNAs can control the production of target genes by altering the structure of chromatin and epigenetic changes through their binding to DNA. Second, lncRNAs act as molecular sponges, communicating with miRNAs and mRNAs to alter the translation of mRNAs as well as the binding or stability of their targets. Thirdly, lncRNAs can bind to proteins and control various aspects of their functions, such as their conformation, stability, localization, and formation or dissociation of protein complexes.

4.3 MECHANISM OF NON-CODING RNA-MEDIATED CANCER RESISTANCE

There are two categories of drug resistance: drug resistance that is both single- and multidrug-resistant (MDR). Most of these patient deaths are related to MDR. According to recent studies, ncRNAs and cancer treatment resistance are strongly correlated [49]. Non-coding RNAs, also known as ncRNAs can be classified into different categories primarily according to their size. Among the important small ncRNAs in cancer are piRNAs, circRNAs, tsRNAs, and miRNAs as shown in Figure 4.2 [50].

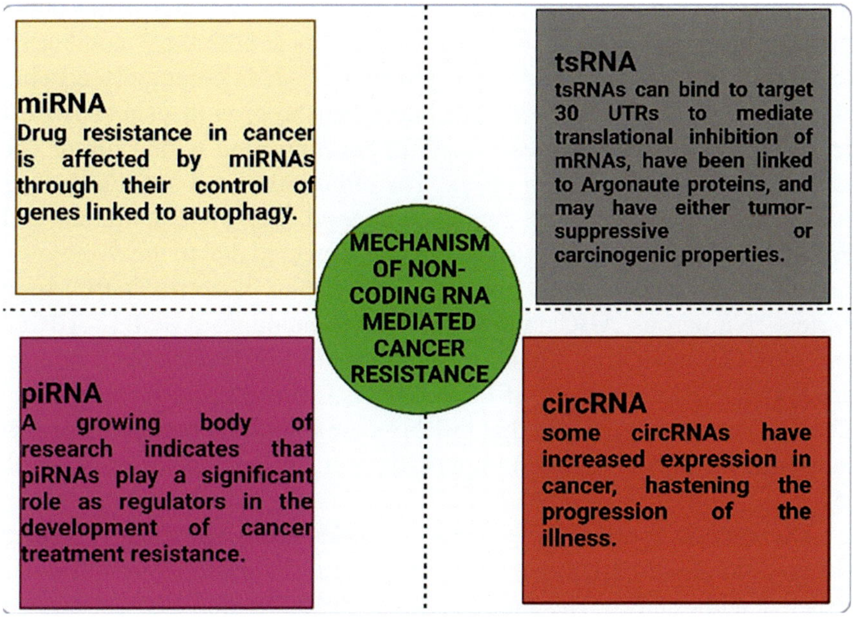

FIGURE 4.2 Various mechanisms of non-coding mediated cancer resistance.

4.3.1 miRNA

MicroRNAs (miRNAs) are a class of ncRNAs that are composed of 22 nucleotides. These molecules carry out their regulatory role by binding to specific sequences in target RNAs, which exhibit complementarity to the miRNA's 5′ end. This binding mechanism allows miRNAs to modulate the production of various RNA molecules, with a particular emphasis on messenger RNAs (mRNAs). The RNA polymerase II (Pol 2) is responsible for transcribing the genes that encode miRNAs, and it carries out this process through a process that has been maintained across evolutionary time. Within the canonical processing pathways, a lengthier primary transcript, commonly known as the prior-miRNA, undergoes cleavage to form a pre-miRNA. The pre-miRNA molecule is subsequently translocated to the cytoplasm via the concerted activity of Exportin 5 and the Ran-GTP, which interact to form a complex. The microprocessor complex, consisting of Drosha and DGCR8, demonstrates the ability to recognize the pri-miRNA as a distinct hairpin structure. Subsequently, the investigator proceeds to cleave the termini of the precursor microRNA (pre-miRNA), thereby generating a microRNA duplex. This duplex structure exhibits two nucleotide (nt) overhangs at both the 3′ and 5′ ends, accompanied by a total of 50 phosphates [51]. It is commonly accepted that one of the main factors contributing to the growth of resistance to drugs in cancer is the decrease in drug concentration within tumor cells as a result of excessive drug efflux. The effectiveness of anticancer drugs is significantly hampered by this phenomenon. Reports that are currently available indicate that drugs are excessively ejected due to the overexpression of drug efflux pumps, namely ATP-binding cassettes (ABC) transporters. Numerous ABC family members, including ABCB1, ABCC2, and ABCG2, have been linked to the formation of resistance to multiple drugs (MDR) in a variety of cancer types, according to prior research. There is mounting evidence that miRNAs are important regulators of ABC transporter expression, which impacts drug efflux in cancerous tumor cells [52–54].

Therapeutic interventions aimed at modulating autophagy have the potential to ameliorate the unfavorable prognosis observed in individuals afflicted with cancer. The modulation of miRNAs impacts resistance to drugs in cancer by regulating genes associated with autophagy. In this instance, it was observed by researchers that the OC lines of cells A2780 as well as SKOV3, which were resistant to cisplatin (CDDP), exhibited notably diminished levels of miR-133a. The researchers observed a significant enhancement in the susceptibility to cisplatin (CDDP) in cisplatin-resistant A2780 or SKOV3 cells through the overexpression of miR-133a, which directly targets YES1. The achievement was attained by inhibiting the process of autophagy [55]. Dysregulated inflammatory processes influence the biological behaviors of cancer cells, including cellular invasion, proliferation, angiogenesis, metastasis, and resistance to treatment agents. These processes can be triggered by persistent inflammation resulting from infections, abnormal immune responses, and external factors. The main effector cells in the immune system are T cells. They contribute to inflammation by generating cytokines during immune reactions. It has been demonstrated that the primary drivers of the development of drug resistance are immune avoidance and immune tolerance brought on by T cell function dysregulation. As a result, improving drug sensitivity for individuals with cancer can be achieved by specifically targeting T cells. Growing research indicates that miRNAs are essential for controlling T cell functions [56, 57].

4.3.2 tsRNAs

The term "tRNA-derived small RNAs," also known as mRNAs, refers to a novel category of noncoding RNAs that possess medical significance. These RNAs are derived from transfer RNAs (tRNAs). TiRNAs (tRNA-derived stress-induced RNAs) or tRNA fragments (tRFs) are other names for these molecules. There are still a lot of things to learn about their biogenesis and downstream mechanisms of action in addition to creating a universal nomenclature system. Ribonucleic acid (RNA) RNA polymerase III (Pol III) is responsible for transcribing transfer RNAs (tRNAs) in the form of precursor tRNAs (pre-tRNAs). These pre-tRNAs undergo subsequent modifications and processing steps to generate mature tRNAs. Various types of transfer RNA (tRNA) molecules can produce diverse forms of tRNA-derived small RNAs (mRNAs) depending on the site of cleavage and whether it takes place in the mature tRNA or pre-tRNA transcript. The precise functions of the enzymes responsible for producing mRNAs remain unclear; however, certain ribonucleases such as angiogenin, Dicer, or RNase Z have been sporadically detected in this process [58]. Despite considerable heterogeneity of distinct transfer RNA-derived small RNA (dsRNA) molecules identified in neoplastic cells and their diverse mechanisms of action, tsRNAs and microRNAs (miRNAs) exhibit certain common characteristics. Just like microRNAs (miRNAs), transfer RNA-derived small RNAs (tsRNAs) have been associated with Argonaute proteins, enabling them to interact with the 30 untranslated regions (UTRs) of target mRNAs, thereby facilitating translational repression. Moreover, tsRNAs possess the capacity to exhibit both tumor-suppressive and carcinogenic properties [59].

4.3.3 piRNA

A group of short RNAs with lengths ranging from 21 to 35 nt is known as piRNAs (piwi-interacting RNA). Transposon suppression during germline development or the PIWI subfamily of protein Argonaute are commonly associated with each other. The production of piRNA precursors is facilitated by pathways that are specific to each species, and it is observed that piRNA sequences do not exhibit a high degree of conservation. The human genome contains a substantial number of piRNAs, which undergo transcription by RNA Pol II and are distributed across various genomic loci. piRNAs are generated from long, unpaired transcripts [60]. An increasing amount of research suggests that piRNAs are essential for controlling treatment resistance as cancer develops. For example, in breast cancer tissues, researchers found that there was a notable downregulation of piRNA-36,712. PiRNA-36,712 overexpression significantly raised the susceptibility of MCF-7 and ZR75-1 cells to paclitaxel and doxorubicin. In line with this, the knockdown of piRNA-36,712 produced conflicting results. This chapter demonstrates that piRNA-36,712 and SEPW1P RNAs (SEPW1 pseudogene) engage in direct interactions, facilitating the mechanistic targeting of SEPW1 RNA by miR-7 and miR-324. This targeting event leads to a reduction in SEPW1 expression, consequently enhancing the susceptibility of breast cancer cells to PTX and DOX [61–63].

4.3.4 CircRNA

In cells that are proliferation-stable or terminally differentiated, circRNAs (circular RNA) are typically highly expressed. Yet, a few circRNAs strangely exhibit elevated expression in cancer, which accelerates the disease's development. CircRNAs can function as miRNA sponges, thereby inhibiting the expression of miRNAs. In addition, the expression of let-7 is downregulated by circ-CPA4, a molecule that exhibits high levels of expression in non-small cell lung cancer (NSCLC) cells. The circ-CPA4 molecule can enhance the expression of programmed cell death ligand 1 (PD-L1), which is a target of let-7, via the circ-CPA4/let-7 axis. This promotes resistance to drugs and stemness in cells [64, 65]. At first, circular RNAs (circRNAs) were hypothesized to arise from RNA splicing events or mislocalization, primarily due to their relatively low abundance. Nevertheless, their existence within the eukaryotic phylogenetic tree was subsequently revealed. Multiple recent studies have presented empirical evidence concerning the substantial contributions of RNAs that are circular (circRNAs) in diverse facets of cancer, encompassing its progression, dissemination, and pluripotency. These entities play a role in the initiation, dissemination, and advancement of neoplasms and have the potential to serve as biomarkers for the diagnosis and prognosis of head and neck cancer (HNC). In recent years, there has been a growing body of evidence linking circular RNAs (circRNAs) to the development of medication resistance in tumors. Circular RNA MTO1 was found to enhance the susceptibility of bladder cancer cells to monastrol, whereas circular RNA PVT1 was associated with resistance to chemotherapy and reduced overall survival in osteosarcoma. Nevertheless, the existing body of literature does not provide sufficient data pertaining to the precise role of circular RNAs (circRNAs) in the progression of drug resistance in HNCs. In the near future, there is a strong possibility that circular RNAs (circRNAs) will be recognized as significant regulators in the underlying molecular processes of tumor tolerance in HNCs [66–71].

4.4 THERAPEUTIC STRATEGIES TARGETING NON-CODING RNA

The biggest challenges facing clinical cancer treatment remain to be drug resistance and patient response to chemotherapy. Multiple studies have substantiated the pivotal functions that ncRNAs assume in the emergence of drug resistance in cancer. These genes can display either tumor suppressor or oncogenic properties, depending on their specific downstream targets, resulting in divergent impacts on the growth of cancer. The aforementioned characteristics render ncRNAs highly auspicious as potential targets or agents for therapeutic intervention in the battle against cancer. The targeted treatment of cancer patients, especially those who are not responding well to chemotherapy, may greatly benefit from therapeutic approaches that use ncRNAs or directly target ncRNAs. Enhancing cancer intervention through the targeted delivery of non-coding RNAs (non-coding RNA) possessing tumor-suppressive characteristics to particular cancer cells is a potentially effective approach. For example, it has been noted that adenocarcinoma of the pancreatic duct tissue and cell lines both exhibit downregulation of miRNA-3662 [72,73]. Numerous ncRNAs have been discovered that, through modifying estrogen signaling, either enhance or mitigate cellular resistance to medications. The identification of these ncRNAs, also known as ncRNAs has sparked the creation of potentially ground-breaking therapeutic approaches that may improve a patient's response to hormone treatments. In this specific case, treatment approaches typically involve the delivery of ncRNAs to enhance the effectiveness of medications or the silencing of ncRNAs that impede the response to treatment. Targeting harmful miRNAs can be accomplished through a variety of strategies, such as applying synthetic miRNA sponges or administering anti-miRNA oligonucleotides (antagomiRNAs) [74]. Because ncRNA functions are so complex and because they consistently have pleiotropic effects—regulating several genes, such as tumor suppressor or oncogene genes—targeting or delivering non-coding RNA for therapeutic uses is thought to have a higher risk of producing unfavorable side effects. Therefore, in order to lessen these side effects, it is essential to carefully plan and implement ncRNA-based treatments, as well as to carry out extensive *in vitro* or animal research to confirm their safety. Therefore, the future of this area of study is expected to be shaped by the clinical use of ncRNA-based therapy, which has the potential to significantly improve cancer treatment and overcome treatment resistance [75]. Furthermore, ncRNAs can secrete themselves as actively packed particles (apoptotic bodies, micro-vesicles, and exosomes) and circulate freely in the blood. Their concentrations beneath the blood are nearly identical to those in primary tumors. Additionally, they display a few distinctive qualities like high detectability, high stability, and differently expressed patterns. These characteristics imply that ncRNAs have a great deal of promise as the best biomarkers for prognosis and diagnosis for cancer patients undergoing clinical treatment. Numerous ncRNAs, specifically, prognostic and/or diagnostic markers for cancer have been found for microRNAs (miRNAs) and lncRNAs [76–78].

The targeted treatment of cancer patients, especially those who are not responding well to chemotherapy, may greatly benefit from therapeutic approaches that use ncRNAs or directly target ncRNAs. One potentially promising approach for enhancing cancer intervention involves the administration of tumor-suppressive ncRNAs to specific cancer cells. When it comes to the cancer of the pancreatic ducts (PDAC), it was found that tissues from PDAC and cell lines expressed miRNA-3662 less frequently [79]. Since their original discovery, therapeutic uses of ncRNAs have attracted a great deal of interest. The study of the ncRNAs, including lncRNAs, which are long non-coding RNA and microRNAs (miRNAs), has received a lot of attention in recent years. Although ncRNAs were initially disregarded as transcription noise or artifacts, they have been found to play intricate biological roles. They are important biomarkers for the identification and prognosis of cancer and are involved in the procedures of carcinogenesis or tumor suppression. For instance, earlier research has shown that overexpression of miR-122 causes the expression levels of NOTCH1 or Hes1 in A549 stem cell lines to decrease. Furthermore, it has been shown that A549 stem cells' resistance to gefitinib is lowered by the inhibition of the NOTCH1 pathways caused by miR-122. As a result, the inhibition suppresses the migration and proliferation of cancer cells [80–83].

Even though small ncRNAs have demonstrated promise and efficacy as therapeutic agents *in vitro*, a significant obstacle remains the nucleic acid drugs' low bioavailability *in vivo*. Therefore, there is a pressing need to develop innovative drug delivery strategies. Many small ncRNA carriers, including nanoparticles, ncRNA modification, and off-target effects, have been developed to address the common problems of RNA delivery's limited half-life, low transfection efficiency, and off-target effects [84, 85]. Another useful tactic to increase the accuracy and robustness of small ncRNAs in addressing cancer-related genes is modifying them with lipid and PEG molecules. As a result, siRNAs are altered with lipid and PEG molecules to generate SAMiRNA, which are self-assembled lipid nanoparticles, and siRNAs are chemically attached to carriers to produce carrier-siRNA conjugates. The investigation of GalNac-conjugated siRNAs as a potential treatment for liver cancer is currently underway. Two research groups have collaborated to covalently conjugate specific small interfering RNAs (siRNAs) along with 1-3 acetyl galactosamine (GalNAc) molecules [86]. An additional challenge arises in relation to the cytotoxic characteristics demonstrated by transport agents, such as cationic liposomes, which have the potential to induce inflammation in the lungs and produce reactive oxygen intermediates. For example, the application of TAT-conjugated siRNAs, that contain a cell-penetrating peptide (CPP), has been shown to enhance the efficacy of gene silencing. Nevertheless, this conjugate concurrently stimulates the innate immune system [87]. Furthermore, ncRNAs can be directly targeted due to their spatial configuration, and small-molecule compounds can regulate ncRNAs by supporting complex biological functions. A promising small-molecule molecule that attaches to human ribosomes has been discovered after a thorough screening of three kinases or topoisomerase inhibitors using the "Absorb Array" technique. Therefore, it is thought that ncRNAs are the most alluring prospective targets for cancer therapy [88–90].

4.5 CONCLUSION

Cancer has become more common in low-risk patient populations, particularly those under 45 years of age and without a substance use history. Genetic susceptibility risk prediction has improved, with over 40 hazard-associated single-nucleotide polymorphisms (SNPs) identified. Women who have inherited mutations in either the *BRCA1* or *BRCA2* gene are more genetically susceptible to breast cancer. Non-coding RNAs (ncRNAs) play a crucial role in the control of numerous physiological or pathological mechanisms, including those linked to cancer. Genetic modifications in ncRNAs have the potential to impact the development and advancement of intricate diseases, including cancer. RNA-based therapies have been devised to selectively target and diminish the expression of specific messenger RNAs (mRNAs). However, challenges remain, such as side effects and unintended on-target effects on healthy tissue. RNA-based therapies have demonstrated promise in the treatment of cancer despite these obstacles. To completely comprehend the mechanisms behind drug resistance and create individualized treatment regimens for cancer patients, additional research is still required. Cancer treatment resistance is largely caused by ncRNAs, of which miRNAs, tsRNAs, circRNAs, and piRNAs are important small ncRNAs. MicroRNAs (miRNAs) are a class of ncRNAs that typically consist of approximately 22 nucleotides. They exert regulatory control over the synthesis of other RNAs by binding to specific sequences that are complementary to their own within target RNAs. The enhancement of drug sensitivities in cancer patients can be achieved through the implementation of therapeutic approaches that specifically target autophagy, tsRNAs, and piRNAs. Circular RNAs (circRNAs) have been observed to display increased expression levels within cells that are either actively dividing and stable or in a state of terminal differentiation. These circRNAs have been identified as playing a substantial role in the progression of cancer, metastasis, and the properties of stem cells. Non-coding RNAs (ncRNAs) are highly promising as therapeutic targets in the fight against cancer. Targeting ncRNAs or their delivery can enhance cancer intervention, especially for patients not responding well to chemotherapy. Therapeutic approaches may involve delivering ncRNAs that enhance or mitigate cellular resistance to endocrine therapies. However, ncRNA-based therapeutics must be carefully designed and delivered, and in-depth *in vitro* and animal research is required to confirm their safety.

KEYWORDS

- **long non-coding RNA**
- **microRNA**
- **non-coding RNA**
- **piwi-interacting RNA**
- **t-RNA-derived small RNA**

REFERENCES

1. Gillison, M. L., Chaturvedi, A. K., Anderson, W. F., & Fakhry, C. (2015). Epidemiology of human papillomavirus–positive head and neck squamous cell carcinoma. *Journal of Clinical Oncology, 33*(29), 3235–3242.
2. Mourad, M., Jetmore, T., Jategaonkar, A. A., Moubayed, S., Moshier, E., & Urken, M. L. (2017). Epidemiological trends of head and neck cancer in the United States: a SEER population study. *Journal of Oral and Maxillofacial Surgery, 75*(12), 2562–2572.
3. Patel, S. C., Carpenter, W. R., Tyree, S., Couch, M. E., Weissler, M., Hackman, T., Hayes, D. N., Shores, C., & Chera, B. S. (2011). Increasing incidence of oral tongue squamous cell carcinoma in young white women, age 18 to 44 years. *Journal of Clinical Oncology, 29*(11), 1488–1494.
4. Harris, S. L., Kimple, R. J., Hayes, D. N., Couch, M. E., & Rosenman, J. G. (2010). Never-smokers, never-drinkers: unique clinical subgroup of young patients with head and neck squamous cell cancers. *Head & Neck: Journal for the Sciences and Specialties of the Head and Neck, 32*(4), 499–503.
5. Zafereo, M. E., Xu, L., Dahlstrom, K. R., Viamonte, C. A., El-Naggar, A. K., Wei, Q., Li, G., & Sturgis, E. M. (2016). Squamous cell carcinoma of the oral cavity often overexpresses p16 but is rarely driven by human papillomavirus. *Oral Oncology, 56*, 47–53.
6. Patel, S. C., Carpenter, W. R., Tyree, S., Couch, M. E., Weissler, M., Hackman, T., Hayes, D. N., Shores, C., & Chera, B. S. (2011). Increasing incidence of oral tongue squamous cell carcinoma in young white women, age 18 to 44 years. *Journal of Clinical Oncology, 29*(11), 1488–1494.
7. Verschuur, H. P., Irish, J. C., O'Sullivan, B., Goh, C., Gullane, P. J., & Pintilie, M. (1999). A matched control study of treatment outcome in young patients with squamous cell carcinoma of the head and neck. *The Laryngoscope, 109*(2), 249–258.
8. Hoeijmakers, J. H. (2001). Genome maintenance mechanisms for preventing cancer. *Nature, 411*(6835), 366–374.

9. Liu, Y., Ao, X., Zhou, X., Du, C., & Kuang, S. (2022). The regulation of PBXs and their emerging role in cancer. *Journal of Cellular and Molecular Medicine, 26*(5), 1363–1379.
10. Zhang, Y., Wei, Y. J., Zhang, Y. F., Liu, H. W., & Zhang, Y. F. (2021). Emerging functions and clinical applications of exosomal ncRNAs in ovarian cancer. *Frontiers in Oncology, 11*, 765458.
11. Najafi, S., Tan, S. C., Raee, P., Rahmati, Y., Asemani, Y., Lee, E. H. C., Hushmandi, K., Zarrabi, A., Aref, A. R., Ashrafizadeh, M., & Kumar, A. P. (2022). Gene regulation by antisense transcription: A focus on neurological and cancer diseases. *Biomedicine & Pharmacotherapy, 145*, 112265.
12. Chen, B., Dragomir, M. P., Yang, C., Li, Q., Horst, D., & Calin, G. A. (2022). Targeting non-coding RNAs to overcome cancer therapy resistance. *Signal Transduction and Targeted Therapy, 7*(1), 121.
13. Jiang, Y., Zhao, L., Wu, Y., Deng, S., Cao, P., Lei, X., & Yang, X. (2022). The role of NcRNAs to regulate immune checkpoints in cancer. *Frontiers in Immunology, 13*, 853480.
14. Anastasiadou, E., Jacob, L. S., & Slack, F. J. (2018). Non-coding RNA networks in cancer. *Nature Reviews Cancer, 18*(1), 5–18.
15. Mattick, J. S., & Makunin, I. V. (2006). Non-coding RNA. *Human Molecular Genetics, 15*(suppl_1), R17–R29.
16. Pavet, V., Portal, M. M., Moulin, J. C., Herbrecht, R., & Gronemeyer, H. (2011). Towards novel paradigms for cancer therapy. *Oncogene, 30*(1), 1–20.
17. Alon, U. (2007). Network motifs: theory and experimental approaches. *Nature Reviews Genetics, 8*(6), 450–461.
18. Winkle, M., El-Daly, S. M., Fabbri, M., & Calin, G. A. (2021). Noncoding RNA therapeutics—challenges and potential solutions. *Nature Reviews Drug Discovery, 20*(8), 629–651.
19. Crooke, S. T. (2017). Molecular mechanisms of antisense oligonucleotides. *Nucleic Acid Therapeutics, 27*(2), 70–77.
20. Bader, A. G., Brown, D., & Winkler, M. (2010). The promise of microRNA replacement therapy. *Cancer Research, 70*(18), 7027–7030.
21. Hong, D. S., Kang, Y. K., Brenner, A. J., Sachdev, J. C., Ejadi, S., Borad, M. J., Kim, T. Y., Lim, H. Y., Park, K., Becerra, C., & Bader, A. G. (2016). MRX34, a liposomal miR-34 mimic, in patients with advanced solid tumors: Final dose-escalation results from a first-in-human phase I trial of microRNA therapy. *Journal of Oncology, 34*, 2508.
22. Luo, H., Zhu, G., Xu, J., Lai, Q., Yan, B., Guo, Y., Fung, T. K., Zeisig, B. B., Cui, Y., Zha, J., & Cogle, C. (2019). HOTTIP lncRNA promotes hematopoietic stem cell self-renewal leading to AML-like disease in mice. *Cancer Cell, 36*(6), 645–659.
23. Wang, Y., He, L., Du, Y., Zhu, P., Huang, G., Luo, J., Yan, X., Ye, B., Li, C., Xia, P., & Zhang, G. (2015). The long noncoding RNA lncTCF7 promotes self-renewal of human liver cancer stem cells through activation of Wnt signaling. *Cell Stem Cell, 16*(4), 413–425.
24. Olivero, C. E., Martínez-Terroba, E., Zimmer, J., Liao, C., Tesfaye, E., Hooshdaran, N., Schofield, J. A., Bendor, J., Fang, D., Simon, M. D., & Zamudio, J. R.

(2020). p53 activates the long noncoding RNA Pvt1b to inhibit Myc and suppress tumorigenesis. *Molecular Cell, 77*(4), 761–774.

25. Coe, E. A., Tan, J. Y., Shapiro, M., Louphrasitthiphol, P., Bassett, A. R., Marques, A. C., Goding, C. R., & Vance, K. W. (2019). The MITF-SOX10 regulated long non-coding RNA DIRC3 is a melanoma tumour suppressor. *PLoS Genetics, 15*(12), e1008501.
26. Wang, Y. Q., Jiang, D. M., Hu, S. S., Zhao, L., Wang, L., Yang, M. H., Ai, M. L., Jiang, H. J., Han, Y., Ding, Y. Q., & Wang, S. (2019). SATB2-AS1 suppresses colorectal carcinoma aggressiveness by inhibiting SATB2-dependent Snail transcription and epithelial–mesenchymal transition. *Cancer Research, 79*(14), 3542–3556.
27. Batista, P. J., & Chang, H. Y. (2013). Long noncoding RNAs: cellular address codes in development and disease. *Cell, 152*(6), 1298–1307.
28. Chen, Q. N., Wei, C. C., Wang, Z. X., & Sun, M. (2017). Long non-coding RNAs in anti-cancer drug resistance. *Oncotarget, 8*(1), 1925.
29. Shi, Y., Liu, N., Lai, W., Yan, B., Chen, L., Liu, S., Liu, S., Wang, X., Xiao, D., Liu, X., & Mao, C. (2018). Nuclear EGFR-PKM2 axis induces cancer stem cell-like characteristics in irradiation-resistant cells. *Cancer Letters, 422*, 81–93.
30. Delaney, G., Jacob, S., Featherstone, C., & Barton, M. (2005). The role of radiotherapy in cancer treatment: estimating optimal utilization from a review of evidence-based clinical guidelines. *Cancer: Interdisciplinary International Journal of the American Cancer Society, 104*(6), 1129–1137.
31. Fabbri, M., Girnita, L., Varani, G., & Calin, G. A. (2019). Decrypting noncoding RNA interactions, structures, and functional networks. *Genome Research, 29*(9), 1377–1388.
32. Pisignano, G., Napoli, S., Magistri, M., Mapelli, S. N., Pastori, C., Di Marco, S., Civenni, G., Albino, D., Enriquez, C., Allegrini, S., & Mitra, A. (2017). A promoter-proximal transcript targeted by genetic polymorphism controls E-cadherin silencing in human cancers. *Nature Communications, 8*(1), 15622.
33. Carlevaro-Fita, J., & Johnson, R. (2019). Global positioning system: understanding long noncoding RNAs through subcellular localization. *Molecular Cell, 73*(5), 869–883.
34. Quinn, J. J., & Chang, H. Y. (2016). Unique features of long non-coding RNA biogenesis and function. *Nature Reviews Genetics, 17*(1), 47–62.
35. Dragomir, M. P., Kopetz, S., Ajani, J. A., & Calin, G. A. (2020). Non-coding RNAs in GI cancers: from cancer hallmarks to clinical utility. *Gut, 69*(4), 748–763.
36. Yang, Y., Junjie, P., Sanjun, C., & Ma, Y. (2017). Long non-coding RNAs in colorectal cancer: progression and future directions. *Journal of Cancer, 8*(16), 3212.
37. Ma, Y. L., Wang, C. Y., Guan, Y. J., & Gao, F. M. (2020). Long noncoding RNA ROR promotes proliferation and invasion of colorectal cancer by inhibiting tumor suppressor gene NF2 through interacting with miR-223-3. *European Review for Medical & Pharmacological Sciences, 24*(5), 2401.
38. Ji, P., Diederichs, S., Wang, W., Böing, S., Metzger, R., Schneider, P. M., Tidow, N., Brandt, B., Buerger, H., Bulk, E., & Thomas, M. (2003). MALAT-1, a novel noncoding RNA, and thymosin β4 predict metastasis and survival in early-stage non-small cell lung cancer. *Oncogene, 22*(39), 8031–8041.

39. Zheng, H. T., Shi, D. B., Wang, Y. W., Li, X. X., Xu, Y., Tripathi, P., Gu, W. L., Cai, G. X., & Cai, S. J. (2014). High expression of lncRNA MALAT1 suggests a biomarker of poor prognosis in colorectal cancer. *International Journal of Clinical and Experimental Pathology, 7*(6), 3174.
40. Jiang, W., Kai, J., Li, D., Wei, Z., Wang, Y., & Wang, W. (2020). lncRNA HOXB-AS3 exacerbates proliferation, migration, and invasion of lung cancer via activating the PI3K-AKT pathway. *Journal of Cellular Physiology, 235*(10), 7194–7203.
41. Li, Y., Guo, X. B., & Wei, Y. H. (2020). LncRNA GAS5 affects epithelial-mesenchymal transition and invasion of breast cancer cells by regulating miR-216b. *European Review for Medical & Pharmacological Sciences, 24*(9), 4873.
42. Lan, Y., Xiao, X., He, Z., Luo, Y., Wu, C., Li, L., & Song, X. (2018). Long noncoding RNA OCC-1 suppresses cell growth through destabilizing HuR protein in colorectal cancer. *Nucleic Acids Research, 46*(11), 5809–5821.
43. Liu, K., Gao, L., Ma, X., Huang, J. J., Chen, J., Zeng, L., Ashby, C. R., Zou, C., & Chen, Z. S. (2020). Long non-coding RNAs regulate drug resistance in cancer. *Molecular Cancer, 19*, 1–13.
44. Lian, Y., Wang, J., Feng, J., Ding, J., Ma, Z., Li, J., Peng, P., De, W., & Wang, K. (2016). Long non-coding RNA IRAIN suppresses apoptosis and promotes proliferation by binding to LSD1 and EZH2 in pancreatic cancer. *Tumor Biology, 37*, 14929–14937.
45. Tsuruo, T., Naito, M., Tomida, A., Fujita, N., Mashima, T., Sakamoto, H., & Haga, N. (2003). Molecular targeting therapy of cancer: drug resistance, apoptosis and survival signal. *Cancer Science, 94*(1), 15–21.
46. Zhang, X. W., Bu, P., Liu, L., Zhang, X. Z., & Li, J. (2015). Overexpression of long non-coding RNA PVT1 in gastric cancer cells promotes the development of multidrug resistance. *Biochemical and Biophysical Research Communications, 462*(3), 227–232.
47. Liu, J., Wan, L., Lu, K., Sun, M., Pan, X., Zhang, P., Lu, B., Liu, G., & Wang, Z. (2015). The long noncoding RNA MEG3 contributes to cisplatin resistance of human lung adenocarcinoma. *PloS One, 10*(5), e0114586.
48. Wang, Q., Cheng, N., Li, X., Pan, H., Li, C., Ren, S., Su, C., Cai, W., Zhao, C., Zhang, L., & Zhou, C. (2016). Correlation of long non-coding RNA H19 expression with cisplatin-resistance and clinical outcome in lung adenocarcinoma. *Oncotarget, 8*(2), 2558.
49. Liu, Y., Ao, X., Wang, Y., Li, X., & Wang, J. (2022). Long non-coding RNA in gastric cancer: mechanisms and clinical implications for drug resistance. *Frontiers in Oncology, 12*, 841411.
50. Bartel, D. P. (2018). Metazoan micrornas. *Cell, 173*(1), 20–51.
51. Adhikari, S., Bhattacharya, A., Adhikary, S., Singh, V., Gadad, S. S., Roy, S., & Das, C. (2022). The paradigm of drug resistance in cancer: an epigenetic perspective. *Bioscience Reports, 42*(4), BSR20211812.
52. Robey, R. W., Pluchino, K. M., Hall, M. D., Fojo, A. T., Bates, S. E., & Gottesman, M. M. (2018). Revisiting the role of ABC transporters in multidrug-resistant cancer. *Nature Reviews Cancer, 18*(7), 452–464.
53. Gomes, B. C., Rueff, J., & Rodrigues, A. S. (2016). MicroRNAs and cancer drug resistance. In *Cancer Drug Resistance: Overviews and Methods*, (pp. 137–162).

54. Shahverdi, M., Hajiasgharzadeh, K., Sorkhabi, A. D., Jafarlou, M., Shojaee, M., Tabrizi, N. J., Alizadeh, N., Santarpia, M., Brunetti, O., Safarpour, H., & Silvestris, N. (2022). The regulatory role of autophagy-related miRNAs in lung cancer drug resistance. *Biomedicine & Pharmacotherapy, 148*, 112735.
55. Singh, N., Baby, D., Prasad Rajguru Jagadish, P. P. B., & Thakkannavar Savita, S. Bhojaraj Pujari V. (2019). Inflammation and cancer, *Annals of African Medicine, 18*(3), 121–126.
56. Dong, C. (2021). Cytokine regulation and function in T cells. *Annual Review of Immunology, 39*(1), 51–76.
57. Slack, F. J., & Chinnaiyan, A. M. (2019). The role of non-coding RNAs in oncology. *Cell, 179*(5), 1033–1055.
58. Balatti, V., Pekarsky, Y., & Croce, C. M. (2017). Role of the tRNA-derived small RNAs in cancer: new potential biomarkers and target for therapy. *Advances in Cancer Research, 135*, 173–187.
59. Goodarzi, H., Liu, X., Nguyen, H. C., Zhang, S., Fish, L., & Tavazoie, S. F. (2015). Endogenous tRNA-derived fragments suppress breast cancer progression via YBX1 displacement. *Cell, 161*(4), 790–802.
60. Aravin, A., Gaidatzis, D., Pfeffer, S., Lagos-Quintana, M., Landgraf, P., Iovino, N., Morris, P., Brownstein, M. J., Kuramochi-Miyagawa, S., Nakano, T., & Chien, M. (2006). A novel class of small RNAs bind to MILI protein in mouse testes. *Nature, 442*(7099), 203–207.
61. Tan, L., Mai, D., Zhang, B., Jiang, X., Zhang, J., Bai, R., Ye, Y., Li, M., Pan, L., Su, J., & Zheng, Y. (2019). PIWI-interacting RNA-36712 restrains breast cancer progression and chemoresistance by interaction with SEPW1 pseudogene SEPW1P RNA. *Molecular Cancer, 18*, 1–15.
62. Mai, D., Ding, P., Tan, L., Zhang, J., Pan, Z., Bai, R., Li, C., Li, M., Zhou, Y., Tan, W., & Zhou, Z. (2018). PIWI-interacting RNA-54265 is oncogenic and a potential therapeutic target in colorectal adenocarcinoma. *Theranostics, 8*(19), 5213.
63. Wang, Y., Gable, T., Ma, M. Z., Clark, D., Zhao, J., Zhang, Y., Liu, W., Mao, L., & Mei, Y. (2017). A piRNA-like small RNA induces chemoresistance to cisplatin-based therapy by inhibiting apoptosis in lung squamous cell carcinoma. *Molecular Therapy-Nucleic Acids, 6*, 269–278.
64. Wang, Y., Xu, R., Zhang, D., Lu, T., Yu, W., Wo, Y., Liu, A., Sui, T., Cui, J., Qin, Y., & Dong, Y. (2019). Circ-ZKSCAN1 regulates FAM83A expression and inactivates MAPK signaling by targeting miR-330-5p to promote non-small cell lung cancer progression. *Translational Lung Cancer Research, 8*(6), 862.
65. Hong, W., Xue, M., Jiang, J., Zhang, Y., & Gao, X. (2020). Circular RNA circ-CPA4/let-7 miRNA/PD-L1 axis regulates cell growth, stemness, drug resistance and immune evasion in non-small cell lung cancer (NSCLC). *Journal of Experimental & Clinical Cancer Research, 39*, 1–19.
66. Sanger, H. L., Klotz, G., Riesner, D., Gross, H. J., & Kleinschmidt, A. K. (1976). Viroids are single-stranded covalently closed circular RNA molecules existing as highly base-paired rod-like structures. *Proceedings of the National Academy of Sciences, 73*(11), 3852–3856.

67. Wang, P. L., Bao, Y., Yee, M. C., Barrett, S. P., Hogan, G. J., Olsen, M. N., Dinneny, J. R., Brown, P. O., & Salzman, J. (2014). Circular RNA is expressed across the eukaryotic tree of life. *PloS One, 9*(3), e90859.
68. Zhang, Y., Liang, W., Zhang, P., Chen, J., Qian, H., Zhang, X., & Xu, W. (2017). Circular RNAs: emerging cancer biomarkers and targets. *Journal of Experimental & Clinical Cancer Research, 36*, 1–13.
69. Geng, Y., Jiang, J., & Wu, C. (2018). Function and clinical significance of circRNAs in solid tumors. *Journal of Hematology & Oncology, 11*, 1–20.
70. Guo, Y., Yang, J., Huang, Q., Hsueh, C., Zheng, J., Wu, C., Chen, H., & Zhou, L. (2019). Circular RNAs and their roles in head and neck cancers. *Molecular Cancer, 18*, 1–18.
71. Liu, Y., Dong, Y., Zhao, L., Su, L., & Luo, J. (2018). Circular RNA-MTO1 suppresses breast cancer cell viability and reverses monastrol resistance through regulating the TRAF4/Eg5 axis. *International Journal of Oncology, 53*(4), 1752–1762.
72. Zhang, X., Xie, K., Zhou, H., Wu, Y., Li, C., Liu, Y., Liu, Z., Xu, Q., Liu, S., Xiao, D., & Tao, Y. (2020). Role of non-coding RNAs and RNA modifiers in cancer therapy resistance. *Molecular Cancer, 19*, 1–26.
73. Yan, H., & Bu, P. (2021). Non-coding RNA in cancer. *Essays in Biochemistry, 65*(4), 625–639.
74. Fu, Z., Wang, L., Li, S., Chen, F., Au-Yeung, K. K. W., & Shi, C. (2021). MicroRNA as an important target for anticancer drug development. *Frontiers in Pharmacology, 12*, 736323.
75. Treeck, O., Haerteis, S., & Ortmann, O. (2023). Non-coding RNAs modulating estrogen signaling and response to endocrine therapy in breast cancer. *Cancers, 15*(6), 1632.
76. Beermann, J., Piccoli, M. T., Viereck, J., & Thum, T. (2016). Non-coding RNAs in development and disease: background, mechanisms, and therapeutic approaches. *Physiological Reviews, 96*(4), 1297–1325.
77. Aurilia, C., Donati, S., Palmini, G., Miglietta, F., Falsetti, I., Iantomasi, T., & Brandi, M. L. (2021). Are non-coding RNAs useful biomarkers in parathyroid tumorigenesis?. *International Journal of Molecular Sciences, 22*(19), 10465.
78. Zhang, L., Zhang, Y., Wang, Y., Zhao, Y., Ding, H., & Li, P. (2020). Circular RNAs: functions and clinical significance in cardiovascular disease. *Frontiers in Cell and Developmental Biology, 8*, 584051.
79. Liu, A., Zhou, Y., Zhao, T., Tang, X., Zhou, B., & Xu, J. (2021). MiRNA-3662 reverses the gemcitabine resistance in pancreatic cancer through regulating the tumor metabolism. *Cancer Chemotherapy and Pharmacology, 88*(2), 343–357.
80. Qian, X., Zhao, J., Yeung, P. Y., Zhang, Q. C., & Kwok, C. K. (2019). Revealing lncRNA structures and interactions by sequencing-based approaches. *Trends in Biochemical Sciences, 44*(1), 33–52.
81. Lu, T. X., & Rothenberg, M. E. (2018). MicroRNA. *Journal of Allergy and Clinical Immunology, 141*(4), 1202–1207.
82. Wu, D., He, X., Wang, W., Hu, X., Wang, K., & Wang, M. (2020). Long noncoding RNA SNHG12 induces proliferation, migration, epithelial–mesenchymal transition, and stemness of esophageal squamous cell carcinoma cells via post-transcriptional regulation of BMI1 and CTNNB1. *Molecular Oncology, 14*(9), 2332–2351.

83. Li, Y., Guo, D., Lu, G., Mohiuddin Chowdhury, A. T. M., Zhang, D., Ren, M., Chen, Y., Wang, R., & He, S. (2020). LncRNA SNAI3-AS1 promotes PEG10-mediated proliferation and metastasis via decoying of miR-27a-3p and miR-34a-5p in hepatocellular carcinoma. *Cell Death & Disease, 11*(8), 685.
84. Li, Z., & Rana, T. M. (2014). Therapeutic targeting of microRNAs: current status and future challenges. *Nature Reviews Drug Discovery, 13*(8), 622–638.
85. Mah, J. K. (2018). An overview of recent therapeutics advances for Duchenne muscular dystrophy. In *Duchenne Muscular Dystrophy: Methods and Protocols* (pp. 3–17).
86. Nair, J. K., Willoughby, J. L., Chan, A., Charisse, K., Alam, M. R., Wang, Q., Hoekstra, M., Kandasamy, P., Kel'in, A.V., Milstein, S., & Taneja, N. (2014). Multivalent N-acetylgalactosamine-conjugated siRNA localizes in hepatocytes and elicits robust RNAi-mediated gene silencing. *Journal of the American Chemical Society, 136*(49), 16958–16961.
87. Moschos, S. A., Jones, S. W., Perry, M. M., Williams, A. E., Erjefalt, J. S., Turner, J. J., Barnes, P. J., Sproat, B. S., Gait, M. J., & Lindsay, M. A. (2007). Lung delivery studies using siRNA conjugated to TAT (48–60) and penetratin reveal peptide induced reduction in gene expression and induction of innate immunity. *Bioconjugate Chemistry, 18*(5), 1450–1459.
88. Krol, J., Loedige, I., & Filipowicz, W. (2010). The widespread regulation of microRNA biogenesis, function and decay. *Nature Reviews Genetics, 11*(9), 597–610.
89. Lintner, N. G., McClure, K. F., Petersen, D., Londregan, A. T., Piotrowski, D. W., Wei, L., Xiao, J., Bolt, M., Loria, P. M., Maguire, B., & Geoghegan, K. F. (2017). Selective stalling of human translation through small-molecule engagement of the ribosome nascent chain. *PLoS Biology, 15*(3), e2001882.
90. Velagapudi, S. P., Costales, M. G., Vummidi, B. R., Nakai, Y., Angelbello, A. J., Tran, T., Haniff, H. S., Matsumoto, Y., Wang, Z. F., Chatterjee, A. K., & Childs-Disney, J. L. (2018). Approved anti-cancer drugs target oncogenic non-coding RNAs. *Cell Chemical Biology, 25*(9), 1086–1094.

CHAPTER 5

The Role of Splicing as a Therapeutic Target of Cancer

ABSTRACT

The process that regulates RNA splicing requires participation from several different cellular processes, including mitogenic signaling, metabolism, autophagy, inflammatory conditions, and immune response, among others. Splicing is one of these processes that can be done. Splices are a subset of RNA that contain genes with the ability to exert control spanning numerous biological processes, the most important of which are, among others, survival, cell division, assault, and apoptosis. RNA trans-splice is involved in several biological pathways for the survival of cancer cells, because of the multiple investigations that have been conducted on the topic. In this chapter, we study the intricate processes of kinase and synapse activity in cancer cells and discuss possible directions for developing therapeutic interventions that can successfully prevent the development of resistance and reduce the rate of cancer spread. In addition, some possible directions are also mentioned for developing therapeutic interventions that can successfully prevent resistance from developing as quickly and slow the progression of cancer.

5.1 INTRODUCTION

Cancer is a very diverse disease, with variations in the course, pace, and mode of progression as well as natural history even within a single cancer type. A portion of the variability is determined by the host's genetic

DNA- and m-RNA-Based Vaccines: An Immunotherapeutic Approach to Cancer.

Sonali Sundram and Rishabha Malviya (Authors)

DOI: 10.1201/9781774919613-5

makeup, the cancerous tissue's aberrant genetic makeup and metabolism, and the treatment-induced variations in how the tumor responds to various treatments [1, 2]. Tumors behave not like individual species but rather like entire ecosystems due to the complex ecological web of interactions between various cells. Once cancer breaches the barriers to selection that tissue homeostasis and stability of multiple cells is present, it can further modify normal regulatory pathways to its advantage, leading to the emergence of this ecological dimension [3–5]. The adaptive difficulty of cancer growth makes it difficult to develop therapeutic interventions that may successfully halt the development of treatment resistance and stop the spread of cancer. Tumor microenvironment (TME) adaptive dynamics of cellular interactions are impacted by multiple interrelated cellular processes, including mitogenic signaling, metabolism, autophagy, irritation, and immune response. These processes take place within the constantly growing cellular heterogeneity and genetic diversity of the tumor [6–8].

Phosphorylation is a mechanism that can regulate the biochemical activity of splicing factors as well as their subcellular localization. Splicing regulatory protein expression is altered in many types of cancer and may be targeted by anticancer treatments [9]. To create mature mRNAs for protein translation, the splicing of RNA is a sophisticated and tightly controlled process that involves cutting out introns and ligating exons. Small nuclear RNAs (RNAs) and ribonucleoproteins (RNPs) make up the spliceosome, a massive complex that mediates splicing [10]. CDC-like kinases, also known as CLKs; dual specificity tyrosine-regulated kinases, also known as DYRKs; and serine-rich protein kinases, also known as SRPKs are well-known kinases that control alternative splicing and splicing factor localization. A megadalton complex of RNA and proteins, comprising over 200 proteins and 5 small nuclear ribonucleoprotein particles, is responsible for splicing. Numerous spliceosome components have had their structures clarified in several recent studies at previously unheard-of near-angstrom resolution [11–13]. The serine residues that can be discovered in serine-arginine and arginine-serine dipeptide patterns are phosphorylated by SRPKs, a grouping within the serine-threonine kinase family that has been conserved throughout evolution. Homeostatic pathways tightly regulate the expression as well as nuclear/cytoplasmic localization of SRPKs, which are distributed throughout the cell [14]. Moreover, a process called alternative splicing (AS) enables the production of multiple mRNAs from a single gene and protein isoforms by using a variety of different techniques. Some of these techniques include skipping exons, retaining introns, having incompatible exons, and having differential 5′ or 3′ splice sites that have different characteristics and diversify the proteome [15]. Pre-mRNA contains trans-acting splicing factors and cis-acting regulatory elements, which regulate AS. Thus, misregulation specific to cancer can result from either over- or underexpression of trans-acting splicing factors, variations in the intronic/exonic cis-acting regulation regions of the spliced gene, which frequently result in novel splice sites and hence impact splicing, or mutations that may affect their function, copy number variation, potentially functionally significant mutations, or changes to the spliced gene's intronic/exonic cis-acting regulatory patterns [16–19].

5.2 DYSREGULATION OF SPLICING IN CANCER

To date, a very small handful of mutations in splicing regulations have been found that are persistently identified in malignant solid tumors, indicating that hematologic malignancies and solid tumors differ fundamentally in terms of splicing targets and/or regulation [20, 21]. By means of the post-transcriptional regulation of multiple alterations constituents, AS has been linked to cancer and has been shown to affect cellular processes that are regarded as "hallmarks" of the disease. These include angiogenesis, invasion, metabolism, cell division, and cell death. Still, more research is needed to fully understand the biological consequences of these pervasive changes to AS [22].

5.2.1 SERINE/ARGININE-RICH SPLICING FACTOR-1 (SRSF1)

The intrinsic and AS processes are both influenced by the splicing factor SRSF1, which is the prototypical SR protein. However, it has been connected to a variety of additional functions, including nuclear export, translation, protein simulations, nonsense-mediated mRNA decay (NMD), and control of mRNA transcription. The various roles that SRSF1 plays are determined by its structure, which also affects its ability to bind RNA, shuttle between the nuclear and cytoplasm, and interact with a variety of other proteins. At the N-terminus of SRSF1, the canonical RNA recognition motifs (RRM) is immediately followed by a pseudo-RRM, and the modular domains of the protein are composed of a pair of RRMs in which a C-terminal RS domain that is shorter than the majority of other serine- and arginine-rich (SR) proteins. The pseudo-RRM, or RRM2, is primarily responsible for determining substrate specificity *in vivo*, even though both RRMs are essential for proper binding of RNA and splicing to take place [23–25]. SRSF1 can perform its role as an RNA splicing regulator because it can recognize components of the ESE sequence on its pre-mRNA sites should degenerate. This allows it to promote the definition of exons and the concentration-dependent use of proximal replacement 50 splice sites as well as 30 splice sites [26]. SRSF1 facilitates splice site selection and affects the splicing process during its earliest stages, when the spliceosome is still being assembled upon binding a cognate ESE, partly by recruiting core spliceosomal proteins. At first, it was thought that the RS domain acted as the only mediator of SRSF1's interactions with other proteins. SRSF1 deletion mutants that lack the complete RS domain, however, continue to be able to splice [27, 28]. Interestingly, it appears that p53 tumor suppressor pathway inactivation is necessary for SRSF1-mediated oncogenesis. This finding may be useful in the development of therapies targeting tumors that are driven or dependent on SRSF1. One of the main reactions observed in mouse and human basic fibroblast when SRSF1 is overexpressed is apoptosis is p53 induction, which causes the cells to undergo early cellular senescence [29].

5.2.2 THE SERINE/ARGININE-RICH SPLICING FACTOR-3 (SRSF3)

A crucial and nonoverlapping function of every SR protein during embryonic growth is suggested by the early lethal phenotype that arises from SRSF3 knockout (KO) in mice, indicating that *SRSF3* is an absolutely necessary gene. *SRSF3* is overexpressed in human tumors that include cancers of the ovary, cervical, lung, intestines, breasts, gastrointestinal tract, skin, urinary bladder, thyroid gland, liver, and kidneys [30]. Ironically, it has also been noted that human hepatocellular carcinoma exhibits a lower expression of *SRSF3*. Furthermore, because the gene is responsible for controlling both the expression and the levels of the protein are independent of RNA, the expression of SRSF3 mRNA is not informative A significant fraction of tumors in the COSMIC database exhibits a loss of variety at the SRSF3 locus, and a fraction of bladder, cervix, respiratory, melanoma, colorectal cancer, and prostate cancers are reported to have mutated and eliminated *SRSF3*. Additionally, The Cancer Genome Atlas database (TCGA) reports that SRSF3 is deleted in a fraction of lung cancers. It would anticipate seeing a signature of SRSF3-dependent expression in human head and neck cancer if SRSF3 is lost in the disease [31]. SRSF3 regulates gene expression through binding to different mRNA groups related to neural differentiation. In addition, SRSF3 accumulates in human ovarian cancer, and ovarian cancer cells that have it knocked down undergo apoptosis. These results imply that SRSF3 is involved in biological networks that are essential for controlling the destiny of cells. It has been demonstrated that SRSF3 controls the splicing of HIPK2, which is a homeodomain-interacting protein, which, in turn, regulates the transition from the 8 Δ isoform, which causes cell death, and the full-length isoform [32]. SRSF3 is critical for regulating mouse hepatocyte differentiation and metabolism, as well as the splicing of particular genes involved in the breakdown of fats or carbohydrates [33].

5.2.3 SERINE/ARGININE-RICH SPLICING FACTOR-6 (SRSF6)

The prototypical SR protein, SRSF6, has two RRMs and an RS domain. It can also control AS and shuttle between the cytoplasm and the nucleus. Both the overexpression of the Drosophila homolog of SRSF6, B52, and the loss of function of this gene prevents normal development in the organism. B52 is required for normal development. Another proposed role of SRSF6 is to prevent the creation of a DNA-RNA hybrid known as R loops, which have the potential to harm the genome and cause mutations to accumulate and damage DNA [34–44]. While SRSF6 KD does not inhibit proliferation, it does enhance it. These results suggest that it is not necessary for SRSF6 to be produced normally or lifespan of such cells, however, overlying gene expression could lead to an increase in cell division due to a gain of function. When SRSF6 is overexpressed in mouse respiratory epithelial cells, cell proliferation, and an inhibition of cell death. Both the formation of tumors and the upkeep of colon and lung cancer cells depend on SRSF6. SRSF6 controls INSR splicing in the lung and colon, which results in the synthesis of the insulin receptor's more mitogenic isoform [45]. In addition, LGR6+ stem cell depletion and increased keratinocyte proliferation and response to injury are caused by SRSF6 overexpression. Moreover, the tenascin-C isoforms influence how SRSF6 functions in an *in vitro* wound healing assay. Consequently, aberrant expression of SR protein may disrupt tissue homeostasis [46].

5.2.4 TRA2B-TRANSFORM 2B HOMOLOG

Tra2 proteins are found in all classes of animals. Invertebrates only have one copy of the Tra2 protein, which is known as the fruit fly Tra2 homologe because it has been studied the most thoroughly. Vertebrates, on the other hand, have two distinct protein copies known as Tra2 and Tra2. Therefore, likely, a gene duplication event occurred very early on in the development of vertebrates. giving vertebrates two copies while invertebrates only kept one copy [47, 48]. Proteins with RS domains, or domains included in this category of proteins are the Tra2 family, which is abundant in serine and arginine residues. The N- and C-terminal RS domains, also known as the RS1 and RS2 domains, respectively, are part of the unique modular structure that characterizes Tra2 proteins among these others. Serine within the Tra2 protein's RS domains undergoes phosphorylation and dephosphorylation cycles that alter them. As with other SR proteins, the transport of Tra2 proteins into the nucleus from the cytoplasm is dependent on the kinase SRPK1 phosphorylating proteins in the cytoplasm [49]. Moreover, Tra2 proteins often bind to ESEs and function as splicing activators. Tra2 protein binding to ESE sequences near regulated splice sites stabilizes spliceosome assembly, which improves the utilization of these regulated splice sites [50]. Tra2β expression levels ranging from medium to high are correlated with an unfavorable outcome in cervical cancer, while Tra2β upregulation is linked to invasive breast cancer. While Tra2β expression is linked to cancer cell survival, it is still not entirely clear how this factor plays into the progression of the disease. The promotion of multiple splicing switches, such as CD44, which are linked to the growth of tumors and their metastasis, is made possible by the overexpression of Tra2β [51]. Additionally, Tra2β controls the α splicing-related alteration of the estrogen receptor, reducing the manifestation of the ERa Δ7 isoform expression and improving the prognosis for endometrial cancer [52].

5.3 THERAPEUTIC MODULATION OF SPLICING

Recent advancements in nucleic acid-based therapies and a better understanding of the role of splicing in the pathophysiology of the disease have made splicing a promising target for therapy. As a result, techniques to promote or prevent splicing have been applied in medical settings. Synthetic molecules ranging from 15 to 30 nucleotides in length, known as splice-switch oligonucleotides (SSOs), using Watson–Crick base pairing, attach themselves to splicing regulatory sequences or splice sites. Base pairing of SSOs to RNA changes pre-mRNA splicing by essentially blocking splicing factors from accessing splicing regulatory sites. As a result, the splicing process is altered. SSOs do not, however, cleave mRNA in contrast to oligonucleotides that catalyze the cleavage of RNA through occupancy (like siRNAs) due to the fact that they do not activate Argonaute RISC catalytic component 2 (AGO2) and RNase H. Due to their ability to change splicing without changing mRNA levels and their resistance to nuclease activity, SSOs can maintain their stability *in vivo* through chemical modifications. SSO-assisted splicing modulation depends on splicing being inhibited or activated via direct targeting to the splice location, as well as cis-regulatory components and RNA secondary structures related to splicing [53–56]. This method can also be used to change a gene's splicing such that a therapeutically useful protein isoform is produced [57]. Targeting aberrant RNA splicing is a reasonable strategy that can directly address disease-associated splicing abnormalities despite having any effect on the genome. Alternate strategies involve concentrating on splicing events to interfere with the replication of disease-related proteins or concentrating on exon junctions altered mRNA to disrupt protein-coding to reframe and recover protein expression. Both of these strategies are examples of alternative approaches [58].

SSOs are also involved in another fascinating modulation mechanism known as induced splicing-dependent nonsense-mediated mRNA degradation (FSD-NMD), resulting in an mRNA that experiences NMD and exon skipping. In this instance, exon skipping results in a frameshift that causes NMD to degrade the offending mRNA. Splicing-enhancing proteins can be recruited or splicing inhibitory elements can be blocked by SSOs, which can also be used to activate splicing [59–62]. Although, several treatment approaches that target aberrant splicing factors activity have been created recently, and several of these methods are presently being tested in clinical settings to treat cancer. Small molecules may interact with proteins involved with any phase of spliceosome assembly, target particular aspects of splicing, inhibit the protein kinases of accessory splicing factors, or directly target the accessory splicing factors themselves to either enhance or inhibit splicing. A naturally occurring substance with antitumor activity is called placenolide B. It inhibits the

SF3b subunit SAP130 by directly binding to it [63]. An additional one is oligonucleotides, which are brief single-stranded nucleic acid patterns that use base pairing to attach to the target mRNA. These techniques approach the splicing factor mRNA instead of the splicing factor protein, in contrast to small molecules. The steric blocking action of RNA oligonucleotides, or SSOs, prevents the exonic/intronic particular regulatory sites of the pre-mRNA molecule from being accessed by the spliceosome or particular splicing factors. Because of this, SSOs alter antisense, which modifies the ratio of different isoforms that come from the identical pre-mRNA [64]. Numerous clinical trials are currently assessing oligonucleotides as a potential cancer treatment. For instance, numerous investigations have revealed that SSOs can reroute AS linked to cancer, resulting in tumor shrinkage in xenograft mouse models and apoptosis and cell cycle arrest in lines of cancer cells [65–67].

Splicing factors and other RNA binding proteins bind to a specific motif sequence present in the pre-mRNA molecules of the target gene. It then either attracts spliceosomes to neighboring splice sites or obstructs spliceosome binding. Phosphothioate backbones were also added to oligonucleotides. The RNA binding motif of a particular splicing factor is repeated three to four times in these oligonucleotides. An increase in the number of RNA binding motif repeats was associated with an increased binding affinity [68, 69]. In a study, PTBP1 was taken as a specific splicing factor where one of the main conclusions was that PTBP1 depletion stopped the SASP's effects on tumor growth. In two tumor models, PTBP1 knockdown stopped the growth of tumors brought on by senescent cells. One possible drawback of using SASP targeting as a tumor therapy is the fact that it causes the immune system to clear fewer preneoplastic cells. However, despite decreased immune surveillance, a higher probability of carcinogenesis was not seen upon PTBP1 depletion [70]. Moreover, the presence of cancer-specific neoantigens, which are mainly brought about by acquired variants in disrupted repair genes and an increased tumor mutation load, is a significant factor influencing the likelihood of an effective immune checkpoint therapy response. The subset of neoantigens specific to cancer may also include peptides produced by abnormal RNA splicing and processing as well as non-coding mutations, in addition to neoantigens resulting from somatic variants in coded genes [71, 72]. Pharmacologic splicing modulation has been proposed as a potential source of abnormal mRNAs that code for unique protein molecules, some of which could be translated by MHC I and released as neoepitopes that trigger immunity against tumors. To test it, researchers first treated cancer cells with sub-inhibitory doses of indisulam, the RBM39-degrader. There was minimal impact on growth, but graded RBM39 degradation was the result. *Ex vivo* therapy and pharmaceutical washout produced a long-lasting reduction of RBM39 protein after drug removal in all cell lines, with negligible impact on subsequent growth or apoptosis. The administration of drugs did not significantly alter the expression of death receptors, cytokines, PD-L1, or MHC I/II [73]. With the establishment of the siRNA pathway in 1998 [74], a related technology that can be used to silence gene expression also emerged. The subset of neoantigens specific to cancer may also include peptides produced by abnormal splicing of RNA and processing as well as non-coding mutations. The structures, biological functions, corresponding effector proteins, and origins of these RNA types vary. In a physiological sense, endogenous post-transcriptional gene regulators like miRNAs shield cell genomes from foreign nucleic acids like viruses, transposons, transgenes, and retrotransposons [75]. For therapeutic purposes, aberrant splicing isoforms can be targeted with these siRNA techniques. It has been noted that in the context of cancer, certain splice variants are more common during tumorigenesis and that many malignant cells have aberrant splicing regulatory machinery [76]. A gene-reprogramming technique based on the trans-splicing mechanism called spliceosome-mediated RNA trans-splicing may have uses in medicine. To correct aberrant mRNAs, the trans-splicing method replaces the entire coding sequence downstream as well as upstream of an intended SS. Target mRNA, spliceosome machinery, and pre-trans-splicing molecule (PTM), also known as RNA trans-splicing molecule (RTM), are all three elements that are involved. Cells already contain the first two components; the third needs to be obtained externally [77, 78].

5.4 SPLICING REGULATION AS A CANCER THERAPEUTIC TARGET

RNA splicing, a crucial stage in the synthesis of precursor mRNA, or pre-mRNA, involves the removal of introns and exons. A great diversity of mature mRNA can be generated from just a few genes by alternating the addition and removal of introns as well as exons in pre-mRNA. Through aberrant splicing regulation, cancer cells develop cancer-specific mechanisms that enable them to develop treatment resistance and advance malignancy [79]. Splicing regulatory kinases, serine-arginine Protein

Kinases (SRPKs), and CDC-like kinases (CLKs) (Figure 5.1) are both in charge of phosphorylating SR proteins *in vivo*. Integrating SRPKs and CLKs are the regulators in charge of SR protein phosphorylation *in vivo*. SRPK2 is mostly found in the brain, conversely, the pancreas and testicles are where SRPK1 is primarily expressed. It has been discovered that both are produced in small amounts in the respiratory, liver, and kidney and in moderate amounts in other body tissues like the heart and skeletal muscle. SRPK3 expression appears to be limited to muscle cells and has not yet been connected to cancer. Many cancer types have been demonstrated to overexpress SRPK1 and SRPK2, including gliomas, ovarian, breast, colon, pancreatic, leukemia, non-small cell pulmonary cancer, squamous cells in lung carcinoma, and hepatocellular carcinoma [80–85]. Furthermore, after gemcitabine and cisplatin treatment, small interfering RNA (RNAi) targeting SRPK1 increased apoptotic potential and facilitated cell killing in cell lines from both of these tumors. These results were accompanied by a decrease in the phosphorylation of AKT, MAPK1, and MAPK3. The RNA binding protein RBM4 and excess SRPK1 have been linked to breast cancer cells' susceptibility to apoptosis [86].

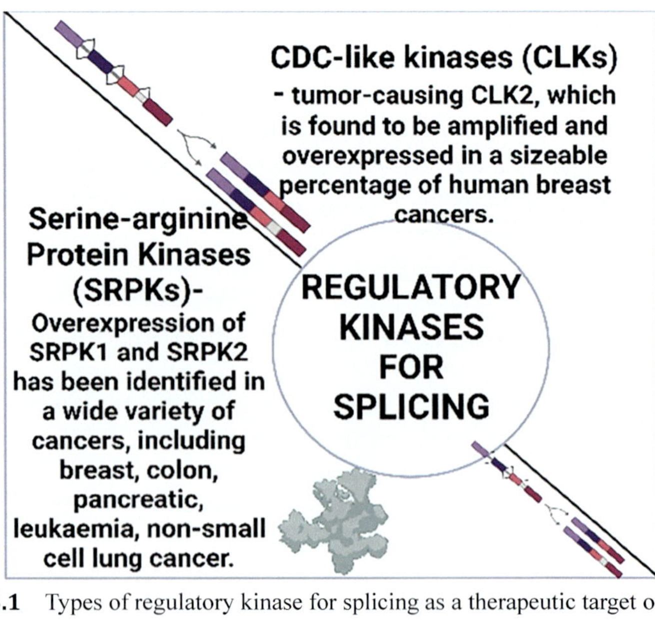

FIGURE 5.1 Types of regulatory kinase for splicing as a therapeutic target of cancer.

However, SR proteins are phosphorylated by CLKs, a nuclear kinase group. This family, which includes the four members CLK1–CLK4, is also connected to the regulation of splicing as opposed to CLK1, CLK2, CLK3, and CLK4 [87]. To facilitate attachment to SR proteins, CLKs' N-terminal RS domain, and the dual specificity C-terminal kinase region of CLKs, which is strikingly similar to serine-threonine kinases are their distinguishing features. In nuclear speckles, SR proteins and CLKs colocalize [88]. Despite having similar substrates, CLKs and SRPKs have distinct specificities and work in tandem to control splicing appropriately [89]. Cancer has also been linked to CLKs. For instance, a different splicing factor 45 (SPF45) is phosphorylated at 8 serine residues by CLK1. In healthy tissues, SPF45 expression is low, but it is elevated in cancer of the breast, ovaries, and prostate. In a manner that depends on CLK1 phosphorylation, the overexpression of SPF45 causes the splicing and phosphorylation of cortactin, a substance that controls actin polymerization, the expression of fibronectin, and the invasion and migration of ovarian cancer cells. Another illustration would be the malignant CLK2, which is overexpressed and magnified in a considerable proportion of human breast cancers [90–92].

Splicing regulation is influenced by a wide range of factors, such as proteins, non-coding RNAs, and DNA sequences at various stages. Spliceosomes are large protein-RNA complexes that quickly alter to catalyze the splicing process. There are two types of spliceosomes: major and minor subunits. Approximately 170 proteins as well as five small nuclear ribonucleoproteins (snRNPs) make up the main spliceosome complex. Its ability to identify most splice sites (ss) is facilitated by this complex, which also contributes to the removal of almost a whole amount of introns [79]. Spliceosomes are formed by spliceosome-forming proteins, non-coding RNAs, snRNAs, and other components. Through their interaction with spliceosomes and binding to pre-mRNA, snRNPs have an impact on splicing efficiency and ss selection. The quantity and degree of snRNP biogenesis, as well as the quantity and mutations of snRNAs, control splicing. For the biogenesis of snRNP, motor neuron (SMN) survival and the survival of a subset of GEMIN proteins are required. These proteins form SMN complexes with snRNAs, which are necessary for the Sm protein's interaction with snRNA in the process of snRNP assembly [93, 94]. Splicing patterns are regulated by post-transcriptional modifications of snRNAs. The two primary post-transcriptional changes of snRNA in eukaryotic cells are 2′-O-methylation and pseudouridine. Methadonosine

N6 (m6A) RNA methylation is an alteration of mRNA (Ψ). Both proteins and small RNAs are responsible for these post-transcriptional changes. In response to intracellular stress, these modifications vary in extent and location. The types and abundances of sno/scaRNA vary depending on the type of cancer. Furthermore, sno/scaRNAs (nucleolus as well as nucleoplasmic cajal bodies) have been shown to exhibit either tumor-suppressive or carcinogenic properties, contingent on the type of cancer. It has also been linked to cellular processes like angiogenesis, development, invasion, spread, cell death, and cancer-related signaling pathways of tumors. Variations in sno/scaRNA expression have been linked to patient outcomes [95–98].

According to recent research, hepatocellular carcinoma and chronic lymphocytic leukemia (CLL) are two tumor types that commonly show adenine>cytosine somatic mutations in the third base of U1 snRNA. Additionally, frequent adenine>guanine alterations at this base are present in about 50% of Sonic Hedgehog medulloblastomas. Uracil-1(U1) snRNA's primary job is to identify the 5′ ss and initiate base pairing. By identifying the ectopic 5′ ss, the altered U1 snRNA stimulates tumorigenesis by creating new splicing sites that alter the splicing sequences of many genes, including those that are known to be cancer-driver genes [99, 100]. In a study of yeast, co-transcriptional activation of the U2 snRNP is facilitated by Gcn5, a histone acetyltransferase present in the SAGA complex. Through interactions with pre-mRNA, the SWI/SNF chromatin remodeling complex in higher eukaryotes controls AS of endogenous genes. Additionally, minigene AS is impacted by therapy with trichostatin A (TSA), a histone deacetylase inhibitor. Furthermore, direct relationships involving splicing factors and modified histones have been observed; however, the importance of these relationships for the regulation of splicing remains unclear. Recent findings from genome-wide nucleosome mapping indicate that nucleosome localization may play a role in exon recognition and correlate with exon positioning. The discovery that AS was impacted by siRNA-induced heterochromatin formation provided evidence for the involvement of nucleosome packing [101–106].

5.5 CONCLUSION

When it comes to behavior and progression patterns, cancer is a very heterogeneous disease. Cancer cell genetic abnormalities, treatment responses, and the genetic makeup of the host all affect these variations. With complex interactions between various cell types, cancer cells function like ecosystems. An ecological dimension can be created by cancer once it has upset tissue equilibrium and stable multicellularity. It can then alter normal pathways to its benefit. The tightly controlled process of RNA splicing, which creates mature mRNA for protein translation by joining exons and removing introns, is an important stage in the development of cancer. A structure known as the spliceosome controls RNA splicing. Different mRNA and protein isoforms that are produced by aberrant splicing have been associated with cancer. Tra2β, SRSF1, SRSF3, SRSF6, and other splicing factors are important in cancer. Cancer-specific splicing patterns linked to drug resistance and malignancy can result from the dysregulation of these factors. Small molecules that obstruct splicing factors, SSOs that target particular splicing sites, and siRNA-based methods to silence aberrant splicing factors are therapeutic approaches to modulate splicing. Correcting splicing abnormalities may change the course of the disease, which is the goal of these approaches. Cancer progression may also be impacted by controlling splicing factors like CLKs and SRPKs. By phosphorylating splicing factors, these kinases affect AS that occurs. Different cancer types have been associated with aberrant kinase activity; therefore, targeting these kinases may have therapeutic benefits. Non-coding RNAs, post-transcriptional changes, and histone interactions also have an impact on the regulation of splicing. Tumorigenesis can be aided by U1 snRNA mutations that cause different splicing patterns. Promising avenues for cancer therapy exist when one understands and targets the complex processes of RNA splicing and splicing factors. This has the potential to improve treatment outcomes, correct splicing abnormalities, and prevent cancer from progressing.

KEYWORDS

- **cancer**
- **dysregulation**
- **modulation**
- **regulatory kinase**
- **splicing**
- **treatment**

REFERENCES

1. Lawrence, M. S., Stojanov, P., Polak, P., Kryukov, G. V., Cibulskis, K., Sivachenko, A., Carter, S. L., Stewart, C., Mermel, C. H., Roberts, S. A, & Kiezun, A. (2013). Mutational heterogeneity in cancer and the search for new cancer-associated genes. *Nature, 499*(7457), 214–218.
2. Yersal, O., & Barutca, S. (2014). Biological subtypes of breast cancer: Prognostic and therapeutic implications. *World Journal of Clinical Oncology, 5*(3), 412.
3. Camacho, D. F., & Pienta, K. J. (2012). Disrupting the networks of cancer. *Clinical Cancer Research, 18*(10), 2801–2808.
4. Basanta, D., & Anderson, A. R. (2013). Exploiting ecological principles to better understand cancer progression and treatment. *Interface Focus, 3*(4), 20130020.
5. Basanta, D., & Anderson, A. R. (2013). Exploiting ecological principles to better understand cancer progression and treatment. *Interface Focus, 3*(4), 20130020.
6. Casanovas, O. (2012). Limitations of therapies exposed. *Nature, 484*(7392), 44–46.
7. Zugazagoitia, J., Guedes, C., Ponce, S., Ferrer, I., Molina-Pinelo, S., & Paz-Ares, L. (2016). Current challenges in cancer treatment. *Clinical Therapeutics, 38*(7), 1551–1566.
8. Ventola, C. L. (2017). Cancer immunotherapy, part 3: challenges and future trends. *Pharmacy and Therapeutics, 42*(8), 514.
9. Nguyen, T. H. D., Galej, W. P., Bai, X. C., Savva, C. G., Newman, A. J., Scheres, S. H., & Nagai, K. (2015). The architecture of the spliceosomal U4/U6. U5 tri-snRNP. *Nature, 523*(7558), 47–52.
10. Wilkinson, M. E., Charenton, C., & Nagai, K. (2020). RNA splicing by the spliceosome. *Annual Review of Biochemistry, 89*(1), 359–388.
11. Yan, C., Hang, J., Wan, R., Huang, M., Wong, C. C., & Shi, Y. (2015). Structure of a yeast spliceosome at 3.6-angstrom resolution. *Science, 349*(6253), 1182–1191.
12. Nguyen, T. H. D., Galej, W. P., Bai, X. C., Oubridge, C., Newman, A. J., Scheres, S. H., & Nagai, K. (2016). Cryo-EM structure of the yeast U4/U6. U5 tri-snRNP at 3.7 Å resolution. *Nature, 530*(7590), 298–302.
13. Wan, R., Yan, C., Bai, R., Wang, L., Huang, M., Wong, C. C., & Shi, Y. (2016). The 3.8 Å structure of the U4/U6. U5 tri-snRNP: Insights into spliceosome assembly and catalysis. *Science, 351*(6272), 466–475.
14. Giannakouros, T., Nikolakaki, E., Mylonis, I., & Georgatsou, E. (2011). Serine-arginine protein kinases: a small protein kinase family with a large cellular presence. *The FEBS Journal, 278*(4), 570–586.
15. Zhang, Y., Qian, J., Gu, C., & Yang, Y. (2021). Alternative splicing and cancer: a systematic review. *Signal Transduction and Targeted Therapy, 6*(1), 78.
16. Roca, X., Krainer, A. R., & Eperon, I. C. (2013). Pick one, but be quick: 5′ splice sites and the problems of too many choices. *Genes & Development, 27*(2), 129–144.
17. Supek, F., Miñana, B., Valcárcel, J., Gabaldón, T., & Lehner, B. (2014). Synonymous mutations frequently act as driver mutations in human cancers. *Cell, 156*(6), 1324–1335.
18. Frampton, G. M., Ali, S. M., Rosenzweig, M., Chmielecki, J., Lu, X., Bauer, T. M., Akimov, M., Bufill, J. A., Lee, C., Jentz, D, & Hoover, R. (2015). Activation of MET

via diverse exon 14 splicing alterations occurs in multiple tumor types and confers clinical sensitivity to MET inhibitors. *Cancer Discovery, 5*(8), 850–859.

19. Jung, H., Lee, D., Lee, J., Park, D., Kim, Y. J., Park, W. Y., Hong, D., Park, P. J, & Lee, E. (2015). Intron retention is a widespread mechanism of tumor-suppressor inactivation. *Nature Genetics, 47*(11), 1242–1248.
20. Ellis, M. J., Ding, L., Shen, D., Luo, J., Suman, V. J., Wallis, J. W., Van Tine, B. A., Hoog, J., Goiffon, R. J., Goldstein, T. C, & Ng, S. (2012). Whole-genome analysis informs breast cancer response to aromatase inhibition. *Nature, 486*(7403), 353–360.
21. Maguire, S. L., Leonidou, A., Wai, P., Marchiò, C., Ng, C. K., Sapino, A., Salomon, A. V., Reis-Filho, J. S., Weigelt, B, & Natrajan, R. C. (2015). SF3B1 mutations constitute a novel therapeutic target in breast cancer. *The Journal of Pathology, 235*(4), 571–580.
22. David, C. J., & Manley, J. L. (2010). Alternative pre-mRNA splicing regulation in cancer: pathways and programs unhinged. *Genes & Development, 24*(21), 2343–2364.
23. Caceres, J. F., & Krainer, A. R. (1993). Functional analysis of pre-mRNA splicing factor SF2/ASF structural domains. *The EMBO Journal, 12*(12), 4715–4726.
24. Zuo, P., & Manley, J. L. (1993). Functional domains of the human splicing factor ASF/SF2. *The EMBO Journal, 12*(12), 4727–4737.
25. Cáceres, J. F., Misteli, T., Screaton, G. R., Spector, D. L., & Krainer, A. R. (1997). Role of the modular domains of SR proteins in subnuclear localization and alternative splicing specificity. *The Journal of Cell Biology, 138*(2), 225–238.
26. Pandit, S., Zhou, Y., Shiue, L., Coutinho-Mansfield, G., Li, H., Qiu, J., Huang, J., Yeo, G. W., Ares, M, & Fu, X. D. (2013). Genome-wide analysis reveals SR protein cooperation and competition in regulated splicing. *Molecular Cell, 50*(2), 223–235.
27. Zhu, J., & Krainer, A. R. (2000). Pre-mRNA splicing in the absence of an SR protein RS domain. *Genes & Development, 14*(24), 3166–3178.
28. Shaw, S. D., Chakrabarti, S., Ghosh, G., & Krainer, A. R. (2007). Deletion of the N-terminus of SF2/ASF permits RS-domain-independent pre-mRNA splicing. *PloS One, 2*(9), e854.
29. Fregoso, O. I., Das, S., Akerman, M., & Krainer, A. R. (2013). Splicing-factor oncoprotein SRSF1 stabilizes p53 via RPL5 and induces cellular senescence. *Molecular Cell, 50*(1), 56–66.
30. Iborra, S., Hirschfeld, M., Jaeger, M., Zur Hausen, A., Braicu, I., Sehouli, J., Gitsch, G, & Stickeler, E. (2013). Alterations in expression pattern of splicing factors in epithelial ovarian cancer and its clinical impact. *International Journal of Gynecologic Cancer, 23*(6).
31. Sen, S., Langiewicz, M., Jumaa, H., & Webster, N. J. (2015). Deletion of serine/arginine-rich splicing factor 3 in hepatocytes predisposes to hepatocellular carcinoma in mice. *Hepatology, 61*(1), 171–183.
32. Kurokawa, K., Akaike, Y., Masuda, K., Kuwano, Y., Nishida, K., Yamagishi, N., Kajita, K., Tanahashi, T, & Rokutan, K. (2014). Downregulation of serine/arginine-rich splicing factor 3 induces G1 cell cycle arrest and apoptosis in colon cancer cells. *Oncogene, 33*(11), 1407–1417.
33. Sen, S., Jumaa, H., & Webster, N. J. (2013). Splicing factor SRSF3 is crucial for hepatocyte differentiation and metabolic function. *Nature Communications, 4*(1), 1336.
34. Screaton, G. R., Caceres, J. F., Mayeda, A., Bell, M. V., Plebanski, M., Jackson, D. G., Bell, J. I., & Krainer, A. R. (1995). Identification and characterization of

three members of the human SR family of pre-mRNA splicing factors. *The EMBO Journal, 14*(17), 4336–4349.
35. Nagel, R. J., Lancaster, A. M., & Zahler, A. M. (1998). Specific binding of an exonic splicing enhancer by the pre-mRNA splicing factor SRp55. *RNA, 4*(1), 11.
36. Cáceres, J. F., Screaton, G. R., & Krainer, A. R. (1998). A specific subset of SR proteins shuttles continuously between the nucleus and the cytoplasm. *Genes & Development, 12*(1), 55–66.
37. Tran, Q., & Roesser, J. R. (2003). SRp55 is a regulator of calcitonin/CGRP alternative RNA splicing. *Biochemistry, 42*(4), 951–957.
38. Fic, W., Juge, F., Soret, J., & Tazi, J. (2007). Eye development under the control of SRp55/B52-mediated alternative splicing of eyeless. *PloS One, 2*(2), e253.
39. Juge, F., Fernando, C., Fic, W., & Tazi, J. (2010). The SR protein B52/SRp55 is required for DNA topoisomerase I recruitment to chromatin, mRNA release and transcription shutdown. *PLoS Genetics, 6*(9), e1001124.
40. Ring, H. Z., & Lis, J. T. (1994). The SR protein B52/SRp55 is essential for Drosophila development. *Molecular and Cellular Biology, 14*(11), 7499–7506.
41. Gabut, M., Dejardin, J., Tazi, J., & Soret, J. (2007). The SR family proteins B52 and dASF/SF2 modulate development of the Drosophila visual system by regulating specific RNA targets. *Molecular and Cellular Biology, 27*, 3087–3097.
42. Rasheva, V. I., Knight, D., Bozko, P., Marsh, K., & Frolov, M. V. (2006). Specific role of the SR protein splicing factor B52 in cell cycle control in Drosophila. *Molecular and Cellular Biology, 26*(9), 3468–3477.
43. Aguilera, A., & García-Muse, T. (2012). R loops: from transcription byproducts to threats to genome stability. *Molecular Cell, 46*(2), 115–124.
44. Jiang, C. C., Lai, F., Tay, K. H., Croft, A., Rizos, H., Becker, T. M., Yang, F., Liu, H., Thorne, R. F., Hersey, P, & Zhang, X. D. (2010). Apoptosis of human melanoma cells induced by inhibition of B-RAFV600E involves preferential splicing of bimS. *Cell Death & Disease, 1*(9), e69.
45. Cohen-Eliav, M., Golan-Gerstl, R., Siegfried, Z., Andersen, C. L., Thorsen, K., Ørntoft, T. F., Mu, D, & Karni, R. (2013). The splicing factor SRSF6 is amplified and is an oncoprotein in lung and colon cancers. *The Journal of Pathology, 229*(4), 630–639.
46. Jensen, M. A., Wilkinson, J. E., & Krainer, A. R. (2014). Splicing factor SRSF6 promotes hyperplasia of sensitized skin. *Nature Structural & Molecular Biology, 21*(2), 189–197.
47. Baker, B. S. (1989). Sex in flies: the splice of life. *Nature, 340*(6234), 521–524.
48. Belote, J. M., & Baker, B. S. (1983). The dual functions of a sex determination gene in Drosophila melanogaster. *Developmental Biology, 95*(2), 512–517.
49. Aubol, B. E., Jamros, M. A., McGlone, M. L., & Adams, J. A. (2013). Splicing kinase SRPK1 conforms to the landscape of its SR protein substrate. *Biochemistry, 52*(43), 7595–7605.
50. Lam, B. J., Bakshi, A., Ekinci, F. Y., Webb, J., Graveley, B. R., & Hertel, K. J. (2003). Enhancer-dependent 5′-splice site control of fruitless pre-mRNA splicing. *Journal of Biological Chemistry, 278*(25), 22740–22747.
51. Iborra, S., Hirschfeld, M., Jaeger, M., Zur Hausen, A., Braicu, I., Sehouli, J., Gitsch, G, & Stickeler, E. (2013). Alterations in expression pattern of splicing factors in

epithelial ovarian cancer and its clinical impact. *International Journal of Gynecologic Cancer, 23*(6).

52. Iborra, S., Hirschfeld, M., Jaeger, M., Zur Hausen, A., Braicu, I., Sehouli, J., Gitsch, G, & Stickeler, E. (2013). Alterations in expression pattern of splicing factors in epithelial ovarian cancer and its clinical impact. *International Journal of Gynecologic Cancer, 23*(6).
53. Suñé-Pou, M., Limeres, M. J., Moreno-Castro, C., Hernández-Munain, C., Suñé-Negre, J. M., Cuestas, M. L., & Suñé, C. (2020). Innovative therapeutic and delivery approaches using nanotechnology to correct splicing defects underlying disease. *Frontiers in Genetics, 11*, 731.
54. Havens, M. A., & Hastings, M. L. (2016). Splice-switching antisense oligonucleotides as therapeutic drugs. *Nucleic Acids Research, 44*(14), 6549–6563.
55. Rigo, F., Seth, P. P., & Bennett, C. F. (2014). Antisense oligonucleotide-based therapies for diseases caused by pre-mRNA processing defects. In *Systems biology of RNA binding proteins* (pp. 303–352).
56. Bauman, J., Jearawiriyapaisarn, N., & Kole, R. (2009). Therapeutic potential of splice-switching oligonucleotides. *Oligonucleotides, 19*(1), 1–13.
57. Du, L., & Gatti, R. A. (2009). Progress toward therapy with antisense-mediated splicing modulation. *Current Opinion in Molecular Therapeutics, 11*(2), 116.
58. Havens, M. A., Duelli, D. M., & Hastings, M. L. (2013). Targeting RNA splicing for disease therapy. *Wiley Interdisciplinary Reviews: RNA, 4*(3), 247–266.
59. Zammarchi, F., De Stanchina, E., Bournazou, E., Supakorndej, T., Martires, K., Riedel, E., Corben, A. D., Bromberg, J. F, & Cartegni, L. (2011). Antitumorigenic potential of STAT3 alternative splicing modulation. *Proceedings of the National Academy of Sciences, 108*(43), 17779–17784.
60. Stepniak-Konieczna, E., Konieczny, P., Cywoniuk, P., Dluzewska, J., & Sobczak, K. (2020). AON-induced splice-switching and DMPK pre-mRNA degradation as potential therapeutic approaches for Myotonic Dystrophy type 1. *Nucleic Acids Research, 48*(5), 2531–2543.
61. LeFave, C. V. M. (2010). *HnRNP H drives an oncogenic splicing switch in Gliomas* (Doctoral dissertation, Cornell University).
62. Ward, A. J., Norrbom, M., Chun, S., Bennett, C. F., & Rigo, F. (2014). Nonsense-mediated decay as a terminating mechanism for antisense oligonucleotides. *Nucleic Acids Research, 42*(9), 5871–5879.
63. Kotake, Y., Sagane, K., Owa, T., Mimori-Kiyosue, Y., Shimizu, H., Uesugi, M., Ishihama, Y., Iwata, M, & Mizui, Y. (2007). Splicing factor SF3b as a target of the antitumor natural product pladienolide. *Nature Chemical Biology, 3*(9), 570–575.
64. Havens, M. A., & Hastings, M. L. (2016). Splice-switching antisense oligonucleotides as therapeutic drugs. *Nucleic Acids Research, 44*(14), 6549–6563.
65. Mogilevsky, M., Shimshon, O., Kumar, S., Mogilevsky, A., Keshet, E., Yavin, E., Heyd, F, & Karni, R. (2018). Modulation of MKNK2 alternative splicing by splice-switching oligonucleotides as a novel approach for glioblastoma treatment. *Nucleic Acids Research, 46*(21), 11396–11404.
66. Nielsen, T. O., Sorensen, S., Dagnæs-Hansen, F., Kjems, J., & Sorensen, B. S. (2013). Directing HER4 mRNA expression towards the CYT2 isoform by antisense

oligonucleotide decreases growth of breast cancer cells in vitro and in vivo. *British Journal of Cancer, 108*(11), 2291–2298.

67. Khurshid, S., Montes, M., Sanford, B., Brown, C., Comiskey, D., Rigo, F., Houghton, P, & Chandler, D. (2018). ASO screen uncovers splicing as a therapeutic vulnerability in theinsulin-like growth factor (IGF) signaling pathway. *Cancer Research, 78*(13_Supplement), 4132–4132.
68. Cartegni, L., Chew, S. L., & Krainer, A. R. (2002). Listening to silence and understanding nonsense: exonic mutations that affect splicing. *Nature Reviews Genetics, 3*(4), 285–298.
69. Denichenko, P., Mogilevsky, M., Cléry, A., Welte, T., Biran, J., Shimshon, O., Barnabas, G. D., Danan-Gotthold, M., Kumar, S., Yavin, E, & Levanon, E. Y. (2019). Specific inhibition of splicing factor activity by decoy RNA oligonucleotides. *Nature Communications, 10*(1), 1590.
70. Georgilis, A., Klotz, S., Hanley, C. J., Herranz, N., Weirich, B., Morancho, B., Leote, A. C., D'Artista, L., Gallage, S., Seehawer, M, & Carroll, T. (2018). PTBP1-mediated alternative splicing regulates the inflammatory secretome and the pro-tumorigenic effects of senescent cells. *Cancer Cell, 34*(1), 85–102.
71. Jayasinghe, R. G., Cao, S., Gao, Q., Wendl, M. C., Vo, N. S., Reynolds, S. M., Zhao, Y., Climente-González, H., Chai, S., Wang, F, & Varghese, R. (2018). Systematic analysis of splice-site-creating mutations in cancer. *Cell Reports, 23*(1), 270–281.
72. Kahles, A., Lehmann, K. V., Toussaint, N. C., Hüser, M., Stark, S. G., Sachsenberg, T., Stegle, O., Kohlbacher, O., Sander, C., Caesar-Johnson, S. J, & Demchok, J. A. (2018). Comprehensive analysis of alternative splicing across tumors from 8,705 patients. *Cancer Cell, 34*(2), 211–224.
73. Lu, S. X., De Neef, E., Thomas, J. D., Sabio, E., Rousseau, B., Gigoux, M., Knorr, D. A., Greenbaum, B., Elhanati, Y., Hogg, S. J, & Chow, A. (2021). Pharmacologic modulation of RNA splicing enhances anti-tumor immunity. *Cell, 184*(15), 4032–4047.
74. Fire, A., Xu, S., Montgomery, M. K., Kostas, S. A., Driver, S. E., & Mello, C. C. (1998). Potent and specific genetic interference by double-stranded RNA in Caenorhabditis elegans. *Nature, 391*(6669), 806–811.
75. Dana, H., Chalbatani, G. M., Mahmoodzadeh, H., Karimloo, R., Rezaiean, O., Moradzadeh, A., Mehmandoost, N., Moazzen, F., Mazraeh, A., Marmari, V, & Ebrahimi, M. (2017). Molecular mechanisms and biological functions of siRNA. *International Journal of Biomedical Science: IJBS, 13*(2), p.48.
76. Hayes, G. M., Carrigan, P. E., Beck, A. M., & Miller, L. J. (2006). Targeting the RNA splicing machinery as a novel treatment strategy for pancreatic carcinoma. *Cancer Research, 66*(7), 3819–3827.
77. Wally, V., Murauer, E. M., & Bauer, J. W. (2012). Spliceosome-mediated trans-splicing: the therapeutic cut and paste. *Journal of Investigative Dermatology, 132*(8), 1959–1966.
78. Berger, A., Maire, S., Gaillard, M. C., Sahel, J. A., Hantraye, P., & Bemelmans, A. P. (2016). m RNA trans-splicing in gene therapy for genetic diseases. *Wiley Interdisciplinary Reviews: RNA, 7*(4), 487–498.
79. Jurica, M. S., & Moore, M. J. (2003). Pre-mRNA splicing: awash in a sea of proteins. *Molecular Cell, 12*(1), 5–14.

80. Nakagawa, O., Arnold, M., Nakagawa, M., Hamada, H., Shelton, J. M., Kusano, H., Harris, T. M., Childs, G., Campbell, K. P., Richardson, J. A, & Nishino, I. (2005). Centronuclear myopathy in mice lacking a novel muscle-specific protein kinase transcriptionally regulated by MEF2. *Genes & Development, 19*(17), 2066–2077.
81. Wang, H. Y., Lin, W., Dyck, J. A., Yeakley, J. M., Songyang, Z., Cantley, L. C., & Fu, X. D. (1998). SRPK2: a differentially expressed SR protein-specific kinase involved in mediating the interaction and localization of pre-mRNA splicing factors in mammalian cells. *The Journal of Cell Biology, 140*(4), 737–750.
82. Gout, S., Brambilla, E., Boudria, A., Drissi, R., Lantuejoul, S., Gazzeri, S., & Eymin, B. (2012). Abnormal expression of the pre-mRNA splicing regulators SRSF1, SRSF2, SRPK1 and SRPK2 in non small cell lung carcinoma.
83. Hayes, G. M., Carrigan, P. E., & Miller, L. J. (2007). Serine-arginine protein kinase 1 overexpression is associated with tumorigenic imbalance in mitogen-activated protein kinase pathways in breast, colonic, and pancreatic carcinomas. *Cancer Research, 67*(5), 2072–2080.
84. Jang, S. W., Yang, S. J., Ehlen, A., Dong, S., Khoury, H., Chen, J., Persson, J. L, & Ye, K. (2008). Serine/arginine protein–specific kinase 2 promotes leukemia cell proliferation by phosphorylating Acinus and regulating Cyclin A1. *Cancer Research, 68*(12), 4559–4570.
85. Wu, Q., Chang, Y., Zhang, L., Zhang, Y., Tian, T., Feng, G., Zhou, S., Zheng, Q., Han, F, & Huang, F. (2013). SRPK1 dissimilarly impacts on the growth, metastasis, chemosensitivity and angiogenesis of glioma in normoxic and hypoxic conditions. *Journal of Cancer, 4*(9), 727.
86. Lin, J. C., Lin, C. Y., Tarn, W. Y., & Li, F. Y. (2014). Elevated SRPK1 lessens apoptosis in breast cancer cells through RBM4-regulated splicing events. *RNA, 20*(10), 1621–1631.
87. Nayler, O., Stamm, S., & Ullrich, A. (1997). Characterization and comparison of four serine-and arginine-rich (SR) protein kinases. *Biochemical Journal, 326*(3), 693–700.
88. Colwill, K., Pawson, T., Andrews, B., Prasad, J., Manley, J. L., Bell, J. C., & Duncan, P. I. (1996). The Clk/Sty protein kinase phosphorylates SR splicing factors and regulates their intranuclear distribution. *The EMBO Journal, 15*(2), 265–275.
89. Colwill, K., Feng, L. L., Yeakley, J. M., Gish, G. D., Cáceres, J. F., Pawson, T., & Fu, X. D. (1996). SRPK1 and Clk/Sty protein kinases show distinct substrate specificities for serine/arginine-rich splicing factors. *Journal of Biological Chemistry, 271*(40), 24569–24575.
90. Sampath, J., Long, P. R., Shepard, R. L., Xia, X., Devanarayan, V., Sandusky, G. E., Perry III, W. L., Dantzig, A. H., Williamson, M., Rolfe, M, & Moore, R. E. (2003). Human SPF45, a splicing factor, has limited expression in normal tissues, is overexpressed in many tumors, and can confer a multidrug-resistant phenotype to cells. *The American Journal of Pathology, 163*(5), 1781–1790.
91. Yoshida, T., Kim, J. H., Carver, K., Su, Y., Weremowicz, S., Mulvey, L., Yamamoto, S., Brennan, C., Mei, S., Long, H, & Yao, J. (2015). CLK2 is an oncogenic kinase and splicing regulator in breast cancer. *Cancer Research, 75*(7), 1516–1526.
92. Vivanco, I., & Sawyers, C. L. (2002). The phosphatidylinositol 3-kinase–AKT pathway in human cancer. *Nature Reviews Cancer, 2*(7), 489–501.

93. Pellizzoni, L., Kataoka, N., Charroux, B., & Dreyfuss, G. (1998). A novel function for SMN, the spinal muscular atrophy disease gene product, in pre-mRNA splicing. *Cell, 95*(5), 615–624.
94. Zhang, Z., Lotti, F., Dittmar, K., Younis, I., Wan, L., Kasim, M., & Dreyfuss, G. (2008). SMN deficiency causes tissue-specific perturbations in the repertoire of snRNAs and widespread defects in splicing. *Cell, 133*(4), 585–600.
95. Adachi, H., & Yu, Y. T. (2014). Insight into the mechanisms and functions of spliceosomal snRNA pseudouridylation. *World Journal of Biological Chemistry, 5*(4), 398.
96. Uddin, M. B., Wang, Z., & Yang, C. (2020). Dysregulations of functional RNA modifications in cancer, cancer stemness and cancer therapeutics. *Theranostics, 10*(7), 3164.
97. Liang, J., Wen, J., Huang, Z., Chen, X. P., Zhang, B. X., & Chu, L. (2019). Small nucleolar RNAs: insight into their function in cancer. *Frontiers in Oncology, 9*, 587.
98. McMahon, M., Contreras, A., Holm, M., Uechi, T., Forester, C. M., Pang, X., Jackson, C., Calvert, M. E., Chen, B., Quigley, D. A, & Luk, J. M. (2019). A single H/ACA small nucleolar RNA mediates tumor suppression downstream of oncogenic RAS. *Elife, 8*, p.e48847.
99. Shuai, S., Suzuki, H., Diaz-Navarro, A., Nadeu, F., Kumar, S. A., Gutierrez-Fernandez, A., Delgado, J., Pinyol, M., López-Otín, C., Puente, X. S, & Taylor, M. D. (2019). The U1 spliceosomal RNA is recurrently mutated in multiple cancers. *Nature, 574*(7780), 712–716.
100. Suzuki, H., Kumar, S. A., Shuai, S., Diaz-Navarro, A., Gutierrez-Fernandez, A., De Antonellis, P., Cavalli, F. M., Juraschka, K., Farooq, H., Shibahara, I, & Vladoiu, M. C. (2019). Recurrent noncoding U1 snRNA mutations drive cryptic splicing in SHH medulloblastoma. *Nature, 574*(7780), 707–711.
101. Batsché, E., Yaniv, M., & Muchardt, C. (2006). The human SWI/SNF subunit Brm is a regulator of alternative splicing. *Nature Structural & Molecular Biology, 13*(1), 22–29.
102. Tyagi, A., Ryme, J., Brodin, D., Östlund Farrants, A. K., & Visa, N. (2009). SWI/SNF associates with nascent pre-mRNPs and regulates alternative pre-mRNA processing. *PLoS Genetics, 5*(5), e1000470.
103. Sims, R. J., Millhouse, S., Chen, C. F., Lewis, B. A., Erdjument-Bromage, H., Tempst, P., Manley, J. L, & Reinberg, D. (2007). Recognition of trimethylated histone H3 lysine 4 facilitates the recruitment of transcription postinitiation factors and pre-mRNA splicing. *Molecular Cell, 28*(4), 665–676.
104. Loomis, R. J., Naoe, Y., Parker, J. B., Savic, V., Bozovsky, M. R., Macfarlan, T., Manley, J. L, & Chakravarti, D. (2009). Chromatin binding of SRp20 and ASF/SF2 and dissociation from mitotic chromosomes is modulated by histone H3 serine 10 phosphorylation. *Molecular Cell, 33*(4), 450–461.
105. Schwartz, S., Meshorer, E., & Ast, G. (2009). Chromatin organization marks exon-intron structure. *Nature Structural & Molecular Biology, 16*(9), 990–995.
106. Tilgner, H., Nikolaou, C., Althammer, S., Sammeth, M., Beato, M., Valcárcel, J., & Guigó, R. (2009). Nucleosome positioning as a determinant of exon recognition. *Nature Structural & Molecular Biology, 16*(9), 996–1001.

CHAPTER 6

Cancer DNA Vaccines: Inducing Efficient Immunity

ABSTRACT

Cancer DNA vaccines are a promising and ground-breaking kind of cancer immunotherapy that uses the immune system's ability to recognize and destroy cancerous cells. This abstract offers a summary of recent advancements in cancer DNA vaccines with a focus on their ability to induce effective and robust protection against distinct cancer types. The key component of cancer DNA vaccines is their capacity to elicit an immunological response from the host by encoding tumor-associated antigens (TAAs) or neoantigens, leading to the induction of a focused and long-lasting immune response. Cancer DNA vaccines are now a possibility for immunotherapy thanks to developments in genetic engineering and immunology that have helped to create safer and more efficient vaccine delivery methods. An in-depth discussion of the processes underpinning cancer DNA vaccines' mode of action, the design and selection of TAAs, the optimization of vaccine distribution, and the crucial part played by the tumor microenvironment in vaccination effectiveness are provided in this chapter. Additionally, it analyzes the clinical developments and outcomes from preclinical and early-phase clinical studies, highlighting cases when cancer DNA vaccines have proven to be remarkably effective in slowing the growth of tumors and enhancing patient survival. This presentation also discusses the field's ongoing issues and constraints, including the need for customized vaccines, how to deal with immune evasion mechanisms, and how to increase production scalability. Next-generation cancer DNA vaccines show enormous promise for developing even more effective and long-lasting anti-cancer immune

DNA- and m-RNA-Based Vaccines: An Immunotherapeutic Approach to Cancer.
Sonali Sundram and Rishabha Malviya (Authors)

DOI: 10.1201/9781774919613-6

responses due to the rapid growth of technologies like CRISPR-Cas9 and the improving understanding of cancer immunology.

6.1 INTRODUCTION AND BACKGROUND

Cancer is a hereditary illness that primarily develops owing to mutagenesis brought on by environmental causes, tumor suppressor gene dysfunction, or oncogene activation [1]. Over 277 different forms of cancer diseases are included in the term "cancer" in its broadest sense. Different stages of cancer are identified by researchers, indicating that the etiology of cancer may be influenced by a variety of gene changes [2]. Chemotherapeutic agents and medicines have been extremely useful during the recent decades and continue to be a primary treatment for stage-specific carcinoma when treatment with radiation or surgery is contraindicated for a variety of conditions [3]. The harmful byproducts of various chemotherapy medications are primarily stored inside the liver, causing toxicity inside the liver, which causes a variety of side symptoms, including anemia, lethargy, hyperthermia, hair loss, and others [4]. The idea that the immune system can be used as a tool against cancer cells sparked interest in cancer immunology. The combined assumptions that tumor cells have an antigenic profile unique from their typical cellular counterparts as well as that the immune system has the ability of identifying these antigenic distinctions are fundamental to the idea of effective cancer immunotherapy [5]. Immune checkpoint inhibitors (ICIs), including anti-CTLA4, anti-PD1, and anti-PDL1, which alter the patient's natural immune system, have produced long-lasting remissions in a range of cancer types [6]. By demonstrating that the adaptive immune system may react to artificially created animal tumors, it has been decisively proven that malignant cells might be amenable to control by the host's immunological network [7]. Tumor microenvironment (TME) is made up of composite networks of cells, which often include regulatory proteins, multiple kinds of cells from the immune system, stromal cells, blood arteries, and cancer cells. As a result of the TME's many strategies for suppressing the immune system, cancer cells are capable of persisting by avoiding immune reactions that are aimed there [8]. Understanding the connection among the immune system with cancer is necessary before we can fully understand the DNA vaccine's function. Immune cells have the capacity to prevent the development and spread of tumors as well as to stimulate their growth, infiltration, and metastasis. Adaptive immune cells (T and B lymphocytes) along with dendritic cells (DCs) and innate immune cells, which include natural killer (NK) cells, neutrophils, macrophages, mast cells, and myeloid-derived suppressor cells, are both present and interact with the tumor either directly or through chemokine as well as cytokine signaling, that affects the cancer cell's behavior along with its response to the treatment. Innate immune cells that recognize an antigen set off an inflammatory cascade that causes DCs and macrophages to convey the antigen to T cells, triggering an adaptive immunological reaction [1]. Innate defense mechanisms particularly recognize cancer-particular antigens onto the exterior of tumor cells in a certain way akin to the detection of external pathogens in cancer. The absence of MHC-I surface molecules on cancer cells is recognized by innate immune cells like NK cells, which then actively attack the cancer cells by producing cytokines that attract other inflammatory cells. [2] After phagocytosing tumor cells, recruited monocytes, which are macrophages and DCs, exhibit cancer cell-associated antigens on their surface [3] that prompt a particular T cell reaction called cytolysis which is targeted toward the tumor [9]. Adoptive cell transfers (ACT), cancer vaccines, antibody treatments, immune checkpoint inhibitors (ICI), and cytokine treatments are only several categories of immunotherapy [10, 11]. An effective method of controlling the immune system is DNA vaccination. Plasmids are DNA vaccinations created to transmit genes encoding TA, boosting or activating the immune system to attack TA-bearing cancer cells. Cancer because of CpG motifs present furthermore the double-stranded structure. By acting as strong "danger signals" that activate numerous DNA-sensing systems within the cytosol of transfected cells, DNA vaccines may be able to stimulate the innate immune response [12]. There are several ways to administer DNA vaccinations, but electroporation, sonoporation, and DNA tattooing, along with gene gun are the best [13]. Compared to other nontargeted medicines, DNA vaccines are safer and more antigen-specific, and they also have fewer adverse effects [14]. When a specific sequence from an antigen's gene is integrated into the vaccine carrier, immunological pathways like cytotoxic T-cell pathways can be activated. T-cell stimulating substances like cytokines and the xenogeneic p53 form of the antigen are some methods to improve this process, along with the suppression of immunological tolerance [15]. Figure 6.1 demonstrates the procedure for the formation of DNA vaccination.

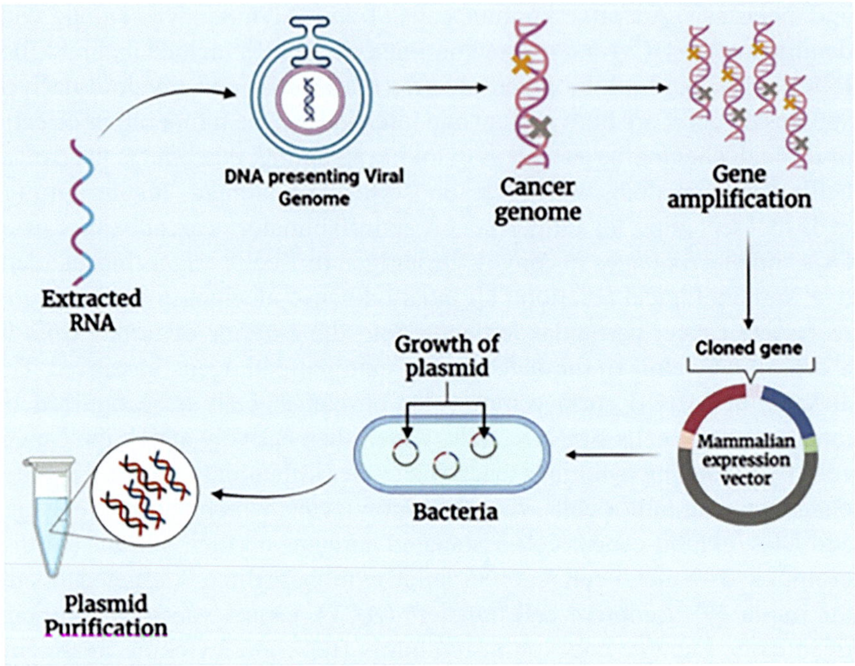

FIGURE 6.1 Process of DNA vaccine formation.

6.2 TYPES OF CANCER DNA VACCINES

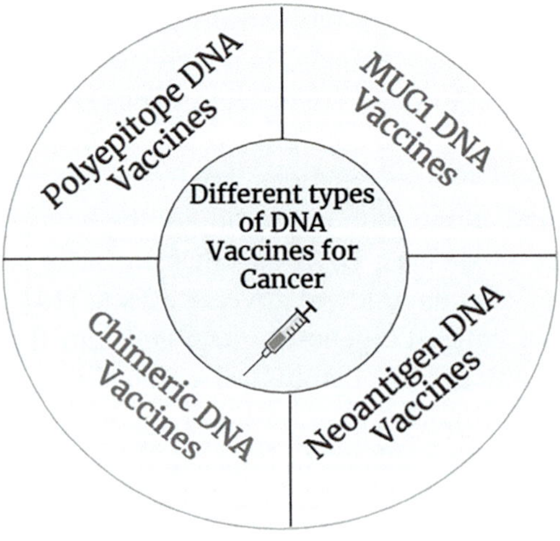

FIGURE 6.2 Different types of cancer DNA vaccines.

6.2.1 POLYEPITOPE DNA VACCINES

The finding that the administration of an epitope-encoding recombinant plasmid may result in epitope generation, exposure to CD8+ T-lymphocytes after processing, as well as the benefit of utilizing a single piece of DNA that encode a number of a few TAAs' epitopes to generate many different types of cytotoxic T-lymphocytes, have prompted the establishment of a number of tactics with the goal of boosting immunogenicity of DNA-based TAA polyepitope vaccines [16]. Peptide-based vaccination has been used to study the utilization of vaccines based on epitope against cancer as the most precise method to activate T lymphocytes as opposed to cancer cells [17]. Unique characteristics of peptide-based cancer vaccines are their ease of preparation for clinical application, low toxicity, and ability to incorporate numerous peptides to avoid immune escape and tumor heterogeneity [18]. In clinical trials in both phases I and II in the therapy of melanoma patients, peptides derived the earliest immunogens were derived from melanoma antigens [19]. The MART-1(27-35) peptide derived from antigen associated with melanoma was also shown to safely increase reactivity of cytotoxic T lymphocytes' (CTL) against epitopes that are frequently expressed in patients' melanoma cells with melanoma when administered *in vivo* [20]. Three HLA-A2-binding NY-ESO-1 peptides administered intradermally to patients having metastatic NY-ESO-1-expressing tumors were also demonstrated to trigger immunological responses [21]. Two general methods have been used to increase epitope immunogenicity. The first seeks to make peptides more affine to class I molecules found in MHC. In fact, a prolonged complex half-life on surfaces of cells as a result of increased affinity increases the likelihood of CTL stimulation. The second tactic tries to enhance the generation and processing of the epitopes [22]. Zaremba et al. changed the CAP-1 peptide's single amino acid to YLSGANLNL among other alterations. The agonist peptide had the ability to produce CD8+ CTL lines, which recognized both the natural CAP-1 sequences, and the agonist, CAP-1, however, was unable to generate CTLs from regular PBMCs. [23]. Loftus et al. identified a number of partial agonists/antagonists of MART1(27-35)-reactive CTL clones generated from tumor-infiltrating lymphocytes (TILs) [24]. The outcomes of a multi-institutional, randomized experiment using a vaccine that is multiepitope peptide, for those patients with metastatic, unresectable melanoma that had previously failed treatment were reported by Kirkwood et al. Three HLA kinds of I-restricted lineages antigen epitopes were administered alone (arm A), with GM-CSF, IFN-2b, or both (arms B, C, and D), or in any other combination (arms E–H). The researchers demonstrated that 6 patients out of 115 had objective therapeutic responses and that 35% of patients had immune responses to a minimum of one melanoma antigen. IFN-2b and GM-CSF did not significantly enhance immune responses [25]. Multiepitope-based vaccinations may be effective treatments for cancer patients eliciting antitumor immune responses [16]. Mateo et al. found that the immunogenicity of the peptides in a tumor-associated polyepitope recombinant vaccine was influenced by their affinity for the MHC [26], in a polyepitope DNA vaccination. The varied MHC affinity of the peptides was demonstrated by Palmowski et al. to be crucial for affecting the immune system's reaction and CTL immunodominance [27].

6.2.2 MUC1 DNA VACCINES

Mucin 1 (MUC1; also referred to as episialin, PEM, H23Ag, EMA, CA15-3, and MCA) is a single pass kind I transmembrane protein with a heavily glycosylated external domain which extends up to 200–500 nm beyond the cell surface [28]. Most human epithelial malignancies overexpress abnormally glycosylated MUC1, which has drawn considerable interest as an oncogenic molecule [29]. MUC1 associated with tumors is distinct from MUC1 expressed in regular cells both in terms of its cellular distribution and its metabolic characteristics [30]. Breast cancer develops spontaneously in Muc1/animals with high amounts of mammary gland polyomavirus intermediate T antigen, but the illness progresses and metastasizes much more slowly than in Muc1$^{+/+}$ mice [31]. Cancer patients' circulatory shed MUC1-N is used to stage cancer and track relapse after therapy as a biomarker [32]. For instance, the identification of breast and pancreatic tumors, respectively, is frequently done using carbohydrate antigen 15.3 (CA 15.3, MUC1) along with carbohydrate antigen 19.9 (CA 19.9, sLea antigen, present on various glycoproteins including MUC1) [33]. Examples of cancer vaccines based on MUC1 include subunit vaccinations, vaccines based on DNA, virus-vected vaccines, dendritic cells (DC) vaccines, as well as glycopeptide vaccines [34]. Subunit vaccinations are crucial in preventing tumor expansion and metastasis

[35]. The MUC1 VNTR peptide and heat shock protein 65 (HSP65) showed anticancer potential in a tumor-challenge mice model by drastically enhancing the immune system's adaptive response, preventing the growth of MUC1+ tumor cells, as well as prolonging the survival of tumor-bearing animals [36]. MUC1 subunit vaccines combined with GM-CSF or SB-AS2 from murine macrophages can increase the ability of MUC1-Transgenic (Tg) mice to reject tumors [37]. L-BLP25, a fascinating MUC1 subunit vaccine candidate, was investigated in a phase II trial on colorectal cancer patients who underwent curative resection [38]. In an animal model, the muscle is directly injected with a recombinant eukaryotic expression vector encoding the *MUC1* gene, resulting in the constitutive expression of a specific MUC1 protein that causes specific humoral along with cellular immunological responses [39]. Adjuvants including dinucleotide motifs as well as the MUC1 DNA vaccine's immunogenicity have been increased often by the use of cytokines [40]. Effective anticancer effects were seen in C57BL/6 mice after receiving a chimeric MUC1 DNA vaccination that contained the human *HSP70* gene alongside the *MUC1* gene that had the transmembrane as well as C-terminal domains removed [41]. Additionally, eukaryotic plasmids co-expressing the MUC1 genome linked to the gene-generating soluble programmed death-1 (PD-1) increased the tumor suppression rate and prolonged longevity in a mouse model of colorectal cancer [42]. A DC is the most efficient antigen-presenting cell (APC). The primary job of DCs is to endocytose external antigens and then deliver antigen fragments to T lymphocytes on the cell surface through MHC molecules. By stimulating induced T cell co-stimulatory ligand molecules, which converse with one another, these cells can subsequently stimulate naive T cells, activate memory T cells, and initiate immunological responses [43]. A DC immunization with a 100-mer version of the MUC1 antigen successfully caused tumor rejection in the transgenic mouse model [44].

6.2.3 CHIMERIC DNA VACCINES

The denial of DNA vaccines against cancer was caused by a number of variables, including the selection of target antigens, the methods used in vaccine formulation, and addressing the problem of tolerance. To get over these limitations, the concept of chimeric DNA vaccinations to attack cancer antigens was put out. Combining the chimeric vaccines with immune modulators may increase their effectiveness [45]. However, it can also be recognized and internalized by B cells. Since DCs may absorb the chimeric protein produced by transfected cells, the T-cell immune response is triggered [46]. Mesothelin (MSLN), a tumor antigen, has been identified in a number of malignancies, particularly ovarian and pancreatic cancers. Immunomodulator epigallocatechin-3-gallate (EGCG) was combined with antigen-specific connective tissue growth factor (CTGF/MSLN), which was coated with mesothelin [47], the simultaneous injection of the CD4 T-cell-inducing peptides and the vaccination. One example of these peptides is the use of long peptides called Pan HLA-DR epitope (PADRE) peptides, which stimulate both CD4 cells and dendritic cells [48]. Quaglino et al. found that the plasmid harboring the chimeric neu-Her-2 antigen was superior to both the fully autologous and the totally xenogeneic vaccines when eliciting a protective anticancer immune response against ErbB2+ tumors [49]. In a study, mice given morphine showed increased tumor development rates and decreased CD8+ T lymphocyte percentages. Findings show that long-term morphine use dose-dependently encourages tumor formation, and a chimeric DNA vaccine may be an effective way to alleviate the serious immunosuppressive effects of long-term morphine use and prevent carcinogenesis [50].

6.2.4 NEOANTIGEN DNA VACCINES

Neoantigen vaccines are constructed using the antigenic regions protein mutations produced in tumor cells as their epitopes. These extremely immunogenic antigens could provoke the body's defenses to attack cancerous cells. Numerous neoantigen vaccination clinical studies on cancer patients have been made possible by advancements in sequencing technology as well as computational techniques [51]. A subset of TSAs known as neoantigens differs from TAAs. Neoantigens are specific to tumor cells whereas TAAs are not. TAAs are made from overexpressed proteins, which are sometimes found in healthy cells [52]. Individualized immunizations against neoantigens may help the immune system learn to identify and destroy cancer cells that express neopeptides. The neoantigen vaccine has other benefits besides inducing immunogenicity, such as the ability to be administered to outpatients and negligible adverse effects

[53]. A DNA vaccination platform was created and improved by Li et al. to target several neoantigens. Model antigens were used to optimize the polyepitope DNA vaccination platform both *in vitro* as well as *in vivo*. In clinical simulations and clinical translation, the polyepitope neoantigen DNA vaccination platform targeted numerous neoantigens and elicited anticancer immune responses [54]. Neoantigen vaccines work best when combined with other treatments, including immune checkpoint inhibitors, treatment with chemotherapy, and radiation therapy. Adjuvant therapy is used to enhance the effects of several neoantigen vaccination types, with poly-ICLC being the most popular adjuvant [55]. The development of next-generation sequencing (NGS) has enabled the rapid sequencing of whole genomes, enabling high-throughput data analysis. Neoantigens can be anticipated in conjunction with cutting-edge bioinformatic analysis methods, and complete personalized vaccination reagents can be made available for delivery in a reasonable amount of time [56]. Numerous recent researches have attempted to understand the fundamental biological components and mechanisms that may impact the overall efficacy of neoantigen vaccines. One study discovered that despite the presence of sufficient amounts of clonal neoantigens, there were no developed neoantigen-specific T lymphocytes before immunization [57]. With the help of whole-exome sequencing (WES) and RNA-seq, dendritic cell (DC)-based efficiency prevalidation of vaccine candidates, bioinformatic forecasting of neo-epitopes, optimization of the DNA vaccine plus its nanocarrier alongside adjuvant, as well as creation of a liposome-encapsulated multi-epitope DNA vaccine, Yang X. and colleagues developed a framework for a DNA-based vaccine [58].

6.3 MECHANISM OF CANCER DNA VACCINES

When tumor antigens trigger the immune system, APCs are crucial. DCs are the most important because they act as a fundamental connection between innate immunity and adaptive immunity. DCs, the first antigen presenters, may take up antigens as well as display them on their MHC I molecules [59]. Immature DCs excel in identifying and phagocytosing antigens by phagocytosis and micropinocytosis. When the toll-like receptor ligand adjuvants are present, the presence of toll-like receptor ligands within the TME may temporarily boost antigen-specific micropinocytosis via activating immature DCs [60]. Following antigen uptake, MHC I, MHC II, as well as costimulatory molecules are going to be raised on the surface of DCs, and they gradually lose their ability to absorb antigens [61]. The immunosuppressive TME along with T-cell dysfunction are the leading causes of the tumor cells' evading the body's immune system. Myeloid-derived stem cells (MDSCs) and regulatory T-cells (Tregs) are the most well-known immune cells. MDSCs are the immunosuppressive, tumor-infiltrating macrophages that participate in anti-inflammatory actions [62, 63]. Tregs are able to reduce the immune response to tumors by releasing suppressive cytokines as IL-35 as well as transforming growth factor (TGF) [64]. DNA vaccines can selectively activate both Th1 Helper T cells and Th2 Helper T cells and polarize the ensuing immune response in being either humoral or cellular-oriented by using various administration methods and modifying the antigen processing pathways [65]. Figure 6.3 shows the mode of working of cancer DNA vaccines.

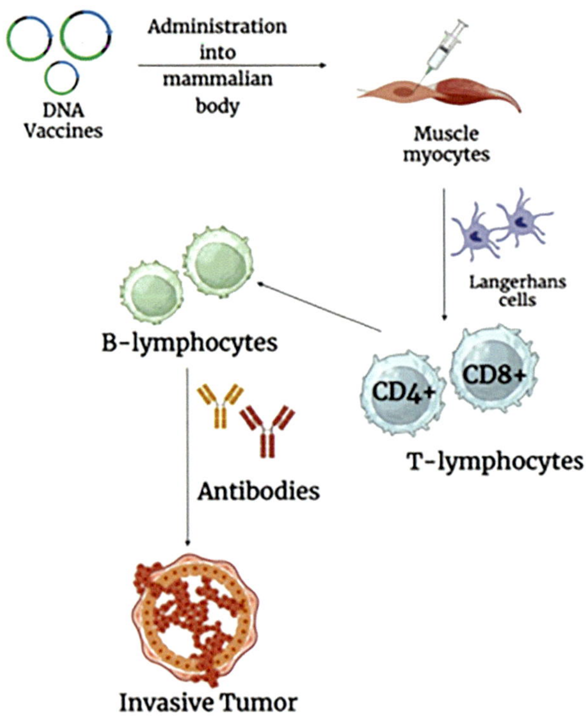

FIGURE 6.3 Cancer DNA vaccines' mode of action.

6.4 DNA VACCINES COMBINED WITH OTHER TREATMENTS

Combining cancer DNA vaccines with other tactics that can both amplify the antigen response and quiet immunosuppression in the TME will increase their effectiveness [66].

6.4.1 COMBINATION WITH CHEMOTHERAPY

Cyclophosphamide and DNA vaccines were used in a preclinical investigation to increase mice longevity and reduce the expression of cytokines that inhibit the immune system including IL-10 and VEGF [67]. DNA vaccines might additionally be used in conjunction with specific treatments that can promote T cell priming and mediate tumor cell antigen release. The multitargeted tyrosine kinase receptor inhibitor sunitinib was observed to decrease Tregs and MDSCs and increase INF-producing T cells in individuals with renal cell cancer [68]. Through TLR4 simulation, it has been proven that chemotherapy treatment recovered sensitivity to checkpoint blockage [69]. Preclinical animal studies along with early-stage clinical trials have evaluated the efficacy of such a strategy employing clinically licensed PD-1/PD-L1 and CTLA4 inhibition with cell-based vaccines using Pembrolizumab or Ipilimumab, respectively [70–72].

6.4.2 COMBINATION WITH RADIOTHERAPY

In conjunction with passive administration of tumor-specific cytotoxic T lymphocytes (CTLs) and vaccination against cancer-specific antigens, sublethal dosages of chemotherapy and radiation have been shown to be effective. Epithelial cells altered with HPV E6/E7 plus activated Ras oncogene have been used as a preclinical cervical cancer model to investigate the pairing of low-dose RT and DNA vaccination [73]. By including radioiodine gene treatment into a cancer in animal models, Jeon H and colleagues showed how combination therapy can be used to get around the drawbacks of cancer DNA vaccines. They developed an established cell line (CT26/hMUC1-hNIS-Fluc: CMNF) which produces the *hMUC1*, *hNIS*, and *Fluc* genes using a retro- and lentivirus system. This work demonstrates that radioiodine gene treatment using iodide-to-sodium symporter can overcome the ineffective preventative effects of cancer DNA vaccination [74]. When combined with therapeutic HPV DNA vaccines, methods that promote tumor cell apoptosis, such as low-dose radiation and death receptor 5 monoclonal antibodies, have also improved cytotoxic T cell immunity specific to the HPV antigen against E7-expressing tumors [73]. Together, our findings show that therapeutic DNA vaccines may be more effective when tumors are treated with radiotherapy that might accelerate tumor cell apoptosis.

6.4.3 COMBINATION WITH IMMUNE CHECKPOINT BLOCKADE

In multiple investigations, *in vivo* CTLA-4 inhibition reduced tumor expansion in animal models while encouraging tumor rejection in melanoma patients [75]. This also led to protection against a subsequent exposure to tumor cells, indicating that anti-CTLA-4 antibodies may be able to trigger the immune system's memory component [76]. Sixty-four patients having advanced melanoma were sequenced by Snyder et al., who discovered a substantial correlation between the somatic mutation burden and the patient's clinical response to anti-CTLA4 therapy [77]. In preclinical and clinical research, combinations of ICB with other techniques were attempted for various kinds of malignancies in order to increase T cell proliferation in the TME as well as the proportion of patients that respond to ICB [78]. Pairing with cancer in order to combine the advantages of ICB with vaccines' capacity to stimulate the antigen-specific CTL response, DNA vaccination appears to hold some promise [79]. The combination of pEMS-OVA and pVAX-PD-1 therapies improved survival and slowed tumor growth. The potential of DNA vaccines along with ICBs to activate T cells to target certain cancer antigens, hence enhancing the activity of T-cell and tumor invasion, is the source of this synergistic impact. ICB thus produces a favorable milieu for the activation of tumor-specific DNA vaccines [80].

6.5 CHALLENGES ASSOCIATED WITH CANCER DNA VACCINES

The majority of the critical challenges raised by the cancer-specific DNA vaccine can eventually only be successfully addressed in clinical settings because it is so challenging to convert knowledge from animal studies. This is because human and animal immune systems function differently and because tumors have various features [81]. Until recently, vaccinations were only employed as a last resort. Knowing when to administer them is essential if you want to incorporate them into your standard of care treatment. When making this decision, it is important to consider the time frame for the immune system's creation of a specific immunological response to the given antigen, the need for several administration dosages, and the interaction of the combined therapy. For instance, numerous studies demonstrated that providing ICB after the peptide/RNA vaccine treatment led to a long-lasting remission with no signs of a disease recurrence [82]. Most tumors have relevant TAAs, although immune tolerance may reduce their effectiveness. Neoantigen detection is time- and resource-intensive, and it does not accurately reflect the tumor heterogeneity within a particular patient (for instance, in metastasis). Second, how many antigens should be encoded on a single plasmid? Which antigens are preferable to one another when it comes to the frequency of an immune system reaction or a clinical result is still up for debate [83]. Immunotherapies frequently cause side effects and have a varying reaction rate from patient to patient. Because of this, it's critical to find biomarkers that can forecast how a patient will react to a certain medication and standardize the therapy in accordance with the projected biomarker. However, because of the intricate relationships between tumors and the immune system as well as the diversity of the host and the tumor, the conversion of biological data into prognostic or predictive biomarkers is challenging. Numerous research are predicting distinct tumor signatures using bioinformatics techniques and cutting-edge genomic and proteomic technologies, creating complex datasets that present analytical hurdles [69].

6.6 ADVANTAGES AND DISADVANTAGES OF USING DNA VACCINES

Long-term immunogenicity persistence and *in vivo* expression, which guarantees that the protein mimics the normal eukaryotic one, are two benefits of utilizing DNA vaccines [84]. A broad-spectrum vaccine can be formulated by using a mixture of plasmids [85]. A further benefit of DNA vaccines for the treatment of cancer is the selective immune response to the target antigen [86]. DNA vaccines offer great merits of being thermally stable as well as inexpensive [87]. These vaccines are more stable, dependable, and manageable [88]. They activate cellular and humoral immune defenses [89]. When you consider the costs of mass production and storage, these vaccinations are very expensive [90]. Rapid changes in antigens are made easier by recombinant DNA technologies [91]. They support the proper handling and presentation of the necessary gene targets, with the antigen's *in vivo* presentation and internal post-translational changes as seen with infectious diseases as a contributing factor [92]. Along with these various advantages, there are some drawbacks to DNA vaccines that have prevented their use in treating human cancer. The poor immunogenicity of DNA vaccines is one of their main drawbacks. Larger doses of around 5–10 mg are necessary for the mild stimulation of the immune system [93]. By expressing antigens within the host body, these might induce immunologic tolerance [85].

6.7 CONCLUSION AND FUTURE PROSPECTIVE

In conclusion, the development and use of DNA vaccinations in the therapy of cancer provide a possible and cutting-edge tactic to combat this complex and varied disease. Over the past few decades, significant progress has been made in our knowledge of how the body's immune system detects and eliminates cancer cells. DNA vaccines have proven to be a successful way to make use of the immune system's ability to target and destroy cancer cells with precision. Clinical trials along with preclinical studies have demonstrated the safety and efficacy of DNA vaccines against a variety of cancer types, and they possess the potential to stimulate robust and sustained immune responses. The creation of personalized DNA vaccinations that are catered to a person's particular tumor antigens is now possible thanks to developments in genomics and bioinformatics. These vaccinations may be more effective since they can target particular mutations or proteins found in a patient's tumor. DNA vaccines can be paired with other immunotherapies, including adoptive cell treatments or checkpoint inhibitors, to increase their effectiveness. Combining various cancer immunotherapy techniques may provide synergistic advantages. While DNA vaccines have showed potential in some cancer types, further study is being done to see if they can be used to treat a wider variety of cancers. This covers uncommon tumors and those that are ordinarily thought to be less immunogenic. Immunotherapy resistance is still a major problem in the fight against cancer. Future studies may concentrate on methods to circumvent resistance mechanisms and increase the efficiency of DNA vaccines, maybe through the utilization of combination therapy or genetic alterations. The creation of effective and secure delivery systems for DNA vaccines is essential. Research into cutting-edge delivery methods, such as nanoparticles or electroporation, may increase vaccination uptake and immunological responses. DNA vaccinations for cancer may receive regulatory clearances and establish themselves as a conventional form of treatment, making them more widely available to patients globally as more encouraging clinical trial results become available. To evaluate the durability as well as potential side effects of DNA vaccines over time, the effectiveness and safety of these medicines for cancer patients must be closely monitored.

KEYWORDS

- **cancer**
- **DNA vaccines**
- **immunity**
- **polyepitope**
- **MUC1**

REFERENCES

1. Imran, A., Qamar, H. Y., Qurban, A. L. I., Naeem, H., Mariam, R. I. A. Z., Saima, A. M. I. N., Kanwal, N., Fawad, A. L. I., Sabar, M. F., & Nasir, I. A. (2017). Role of molecular biology in cancer treatment: a review article. *Iranian Journal of Public Health, 46*(11), 1475.
2. Hassanpour, S. H., & Dehghani, M. (2017). Review of cancer from perspective of molecular. *Journal of Cancer Research and Practice, 4*(4), 127–129.
3. Anand, U., Dey, A., Chandel, A. K. S., Sanyal, R., Mishra, A., Pandey, D. K., De Falco, V., Upadhyay, A., Kandimalla, R., Chaudhary, A, & Dhanjal, J. K. (2023). Cancer chemotherapy and beyond: current status, drug candidates, associated risks and progress in targeted therapeutics. *Genes & Diseases, 10*(4), 1367–1401.
4. Mustapha, A., Ismail, A., Abdullahi, S. U., Hassan, O. N., Ugwunnaji, P. I., & Berinyuy, E. B. (2021). Cancer chemotherapy: a review update of the mechanisms

of actions, prospects and associated problems. *BIOMED Natural and Applied Science, 1*(1), 1–19.

5. Pardoll, D. (2015). Cancer and the immune system: basic concepts and targets for intervention. In *Seminars in oncology* (Vol. 42, No. 4, pp. 523–538). WB Saunders.
6. Hiam-Galvez, K. J., Allen, B. M., & Spitzer, M. H. (2021). Systemic immunity in cancer. *Nature Reviews Cancer, 21*(6), 345–359.
7. Baldwin, R. W. (1987, February). Relationship Between the Immune System and Cancer. In *Immunotoxicology: Proceedings of the International Seminar on the Immunological System as a Target for Toxic Damage—Present Status, Open Problems and Future Perspectives* (pp. 24–34). Springer Netherlands.
8. Lokman, N. A., Price, Z. K., Hawkins, E. K., Macpherson, A. M., Oehler, M. K., & Ricciardelli, C. (2019). 4-Methylumbelliferone inhibits cancer stem cell activation and overcomes chemoresistance in ovarian cancer. *Cancers, 11*(8), 1187.
9. Markman, J. L., & Shiao, S. L. (2015). Impact of the immune system and immunotherapy in colorectal cancer. *Journal of Gastrointestinal Oncology, 6*(2), 208.
10. Shell, S. S., Prestwich, E. G., Baek, S. H., Shah, R. R., Sassetti, C. M., Dedon, P. C., & Fortune, S. M. (2013). DNA methylation impacts gene expression and ensures hypoxic survival of Mycobacterium tuberculosis. *PLoS Pathogens, 9*(7), e1003419.
11. Ottaviano, M., De Placido, S., & Ascierto, P. A. (2019). Recent success and limitations of immune checkpoint inhibitors for cancer: a lesson from melanoma. *Virchows Archiv, 474*(4), 421–432.
12. Herrada, A. A., Rojas-Colonelli, N., González-Figueroa, P., Roco, J., Oyarce, C., Ligtenberg, M. A., & Lladser, A. (2012). Harnessing DNA-induced immune responses for improving cancer vaccines. *Human Vaccines & Immunotherapeutics, 8*(11), 1682–1693.
13. Lopes, A., Vandermeulen, G., & Préat, V. (2019). Cancer DNA vaccines: current preclinical and clinical developments and future perspectives. *Journal of Experimental & Clinical Cancer Research, 38*, 1–24.
14. Amara, S., & Tiriveedhi, V. (2017). The five immune forces impacting DNA-based cancer immunotherapeutic strategy. *International Journal of Molecular Sciences, 18*(3), 650.
15. Das, S. S., Moitra, I., Singh, S. K., Verma, P. R. P., & Swain, S. (2022). DNA vaccines for cancer treatment: challenges and promises. In *Nanotherapeutics in cancer vaccination and challenges* (pp. 259–278). Academic Press.
16. Bei, R., & Scardino, A. (2010). TAA polyepitope DNA-based vaccines: a potential tool for cancer therapy. *BioMed Research International, 2010*(1), 102758.
17. Mocellin, S., Pilati, P., & Nitti, D. (2009). Peptide-based anticancer vaccines: recent advances and future perspectives. *Current Medicinal Chemistry, 16*(36), 4779–4796.
18. Pilla, L., Rivoltini, L., Patuzzo, R., Marrari, A., Valdagni, R., & Parmiani, G. (2009). Multipeptide vaccination in cancer patients. *Expert Opinion on Biological Therapy, 9*(8), 1043–1055.
19. Rosenberg, S. A., Yang, J. C., Schwartzentruber, D. J., Hwu, P., Marincola, F. M., Topalian, S. L., Restifo, N. P., Dudley, M. E., Schwarz, S. L., Spiess, P. J., & Parkhurst, M. R. (1998). Immunologic and therapeutic evaluation of a synthetic peptide vaccine for the treatment of patients with metastatic melanoma. *Nature Medicine, 4*(3), 321–327.

20. Cormier, J. N., Salgaller, M. L., Prevette, T., Barracchini, K. C., Rivoltini, L., Restifo, N. P., Rosenberg, S. A., & Marincola, F. M. (1997). Enhancement of cellular immunity in melanoma patients immunized with a peptide from MART-1/Melan A. *The Cancer Journal from Scientific American, 3*(1), 37.
21. Jäger, E., Gnjatic, S., Nagata, Y., Stockert, E., Jäger, D., Karbach, J., Neumann, A., Rieckenberg, J., Chen, Y. T., Ritter, G., & Hoffman, E. (2000). Induction of primary NY-ESO-1 immunity: CD8+ T lymphocyte and antibody responses in peptide-vaccinated patients with NY-ESO-1+ cancers. *Proceedings of the National Academy of Sciences, 97*(22), 12198–12203.
22. Parmiani, G., Castelli, C., Dalerba, P., Mortarini, R., Rivoltini, L., Marincola, F. M., & Anichini, A. (2002). Cancer immunotherapy with peptide-based vaccines: what have we achieved? Where are we going? *Journal of the National Cancer Institute, 94*(11), 805–818.
23. Zaremba, S., Barzaga, E., Zhu, M., Soares, N., Tsang, K. Y., & Schlom, J. (1997). Identification of an enhancer agonist cytotoxic T lymphocyte peptide from human carcinoembryonic antigen. *Cancer Research, 57*(20), 4570–4577.
24. Loftus, D. J., Squarcina, P., Nielsen, M. B., Geisler, C., Castelli, C., Ødum, N., Appella, E., Parmiani, G., & Rivoltini, L. (1998). Peptides derived from self-proteins as partial agonists and antagonists of human CD8+ T-cell clones reactive to melanoma/melanocyte epitope MART127–35. *Cancer Research, 58*(11), 2433–2439.
25. Kirkwood, J. M., Lee, S., Moschos, S. J., Albertini, M. R., Michalak, J. C., Sander, C., Whiteside, T., Butterfield, L. H., & Weiner, L. (2009). Immunogenicity and antitumor effects of vaccination with peptide vaccine+/− granulocyte-monocyte colony-stimulating factor and/or IFN-α2b in advanced metastatic melanoma: eastern cooperative oncology group phase II Trial E1696. *Clinical Cancer Research, 15*(4), 1443–1451.
26. Mateo, L., Gardner, J., Chen, Q., Schmidt, C., Down, M., Elliott, S. L., Pye, S. J., Firat, H., Lemonnier, F. A., Cebon, J., & Suhrbier, A. (1999). An HLA-A2 polyepitope vaccine for melanoma immunotherapy. *The Journal of Immunology, 163*(7), 4058–4063.
27. Palmowski, M. J., Choi, E. M. L., Hermans, I. F., Gilbert, S. C., Chen, J. L., Gileadi, U., Salio, M., Van Pel, A., Man, S., Bonin, E., & Liljestrom, P. (2002). Competition between CTL narrows the immune response induced by prime-boost vaccination protocols. *The Journal of Immunology, 168*(9), 4391–4398.
28. Hattrup, C. L., & Gendler, S. J. (2008). Structure and function of the cell surface (tethered) mucins. *Annual Review of Physiology, 70*(1), 431–457.
29. Lau, S. K., Weiss, L. M., & Chu, P. G. (2004). Differential expression of MUC1, MUC2, and MUC5AC in carcinomas of various sites: an immunohistochemical study. *American Journal of Clinical Pathology, 122*(1), 61–69.
30. Nath, S., & Mukherjee, P. (2014). MUC1: a multifaceted oncoprotein with a key role in cancer progression. *Trends in Molecular Medicine, 20*(6), 332–342.
31. Besmer, D. M., Curry, J. M., Roy, L. D., Tinder, T. L., Sahraei, M., Schettini, J., Hwang, S. I., Lee, Y. Y., Gendler, S. J., & Mukherjee, P. (2011). Pancreatic ductal adenocarcinoma mice lacking mucin 1 have a profound defect in tumor growth and metastasis. *Cancer Research, 71*(13), 4432–4442.

32. Safi, F., Kohler, I., Beger, H. G., & Röttinger, E. (1991). The value of the tumor marker CA 15-3 in diagnosing and monitoring breast cancer. A comparative study with carcinoembryonic antigen. *Cancer, 68*(3), 574–582.
33. Steinberg, W. (1990). The clinical utility of the CA 19-9 tumor-associated antigen. *American Journal of Gastroenterology, 85*(4).
34. Gao, T., Cen, Q., & Lei, H. (2020). A review on development of MUC1-based cancer vaccine. *Biomedicine & Pharmacotherapy, 132*, 110888.
35. Apostolopoulos, V., & McKenzie, I. F. (1994). Cellular mucins: targets for immunotherapy. *Critical Reviews in Immunology, 14*(3–4).
36. Li, D., Li, H., Zhang, P., Wu, X., Wei, H., Wang, L., Wan, M., Deng, P., Zhang, Y., Wang, J., & Liu, Y. (2006). Heat shock fusion protein induces both specific and nonspecific anti-tumor immunity. *European Journal of Immunology, 36*(5), 1324–1336.
37. Tempero, R. M., Rowse, G. J., Gendler, S. J., & Hollingsworth, M. A. (1999). Passively transferred anti-MUC1 antibodies cause neither autoimmune disorders nor immunity against transplanted tumors in MUC1 transgenic mice. *International Journal of Cancer, 80*(4), 595–599.
38. Schimanski, C. C., Möhler, M., Schön, M., Van Cutsem, E., Greil, R., Bechstein, W. O., Hegewisch-Becker, S., von Wichert, G., Vöhringer, M., Heike, M., & Heinemann, V. (2012). LICC: L-BLP25 in patients with colorectal carcinoma after curative resection of hepatic metastases--a randomized, placebo-controlled, multicenter, multinational, double-blinded phase II trial. *BMC Cancer, 12*, 1–9.
39. Rajčáni, J., Moško, T., & Režuchová, I. (2005). Current developments in viral DNA vaccines: shall they solve the unsolved? *Reviews in Medical Virology, 15*(5), 303–325.
40. Shirota, H., Tross, D., & Klinman, D. M. (2015). CpG oligonucleotides as cancer vaccine adjuvants. *Vaccines, 3*(2), 390–407.
41. Choi, D. H., Woo, J. K., Choi, Y., Seo, H. S., & Kim, C. W. (2011). A novel chimeric DNA vaccine: enhancement of preventive and therapeutic efficacy of DNA vaccine by fusion of Mucin 1 to a heat shock protein 70 gene. *Molecular Medicine Reports, 4*(5), 885–890.
42. Choi, D. H., Woo, J. K., Choi, Y., Seo, H. S., & Kim, C. W. (2011). A novel chimeric DNA vaccine: enhancement of preventive and therapeutic efficacy of DNA vaccine by fusion of Mucin 1 to a heat shock protein 70 gene. *Molecular Medicine Reports, 4*(5), 885–890.
43. Steinman, R. M. (1991). The dendritic cell system and its role in immunogenicity. *Annual Review of Immunology, 9*, 271–296.
44. Maehara, Y., Kabashima, A., Tokunaga, E., Hasuda, S., Oki, E., Kakeji, Y., Baba, H., & Sugimachi, K. (1999). Recurrences and relation to tumor growth potential and local immune response in node-negative advanced gastric cancer. *Oncology, 56*(4), 322–327.
45. Pandya, A., Shah, Y., Kothari, N., Postwala, H., Shah, A., Parekh, P., & Chorawala, M. R. (2023). The future of cancer immunotherapy: DNA vaccines leading the way. *Medical Oncology, 40*(7), 200.
46. Riccardo, F., Bolli, E., Macagno, M., Arigoni, M., Cavallo, F., & Quaglino, E. (2017). Chimeric DNA vaccines: an effective way to overcome immune tolerance. *Cancer Vaccines,* 99–122.

47. Chen, Y. L., Chang, M. C., Chiang, Y. C., Lin, H. W., Sun, N. Y., Chen, C. A., Sun, W. Z., & Cheng, W. F. (2018). Immuno-modulators enhance antigen-specific immunity and anti-tumor effects of mesothelin-specific chimeric DNA vaccine through promoting DC maturation. *Cancer Letters, 425*, 152–163.
48. Safavi, A., Kefayat, A., Abiri, A., Mahdevar, E., Behnia, A. H., & Ghahremani, F. (2019). In silico analysis of transmembrane protein 31 (TMEM31) antigen to design novel multiepitope peptide and DNA cancer vaccines against melanoma. *Molecular Immunology, 112*, 93–102.
49. Quaglino, E., Riccardo, F., Macagno, M., Bandini, S., Cojoca, R., Ercole, E., Amici, A., & Cavallo, F. (2011). Chimeric DNA vaccines against ErbB2+ carcinomas: from mice to humans. *Cancers, 3*(3), 3225–3241.
50. Cheng, W. F., Chen, L. K., Chen, C. A., Chang, M. C., Hsiao, P. N., Su, Y. N., Lee, C. N., Jeng, H. J., Hsieh, C. Y., & Sun, W. Z. (2006). Chimeric DNA vaccine reverses morphine-induced immunosuppression and tumorigenesis. *Molecular Therapy, 13*(1), 203–210.
51. Biswas, N., Chakrabarti, S., Padul, V., Jones, L. D., & Ashili, S. (2023). Designing neoantigen cancer vaccines, trials, and outcomes. *Frontiers in Immunology, 14*, 1105420.
52. Peng, M., Mo, Y., Wang, Y., Wu, P., Zhang, Y., Xiong, F., Guo, C., Wu, X., Li, Y., Li, X., & Li, G. (2019). Neoantigen vaccine: an emerging tumor immunotherapy. *Molecular Cancer, 18*, 1–14.
53. Rosenberg, S. A., Yang, J. C., & Restifo, N. P. (2004). Cancer immunotherapy: moving beyond current vaccines. *Nature Medicine, 10*(9), 909–915.
54. Li, L., Zhang, X., Wang, X., Kim, S. W., Herndon, J. M., Becker-Hapak, M. K., Carreno, B. M., Myers, N. B., Sturmoski, M. A., McLellan, M. D., & Miller, C. A. (2021). Optimized polyepitope neoantigen DNA vaccines elicit neoantigen-specific immune responses in preclinical models and in clinical translation. *Genome Medicine, 13*, 1–13.
55. Niemi, J. V. L., Sokolov, A. V., & Schiöth, H. B. (2022). Neoantigen vaccines; clinical trials, classes, indications, adjuvants and combinatorial treatments. *Cancers, 14*(20), 5163.
56. Kreiter, S., Vormehr, M., Van de Roemer, N., Diken, M., Löwer, M., Diekmann, J., Boegel, S., Schrörs, B., Vascotto, F., Castle, J. C., & Tadmor, A. D. (2015). Mutant MHC class II epitopes drive therapeutic immune responses to cancer. *Nature, 520*(7549), 692–696.
57. Linette, G. P., Becker-Hapak, M., Skidmore, Z. L., Baroja, M. L., Xu, C., Hundal, J., Spencer, D. H., Fu, W., Cummins, C., Robnett, M., & Kaabinejadian, S. (2019). Immunological ignorance is an enabling feature of the oligo-clonal T cell response to melanoma neoantigens. *Proceedings of the National Academy of Sciences, 116*(47), 23662–23670.
58. Yang, X., Fan, J., Wu, Y., Ma, Z., Huang, J., Zhang, Y., Zhou, Z., Mo, F., Liu, X., Yuan, H., & Xu, Y. (2021). Synthetic multiepitope neoantigen DNA vaccine for personalized cancer immunotherapy. *Nanomedicine: Nanotechnology, Biology and Medicine, 37*, p.102443.
59. Itano, A. A., McSorley, S. J., Reinhardt, R. L., Ehst, B. D., Ingulli, E., Rudensky, A. Y., & Jenkins, M. K. (2003). Distinct dendritic cell populations sequentially

present antigen to CD4 T cells and stimulate different aspects of cell-mediated immunity. *Immunity, 19*(1), 47–57.
60. West, M. A., Wallin, R. P., Matthews, S. P., Svensson, H. G., Zaru, R., Ljunggren, H. G., Prescott, A. R., & Watts, C. (2004). Enhanced dendritic cell antigen capture via toll-like receptor-induced actin remodeling. *Science, 305*(5687), 1153–1157.
61. Sallusto, F., Cella, M., Danieli, C., & Lanzavecchia, A. (1995). Dendritic cells use macropinocytosis and the mannose receptor to concentrate macromolecules in the major histocompatibility complex class II compartment: downregulation by cytokines and bacterial products. *The Journal of Experimental Medicine, 182*(2), 389–400.
62. Fioretti, D., Iurescia, S., Fazio, V. M., & Rinaldi, M. (2010). DNA vaccines: developing new strategies against cancer. *BioMed Research International, 2010*(1), 174378.
63. Sica, A., & Bronte, V. (2007). Altered macrophage differentiation and immune dysfunction in tumor development. *The Journal of Clinical Investigation, 117*(5), 1155–1166.
64. Collison, L. W., Workman, C. J., Kuo, T. T., Boyd, K., Wang, Y., Vignali, K. M., Cross, R., Sehy, D., Blumberg, R. S., & Vignali, D. A. (2007). The inhibitory cytokine IL-35 contributes to regulatory T-cell function. *Nature, 450*(7169), 566–569.
65. Anderson, R. J., & Schneider, J. (2007). Plasmid DNA and viral vector-based vaccines for the treatment of cancer. *Vaccine, 25*, B24–B34.
66. Melero, I., Berman, D. M., Aznar, M. A., Korman, A. J., Gracia, J. L. P., & Haanen, J. (2015). Evolving synergistic combinations of targeted immunotherapies to combat cancer. *Nature Reviews Cancer, 15*(8), 457–472.
67. Xia, Q., Geng, F., Zhang, F. F., Liu, C. L., Xu, P., Lu, Z. Z., Xie, Y., Sun, B., Wu, H., Yu, B., & Kong, W. (2017). Cyclophosphamide enhances anti-tumor effects of a fibroblast activation protein α-based DNA vaccine in tumor-bearing mice with murine breast carcinoma. *Immunopharmacology and Immunotoxicology, 39*(1), 37–44.
68. Finke, J. H., Rini, B., Ireland, J., Rayman, P., Richmond, A., Golshayan, A., Wood, L., Elson, P., Garcia, J., Dreicer, R., & Bukowski, R. (2008). Sunitinib reverses type-1 immune suppression and decreases T-regulatory cells in renal cell carcinoma patients. *Clinical Cancer Research, 14*(20), 6674–6682.
69. Lopes, A., Vandermeulen, G., & Préat, V. (2019). Cancer DNA vaccines: current preclinical and clinical developments and future perspectives. *Journal of Experimental & Clinical Cancer Research, 38*, 1–24.
70. Li, B., VanRoey, M., Wang, C., Chen, T. H. T., Korman, A., & Jooss, K. (2009). Anti–programmed death-1 synergizes with granulocyte macrophage colony-stimulating factor–secreting tumor cell immunotherapy providing therapeutic benefit to mice with established tumors. *Clinical Cancer Research, 15*(5), 1623–1634.
71. Santos, P. M., Adamik, J., Howes, T. R., Du, S., Vujanovic, L., Warren, S., Gambotto, A., Kirkwood, J. M., & Butterfield, L. H. (2020). Impact of checkpoint blockade on cancer vaccine–activated CD8+ T cell responses. *Journal of Experimental Medicine, 217*(7).
72. Duraiswamy, J., Kaluza, K. M., Freeman, G. J., & Coukos, G. (2013). Dual blockade of PD-1 and CTLA-4 combined with tumor vaccine effectively restores T-cell rejection function in tumors. *Cancer Research, 73*(12), 3591–3603.

73. Tseng, C. W., Trimble, C., Zeng, Q., Monie, A., Alvarez, R. D., Huh, W. K., Hoory, T., Wang, M. C., Hung, C. F., & Wu, T. C. (2009). Low-dose radiation enhances therapeutic HPV DNA vaccination in tumor-bearing hosts. *Cancer Immunology, Immunotherapy, 58*, 737–748.
74. Jeon, Y. H., Choi, Y., Kim, H. J., Kim, C. W., Jeong, J. M., Lee, D. S., & Chung, J. K. (2007). Human sodium iodide symporter gene adjunctive radiotherapy to enhance the preventive effect of hMUC1 DNA vaccine. *International Journal of Cancer, 121*(7), 1593–1599.
75. Puzanov, I., Milhem, M. M., Andtbacka, R. H. I., Minor, D. R., Hamid, O., Li, A., Chastain, M., Gorski, K., Anderson, A., Vanderwalde, A. M., & Chou, J. (2014). Primary analysis of a phase 1b multicenter trial to evaluate safety and efficacy of talimogene laherparepvec (T-VEC) and ipilimumab (ipi) in previously untreated, unresected stage IIIB-IV melanoma.
76. Gao, Y., Whitaker-Dowling, P., Griffin, J. A., Barmada, M. A., & Bergman, I. (2009). Recombinant vesicular stomatitis virus targeted to Her2/neu combined with anti-CTLA4 antibody eliminates implanted mammary tumors. *Cancer Gene Therapy, 16*(1), 44–52.
77. Snyder, A., Makarov, V., Merghoub, T., Yuan, J., Zaretsky, J. M., Desrichard, A., Walsh, L. A., Postow, M. A., Wong, P., Ho, T. S., & Hollmann, T. J. (2014). Genetic basis for clinical response to CTLA-4 blockade in melanoma. *New England Journal of Medicine, 371*(23), 2189–2199.
78. Cunha, L. L., Marcello, M. A., Rocha-Santos, V., & Ward, L. S. (2017). Immunotherapy against endocrine malignancies: immune checkpoint inhibitors lead the way. *Endocrine-Related Cancer, 24*(12), T261–T281.
79. Ahrends, T., Bąbała, N., Xiao, Y., Yagita, H., Van Eenennaam, H., & Borst, J. (2016). CD27 agonism plus PD-1 blockade recapitulates CD4+ T-cell help in therapeutic anticancer vaccination. *Cancer Research, 76*(10), 2921–2931.
80. Liu, X., Yang, Y., Zheng, X., Liu, M., & Wang, G. (2023). Enhancedanti-tumor efficacy through a combination of intramuscularly expressed DNA vaccine and plasmid-encoded PD-1 antibody. *Frontiers in Immunology, 14*, 1169850.
81. Overgaard, N. H., Fan, T. M., Schachtschneider, K. M., Principe, D. R., Schook, L. B., & Jungersen, G. (2018). Of mice, dogs, pigs, and men: choosing the appropriate model for immuno-oncology research. *ILAR Journal, 59*(3), 247–262.
82. Sahin, U., Derhovanessian, E., Miller, M., Kloke, B. P., Simon, P., Löwer, M., Bukur, V., Tadmor, A. D., Luxemburger, U., Schrörs, B., & Omokoko, T. (2017). Personalized RNA mutanome vaccines mobilize poly-specific therapeutic immunity against cancer. *Nature, 547*(7662), 222–226.
83. Cheever, M. A., Allison, J. P., Ferris, A. S., Finn, O. J., Hastings, B. M., Hecht, T. T., Mellman, I., Prindiville, S. A., Viner, J. L., Weiner, L. M., & Matrisian, L. M. (2009). The prioritization of cancer antigens: a national cancer institute pilot project for the acceleration of translational research. *Clinical Cancer Research, 15*(17), 5323–5337.
84. Alarcon, J. B., Waine, G. W., & McManus, D. P. (1999). DNA vaccines: technology and application as anti-parasite and anti-microbial agents. *Advances in Parasitology, 42*, 343–410.
85. Khan, F. H., & Khan, F. (2009). *The elements of immunology*. Pearson Education India.

86. Kindt, T. J., Goldsby, R. A., & Osborne, B. A. (2007). *Kuby Immunology* (pp. 475–92). W.H Freeman and Co.
87. Sasaki, S., Takeshita, F., Xin, K. Q., Ishii, N., & Okuda, K. (2003). Adjuvant formulations and delivery systems for DNA vaccines. *Methods, 31*(3), 243–254.
88. Sun, Y., Hu, Y. H., Liu, C. S., & Sun, L. (2010). Construction and analysis of an experimental Streptococcus iniae DNA vaccine. *Vaccine, 28*(23), 3905–3912.
89. Fowler, V. L., & Barnett, P. V. (2012). Progress in the development of DNA vaccines against foot-and-mouth disease. *Expert Review of Vaccines, 11*(4), 481–493.
90. Rezaei, T., Davoudian, E., Khalili, S., Amini, M., Hejazi, M., de la Guardia, M., & Mokhtarzadeh, A. (2021). Strategies in DNA vaccine for melanoma cancer. *Pigment Cell & Melanoma Research, 34*(5), 869–891.
91. Stachyra, A., Góra-Sochacka, A., & Sirko, A. (2014). DNA vaccines against influenza. *Acta Biochimica Polonica, 61*(3), 515–522.
92. Li, L., & Petrovsky, N. (2016). Molecular mechanisms for enhanced DNA vaccine immunogenicity. *Expert Review of Vaccines, 15*(3), 313–329.
93. Anderson, R. J., & Schneider, J. (2007). Plasmid DNA and viral vector-based vaccines for the treatment of cancer. *Vaccine, 25*, B24–B34.

CHAPTER 7

Innovative DNA Vaccines that Utilize Pinpoint Precision Technology to Effectively Stimulate the Immune System Against Cancer

ABSTRACT

In recent years, DNA vaccines have emerged as a prominent and innovative approach for generating an effective immune response against cancer. Gene-based vaccines possess an inherent appeal owing to their exceptional molecular precision, which enables the intentional incorporation of supplementary genes to augment their protective efficacy. However, the initial sense of positivity was replaced by the seemingly enormous challenge of effectively translating encouraging preclinical results into tangible clinical advancements. Fortunately, recent advancements in the field of delivery techniques, particularly electroporation, have provided a pathway for addressing the challenges associated with translation. This chapter explores the origins, present achievements, and limitless possibilities of DNA vaccines in the field of cancer treatment, indicating a forthcoming era characterized by accurate and effective stimulation of the immune system.

7.1 INTRODUCTION

Traditional vaccinations were designed with a limited understanding of immune systems to protect people from illness. The efficacy of the

DNA- and m-RNA-Based Vaccines: An Immunotherapeutic Approach to Cancer.
Sonali Sundram and Rishabha Malviya (Authors)

DOI: 10.1201/9781774919613-7

treatment was measured by a decrease in the incidence of infection with minimum adverse effects. These challenges persist for modern preventive vaccinations, which are needed for more complex infectious species, but they can be overcome, thanks to advances in immunology and new technological developments [1]. The vaccination for recombinant virus-like particles against human papillomavirus is an example of this.

The elimination of persistent infections and the defeat of malignant tumors are further targets. The therapeutic value of passive immunotherapy in the management of cancer has been established. Antibody treatment (including anti-CD20 antibodies for tumors originating in B cells [2] and antibodies targeting HER-2s (also known as ERBB2) for some cases of breast cancer [3]. and the use of transplanted CD8+ T lymphocytes to initiate a graft-versus-leucemia-like activity against tumor cells after allotransplantation [4, 5], are two such examples. To this end, active vaccination seeks to both activate and strengthen preexisting immune effector pathways, and immunological memory to enable long-term surveillance for the emergence of new cancer cells.

Potential antigens are typically very mildly immunogenic, except for malignancies related to viruses being an exception. Genomics and proteomics studies on cancer cells uncover novel target antigens all the time, making generalizations about their nature problematic. Antigens that are unique to tumors or that are commonly found in tumors have been the primary focus of research thus far. Cancer-testis antigens are ideal for recognizing tumors [6] and identifying cancers [7] because they are exclusively found in cancer cells' expression.

Many tumor-associated antigens are derived from normal cells, making their origins and cancer presence transparent. Tumor-associated antigens refer to molecules or proteins that are typically present in normal cells but exhibit abnormal expression or increased levels in cancerous cells. The antigens in question may encompass self-antigens, which are constituents of the organism's own tissues. The significance of their origin from normal cells highlights their pivotal function in the field of cancer immunology [8].

While tumor antigens typically possess immunogenic properties, they may still induce only a restricted degree of self-protection. There are obvious clinical cases in which this reaction is advantageous for tumor management [9] despite the difficulty of investigating it. On the other hand, tolerance might develop as a result of a natural reaction in certain situations. Immune activity is limited and controlled by this natural regulatory system, although vaccinations may be impeded by this system. Tumor infiltrates include regulatory T lymphocytes, which play a role in peripheral tolerance [10, 11]. Antibodies and immunomodulatory drugs are already being used in the clinic to counteract their negative impact on cancer immunity while avoiding unwanted autoimmunity [12, 13]. A possible reason for tumor cells to downregulate their expression of MHC class I and target antigens is indicative of immune system recognition. Cancer cells may stimulate regulatory T-cell activity by creating a tolerogenic milieu that extends to draining lymph nodes. Vaccines must combine ingredients to overcome the difficulties of successfully reversing tolerance and inducing effective immunity [14, 15].

Cancer patients who are in remission and have enough immunological function are great candidates for vaccination. To be effective, a vaccination must activate both innate immunity and specific immunological effector responses, even in this situation. It is possible to combine numerous genes that code for various immunostimulatory molecules into vaccination vectors using DNA fusion gene technology, which may be done within the vector of the vaccination itself, or through a different vector. It is possible to give a wide variety of compounds capable of modulating immune responses. These molecules are antigen-presenting-cell-attracting chemokines [16, 17], cytokine activators [18], costimulatory molecules, antibody targets, and chemicals that change antigen presentation and/or processing [19]. Cell-to-cell protein transfer is facilitated by virus-derived molecules, such as VP22 [20], even though the underlying mechanisms at play are not fully known at this time [21]. Molecules that break down barriers of tolerance are ideal, but since the immune system's job is to fight diseases, they have relied on activating the immune system with foreign antigens instead. Anti-tumor DNA antigens may be delivered in a variety of molecular forms; peptides of varying lengths (from full-length sequences to brief MHC class I- or II-binding peptides) can stimulate T-cell responses. The process of identifying a specific site where an effector antibody or T cell can do its job is straightforward for "liquid" tumors like leukemia but for less accessible solid tumors it is harder. Immune responses in patients may be assessed in pilot clinical trials using a combination of a DNA vaccination that delivers a particular antigen and improved objective tests for assessing specific immune responses. The effectiveness of this vaccination vehicle will be tested in larger clinical studies, which will evaluate whether immune responses are connected to clinical outcomes. Designing a DNA vaccine that can make use of immunological information gained from preclinical models is the subject of this chapter, which will examine how well DNA vaccines function when tested on actual cancer patients.

As long as the full-length sequence necessary to elicit an antibody response is provided by the DNA, tumor antigens may be delivered in any acceptable molecular form for optimal stimulation of T-cell responses. For "liquid" tumors like leukemia, the effector antibody or T cells only need to be activated once; however, finding their target might be problematic in the case of less accessible solid tumors. Translating preclinical findings into human trials has necessitated the development of innovative delivery technologies. DNA vaccines that deliver specific encoded antigens and sophisticated objective testing to generate unique immune reactions in patients are used together in pilot clinical studies to assess vaccine efficacy. Larger trials will be conducted to learn more about the efficacy and safety of this vaccine vehicle. As a result of advances made in preclinical models, immunological information gleaned from DNA vaccine designs is now being put to the ultimate test in clinical trials involving cancer patients.

7.2 DEVELOPING DNA-BASED FUSION GENE VACCINES

DNA-based fusion gene vaccines are an innovative strategy within the field of vaccine development. The development of these novel vaccines involves the construction of fusion genes that combine genetic sequences from various antigens or target molecules. The fusion gene that is produced encodes a chimeric protein that has the ability to enhance the immune response by incorporating multiple antigenic regions, leading to a more comprehensive and robust immune response [22]. The procedure generally entails a meticulous selection of antigens linked to the specific pathogen of interest, the design of a fusion gene, the construction of a plasmid to serve as a carrier for the genetic material, and the production of the DNA vaccine for subsequent administration. Following the introduction of the DNA plasmid, the host cells undergo internalization, resulting in the subsequent synthesis of the chimeric protein and the commencement of an immune reaction. DNA-based fusion gene vaccines possess the advantageous characteristic of adaptability, as they can be customized to specifically target an extensive variety of pathogens [23, 24]. Furthermore, these vaccines have demonstrated considerable potential in conferring durable immunity against infectious diseases. This emerging field has great potential to improve vaccine technology and infectious disease control.

7.3 INTRACELLULAR TRANSLOCATION OF EXPRESSED ANTIGENS

The intracellular translocation of expressed antigens is a complex and essential process in the field of immunology. It is essential to the immune system's ability to recognize and react to foreign invaders, including infections and damaged cells. This process initiates immune responses by presenting antigens and is essential to the adaptive immune system, which protects against infections and cancer. Intracellular translocation begins with the production of antigenic proteins within the host cells. Pathogens like viruses and bacteria or cancer cells may have these proteins as tumor-specific antigens. These antigens must be transported to specific cellular compartments for processing and presentation to immune cells to be recognized by the immune system [24]. The expressed antigen is transported throughout the cell by this method. Adding genes to DNA vaccines can change how antigens are transported within cells, which can then lead to a different immune response. Peptide-specific CD8+ T-cell responses are induced when antigens enter the cytosol and are degraded by the proteasome. Antigens that enter the endoplasmic reticulum (ER), where folding and first glycosylation occur, are thought to be more effective at inducing an antibody response [25]. Incorporating a leader sequence that guides the protein to its final location in the ER may improve antibody induction. There is evidence that using a leader sequence to target proteins for import into the ER can increase CD8+ T-cell responses [26]. Reverse protein transport from the ER into cells is likely to blame for this [27]. In light of this, have decided to include a leader sequence in all of the designs [28]. A wide variety of intracellular locations have been targeted, with varying degrees of success, including the proteasome and the lysosomal-endosomal route. The first step toward gaining entry to the APC is deciphering the encoded antigen [29]. Cross-presentation, potentially through apoptotic cell debris, is the most probable main pathway from muscle locations [30]. The antigen may still be cross presented from keratinocytes even at skin regions where an application of gene guns is to transport DNA to Langerhans cells for direct antigen presentation [31].

7.4 TRANSMISSION OF ANTIGEN TO SKILLED APC

The transfer of antigens to proficient antigen-presenting cells (APCs) is an important phase in the immune response. Specialized APCs, including dendritic cells, macrophages, and B cells, possess the ability to effectively capture, process, and present antigens in order to initiate immune system activation [32]. Antigens can be transferred to these APCs through diverse mechanisms, encompassing phagocytosis, endocytosis, or direct uptake. Upon entering the APC, antigens undergo a process of fragmentation into smaller peptide fragments. These fragments are subsequently bound to major histocompatibility complex (MHC) molecules. The MHC-antigen complex is subsequently displayed on the cellular membrane to facilitate recognition by T cells, thereby initiating the adaptive immune response. The effective delivery of antigens to proficient APCs is crucial for the immune system to accurately identify and mount a robust response against various pathogens and foreign entities, ultimately resulting in immune protection and the establishment of immunological memory [33]. Intramuscular injection of the produced protein, which serves as an antigen stored in DNA vaccines, is the most popular method of administering them. If a protein is released, it may stimulate the body to make more antibodies and cytotoxic T lymphocytes. Given their possibility of elevating the expression of major MHC class I antigens and co-stimulatory molecules as well as cytokine and chemokine production, their possible future function in immune activation is shown. However, it has been proven *in vivo* with vaccines that exogenous immunization is necessary for a robust immune response [34, 35] (Figure 7.1). Since CD8+ T-cell responses are often derived from intracellular antigens and hence are not predicted to be induced in this way, it is believed that antibody and CD4+ T-cell responses are the most effective form of immune system response. However, a recently characterized mechanism has lately been exposed, which indicates that phagosomal material may merge with ER-derived vesicles to enter the MHC class I loading compartment [36]. Because phagosomal breakdown is limited by pH in dendritic cells (DC), it seems that this route is well-suited for DCs [37, 38]. One reason for the effective activation of a similar mechanism of the observed increase in CD8+ T-cell response after intramuscular DNA injection can be explained by the activity of apoptotic vesicles released from transfected muscle cells [33].

After DNA injection, the ratio of antigen cross-presentation to direct presentation has been difficult to establish until recently. Vaccine design may now be manipulated to limit antigen presentation presented either diagonally or head-on by the APC [34]. Vaccine efficacy may be improved by varying the amount and kinetics of the immune response.

7.5 CD4+ T-CELL SUPPORT

CD4+ T-cell support, commonly known as helper T-cell support, plays an essential part in the adaptive immune response. The T cells possess the ability to identify antigens that are presented by APCs. Upon being activated, they undergo differentiation into various subsets, such as Th1 and Th2 cells, each exhibiting unique functions and responsibilities. T-helper 1 (Th1) cells play a crucial role in enhancing the immune response against intracellular pathogens, whereas T-helper 2 (Th2) cells primarily support immune responses directed toward extracellular threats. CD4+ T cells play a crucial role in the establishment of immune memory, thereby rendering them indispensable in the context of vaccine-induced immune responses. The comprehension and utilization of CD4+ T-cell assistance play a crucial role in the development of immunotherapies and vaccines [39]. The depletion of these cells, as evidenced in conditions such as HIV/AIDS, significantly compromises the immune system's capacity to effectively respond to various threats, highlighting their fundamental significance in immune regulation and safeguarding.

When it comes to inducing and maintaining immunological memory, the CD4+ T helper (TH) cells are essential. Regulatory T cells may potentially turn against the body's natural defenses [40–43]. The failure of short peptide vaccinations to produce CD8+ indicates that T cells' inability to stimulate their complementary TH cells is to blame for this phenomenon. In highly immunogenic tumors, anti-CD40 antibodies may be able to fill in for missing TH cells; however, activation of CD40 alone appears to be insufficient to stimulate CD8+ T cells [44], and CD40 is just one of many activating molecule cells in a tolerant environment [45, 46]. Similar dependence on TH cells is also seen in human CD8+ T-cell clones that have been adopted and transplanted against HIV [47]. For CD8+ T lymphocytes to proliferate in a homeostatic manner, they need to be shielded from apoptosis by TH cells [48]. Interleukin 2 (IL2) likely contributes to the way CD4+ T cells impact CD8+ T cell programming for secondary expansion [49]. Upon further stimulation in the absence of TH cells, "helpless" CD8+ T cells die of activation-induced cell death [50]. CD8+ memory T cells, however, do not appear to be self-renewing once activated to need ongoing maintenance from antigen-specific TH [51].

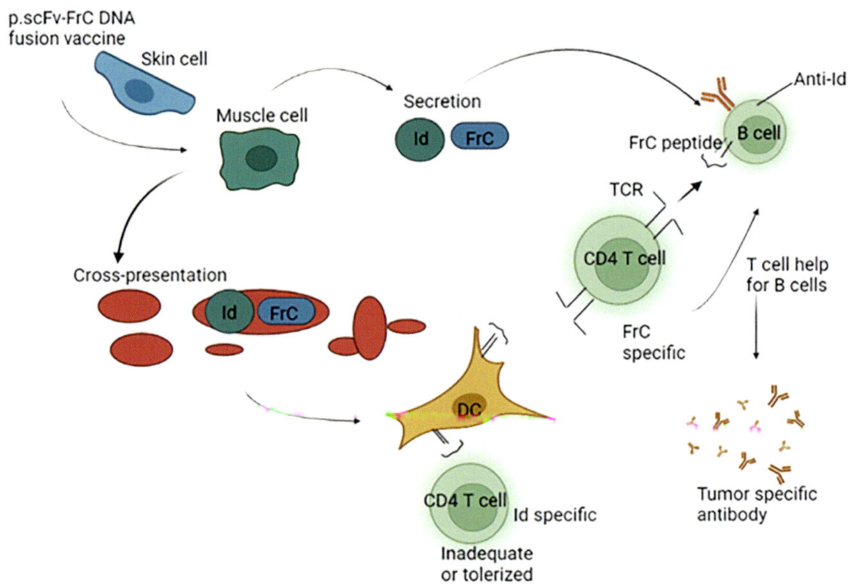

FIGURE 7.1 DNA fusion vaccine has the potential to protect against B-cell lymphoma.

Investigators have successfully stimulated T cells by introducing sequences from the tetanus toxin into the same vector as the tumor antigen. The innovative methodology employed in this study has resulted in the immune system efficiently initiating an attack on the tumor antigen, capitalizing on a wide range of antimicrobial reactions. These sequences combine to use the immune system's memory of past tetanus exposure to better recognize and target tumor cells, resulting in a more potent and comprehensive anti-tumor immune response. This approach demonstrates the potential of integrating pathogen-derived elements with tumor antigens to improve the immune system's response to cancer [52, 53]. Fusion gene vaccines are meant to assist B cells in making antibodies or to help CD8+ T lymphocytes train themselves to kill tumor cells, depending on the target antigen. There have also been attempts to fuse nonself antigens with DNA vaccines, for example, Pseudomonas exotoxin [54], proteins found in the viral coats of plants (including green fluorescent protein [52, 53]. While their mechanisms of action may vary, all of these antigens are not self and contain the ability to stimulate the necessary beneficial T lymphocytes. Immune-targeting molecules may be fused to antigens as another way to boost immunity [19,55]. Activating TH cells may be a desirable side effect of identifying them as non-self-antigens, despite their obvious importance in and of themselves. It's possible that DNA vaccines encoding xenoantigens because of the shared idea of TH cell activation [56, 57], using heterologous antigens (human antigens in preclinical murine models, and vice versa for clinical trials) can generate immunity against the equivalent autologous antigens. The use of a human tyrosine-encoded experimental vaccine on dogs with malignant melanoma has been provisionally approved [56, 58]. Different MHC class II-binding sequences may affect the ability of the foreign sequences to make activating peptides, making it impossible to anticipate whether or not the xenogeneic sequences will yield TH-activating sequences. The CD8+ T-cell response seems to be the most difficult to induce [59]. In theory, once "helped" T cells are generated, they can go after tumor cells on their own. A vaccination that generates tumor-specific CD4+ T lymphocytes, which may be crucial for interferon entrance to solid tumors, is available for recurrent immunizations [59, 60].

7.6 ANTIBODY PRODUCTION TARGETING TUMORS

Cancer cell surface molecules are already being targeted by passive antibodies [61]. Ig produced by lymphoma cells is of unknown identity and was one of the first antibodies to demonstrate the approach's effectiveness [62]. There were therapeutic results from anti-Id antibodies, both polyclonal and monoclonal, but the difficulty of making antibodies that are specific to a given patient dampened enthusiasm [63, 64]. This difficulty is avoided with DNA vaccines since Id determinants may be produced either as a full Ig or as a solitary chain Fv (scFv) by utilizing the variable region genes (Figure 7.2). The scFv sequence, on the other hand, was not very immunogenic on its own [65, 66].

Improved immune response and protection against lymphoma were achieved by fusing a high amount of anti-Id antibodies generated by combining a fragment of tetanus toxin (FrC) with the scFv [66, 67]. (Figure 7.2). Immune responses to low-abundance tumor antigens may be stimulated by employing FrC-specific TH cells, a notion that has been well-established in immunology (Figure 7.3). Expression of a fusion protein made up of Id and FrC is secreted and made possible by the leader sequence, although antigen cross-presentation may occur as well [26, 66]. Anti-FrC TH cells may promote the development of anti-Id B cells by co-presenting FrC peptides on their surface, which is significant (Figure 7.3).

scFv and FrC must thus be related [66, 67]. Antigen provided by the DC activates anti-Id B cells that present FrC peptides to the CD4+ T cell that can identify FrCs. Cytokine production and the CD40-CD40 ligand interaction are related and contribute to the development of anti-Id antibodies. If you think of it as a ruse to get the immune system's attention, this is it. It seems that TH cells are crucial for both priming the B-cell response and maintaining memory B cells [68].

Fusion to FrC or other non-self-antigens may improve the efficacy of DNA immunization against a wide variety of tumor antigens [69]. Patients with follicular lymphoma have been given the scFv-FrC vaccine, and the results have been encouraging. Most patients also experienced adverse reactions to FrC. This is encouraging because previous attempts to treat human patients with nucleic acid alone have failed.

7.7 GENERATE TUMOR-KILLING T LYMPHOCYTES

Cytotoxic CD8+ T lymphocytes' (CTL) function in tumor cell recognition and destruction cannot be overstated. However, the bulk of many tumor antigens are located within cells, where they can only be recognized by surface MHC class I molecules. While antibodies remain active for a long time, infection- or vaccination-induced CTLs grow in number, but eventually die off, leaving just a limited memory population that can respond to the next threat. As a result, immunization is aimed at inducing the maintenance of a memory population and the activation of effector CTL, both of which can increase in number as the malignancy progresses. It needs TH cells [70], and FrC from tetanus toxin [71] is again being used to produce this [72]. The huge number of FrC-specific TH cells is thought to be that TH cells help CD8+ and CD4+ T cells develop by "licensing"

DC70 via the association of ligand-receptor pairs and regional cytokines (Figure 7.2). DCs licensed to present FrC and tumor antigen peptides may thus remain active and resistant to CTL assault, allowing priming and enhancing the response to weak tumor antigens.

To be sure, the immune system's normal CTL responses to infection concentrate on a limited number of immunodominant peptides [73, 74]. Accordingly, it may be crucial to limit the activity of cross-reactive CTL that can cause harm by targeting autoantigens. Competition between dominant CTLs tends to dampen responses to subdominant epitopes, immunodominance is most apparent during priming. As a result, all polyepitope "string of beads" vaccines will likely be less effective at eliciting a universal Inflammatory CD8+ T-cell response. This holds for both mouse and human cell responses [75, 76], demonstrating that the CTL response cannot be expected to function properly unless all epitopes are of comparable strength and target the immunodominant ones. Using the polyepitope design, it is still feasible to elicit antibody production or another type of immunological reaction CD4+ T-cell. Potentially competing with tumor-derived peptides in the fusion gene vaccination strategy are peptides in the FrC that interact with MHC class I. Rather than leaving FrC as a multidomain protein, shrinking it down to a single domain (DOM 1) can still help T cells but is less likely to create competing peptides [35, 77]. The complete tumor sequence can be analyzed and given as potential target epitopes if the full-length antigen is fused to DOM 1. Vaccination with the full-length antigen might, in theory, shield all MHC class I and class II haplotypes in humans. The diagram below illustrates the idea and is presently being researched. However, it seems that moving the target peptide further from the backbone sequence has an extra benefit. It comes as no surprise that substantial quantities of CTL are required to prevent tumor development [78]. To ensure that the tumor-derived peptide has the maximum chance of dominating the CD8+ T-cell response, the sequence encoding the peptide at the 3' terminus of FrC DOM [79]. It has been demonstrated that the pDOM-epitope combination can induce peptide-specific CD8+ T-cell responses in a wide variety of animal species. Examples include its ability to stimulate CD8+ T-cell responses to male HY antigens in mice, hence disrupting tolerance in these animals [80]. As of right now, a pDOM-epitope is used in the diagnostic process for men with prostate cancer. Prostate-specific membrane antigen peptide is encoded by this pDOM-epitope. There are just two potential flaws with this idea, which is a huge plus. About 40%

of the Caucasian population possesses the MHC class I haplotype (HLA-A*0201), making them eligible to receive peptide vaccinations and other peptide-based vaccines. However, with the discovery of peptides that bind to different class I haplotypes, the approach can be applied to a wider variety of peptides. The second possibility is that the target peptide might be lost in the tumor, allowing the cancer to survive. One way to get around this is to create a second vaccination that has an epitope from a different protein or a different part of the same protein. To prevent the negative selection of the immunodominant peptides, this would be supplied at a different location [81]. Immunity may be activated against subdominant peptides, where tolerance may be lower, if this were possible.

7.8 DNA VACCINE MECHANISM

DNA vaccines are commonly delivered via intramuscular or intradermal routes of administration. Both muscle and skin cells have the capacity to accumulate antigens, but they lack the ability to initiate immune responses. The immunogenicity of DNA vaccines is influenced by a minimum of three distinct mechanisms. The presentation of antigenic peptides to CD8 T cells is facilitated by MHC class I molecules [82]. In intramuscular administration, muscle cells absorb most of the vaccine. Plasmid DNA that was fluorescently labeled and internalized by muscle cells in close proximity to the site of injection was subsequently expressed by cells situated along the muscles and in the draining lymph nodes for a duration of several hours. Proteins that have been synthesized undergo secretion or release into the extracellular matrix. Shedlock and Weiner [83] compared DNA vaccine uptake and expression in somatic cells to the virus life cycle. The proteins present within the extracellular matrix undergo endocytosis. The accepted manuscript states that antigens can be processed and presented by APCs using MHC class II molecules. In the presence of costimulatory signals, the CD4 T helper cells that bind antigenic peptides become activated. These cells, depending on their subtype (Th1 or Th2), then activate either cellular or humoral immune responses [83]. B cells that have been activated undergo differentiation and transform into plasma cells, which subsequently release antibodies that specifically bind to antigenic epitopes. The antigenic peptides that persist within the cytoplasm of the target cells are initially presented through major MHC class I molecules, subsequently stimulating cytotoxic CD8 T cells. The introduction of the vaccine via intradermal administration results in the infiltration of DNA into the skin, where dendritic cells, including Langerhans cells, play a crucial role in presenting antigens. Förg and colleagues conducted an investigation into the viability of skeletal muscle, dermis of the abdominal skin, and the ear pinna as potential sites for injection.

7.9 ELECTROPORATION AND VACCINE ADMINISTRATION

Electroporation, an innovative methodology employed in vaccine delivery, serves to augment the absorption and efficacy of DNA-based vaccines. Initially, a DNA vaccine is injected into the target tissue, such as the skin or muscle, in this procedure. Electroporation devices with electrodes are then used to deliver controlled electrical pulses to the injection site. In primates, including humans, DNA vaccines have had a somewhat modest early performance. Particle-mediated administration both of which are implemented via gene gun technology topically, have also been investigated as possible solutions [84]. The pulses transiently enhance the permeability of the cell membrane, thereby facilitating the uptake of the genetic material of the vaccine into the cells of the host. After entering the body, the genetic material contained in the vaccine is processed and then translated into protein antigens, which effectively initiates a robust immune response. The advantages of electroporation are that it can increase the immunogenicity of vaccines, potentially requiring lower doses, extending the duration of protection, and broadening its applicability to various diseases. Low DNA dosages make this ideal for vaccinations that need to be delivered quickly and easily, such as preventative immunizations against infectious illnesses. Seroprotective antibody levels were seen in a recent experiment against the influenza virus [84], and other clinical studies have shown it to be effective. Comparing delivery strategies for cancer vaccines is critically required since there have been few investigations on this method. A fundamental cause for the poor performance in big animals of the intramuscular route has finally been uncovered [85]. The amount of injection was previously apparent from mouse models. In mice, injections of 50 l produce robust immunological responses that progressively wane with decreasing volume. The hydrostatic pressure is likely to produce enough local damage to enhance infection and lead to inflammation. Because it would be inappropriate to have a ratio of 50 l in mice to 100 l in humans, a different strategy was needed.

The prime-boost procedures used in human patients with a vaccine against malaria [86] provided some clues as to what this may be. Naked DNA could not be used to amplify results primed with naked DNA according to one research. Contrast this to using a viral vector to enhance the same gene [86, 87], which resulted in positive results A variety of prime-boost techniques using various viral or bacterial vectors were developed as a result [88]. Using a virus as a vector is thought to increase antigen levels and generate local inflammation, which helps activate the immune system is anticipated to have a role at the time of boost [89, 90]. Even while this strategy has merits for preventative although this is good for most vaccines, it may not be the best choice for cancer vaccines because repeated vaccinations are expected to be required to maintain continuous immunological pressure on a developing tumor [91–93]. The utilization of specialized equipment and the application of expertise are crucial factors in the effective implementation of electroporation, which exhibits significant potential in the advancement of DNA-based vaccine technology. This technology has the capacity to enhance our capabilities in addressing infectious diseases and various other health-related challenges.

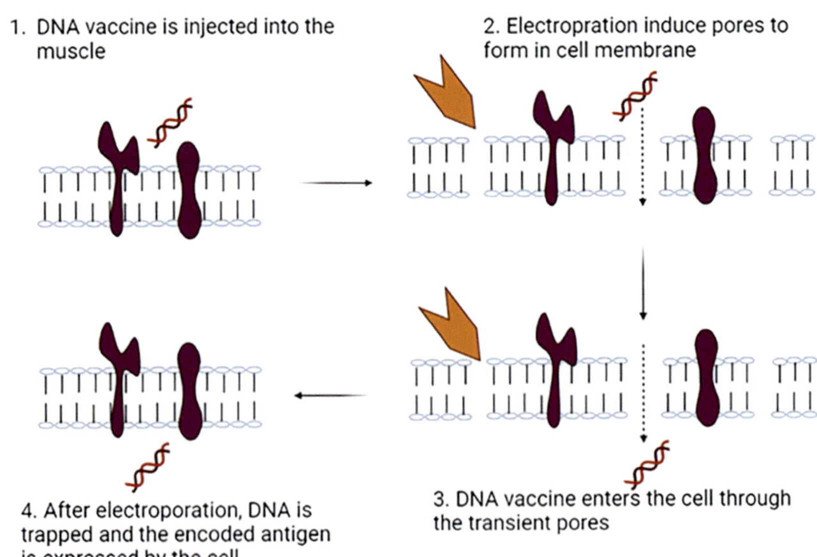

FIGURE 7.2 Electroporation as a model for the mechanism of vaccine delivery.

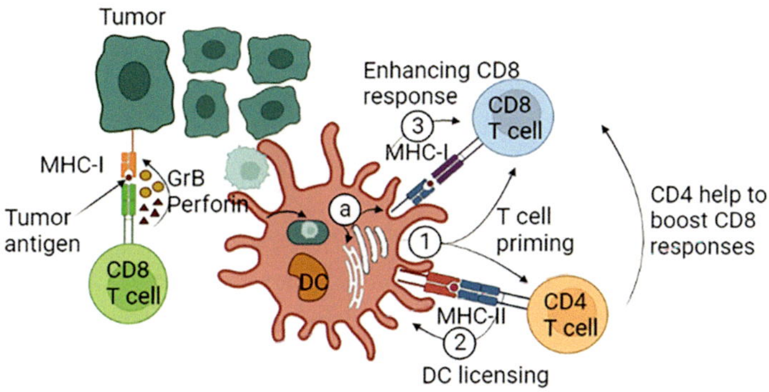

FIGURE 7.3 T-cells have a role in stimulating the body's natural defenses against tumors [95].

Liposomes, microparticles, polymers, nanoparticles, and tattoos are just a few of the physical ways being investigated to overcome this problem [96]. Electroporation (EP) stimulates muscles with generator pulses after DNA-based vaccine injection, a promising technique with a clear clinical path. This procedure temporarily increases cell membrane permeability, allowing for efficient uptake of the vaccine's genetic material. The application of electrical pulses induces the formation of temporary pores within the cells, thereby facilitating the transportation and subsequent activation of vaccine DNA. Consequently, this process elicits a robust and enduring immune response. This methodology signifies a substantial progression in the field of vaccine technology and holds promise for enhancing the durability and effectiveness of immune protection against an extensive array of ailments [97–99]. As a result of increased transfection efficiency, the method enhances antigen expression, which is associated with localized tissue injury and inflammation [100]. The end effect is a boost in immunological responses, both cellular and humoral [85, 101–103].

For mice and other big animals, such as rhesus macaques, EP is effective even when low-volume injection has previously failed to induce immunity [85, 104]. Antibody responses induced by DNA priming followed by an EP boost may be on par with those induced by the protein and increased CTL responses in Complete Freund's Adjuvant [104]. Even though high transfection efficiency increases integration levels, they are still rather small [105]. Prostate cancer patients' DNA vaccines, which use a prime-boost combination like that found with viral vectors, are currently undergoing clinical testing [106]. The patients have had several EPs without requiring general or regional anesthetics and have been proven to have no ill effects on the patient in the long run. For the first time, DNA vaccinations are being tested in humans, and various studies are taking place on infectious illnesses and cancer.

7.10 CONCLUSIONS AND FUTURE DIRECTION

As medical research has advanced, the capacity to modify genes has made it possible to construct gene-based vaccinations. Experts in cancer and infectious illness have come together to work toward a common goal: using immunity to fight against difficult foes. There are two DNA vaccines on the market that have been approved so far and are meant to protect against infectious organisms that are found in fish and horses while early optimism for cancer vaccine clinical trials is encouraging, evolved to dismay as promising vaccine designs from preclinical models seemed to fail to transfer into human participants. EP, a method that has been used effectively *in vitro* to increase transfection, may be able to overcome the delivery of DNA issues. Optimizing vaccine development, enhancing immune recruitment and activation, and identifying optimal antigen targets are all priorities that must be addressed. The primary goal has been to alter the antigen's molecular structure and activate T cells to cause an extreme immunological response to develop and reverse tolerance. Then again, there are a slew of new immunological techniques worth exploring. New and growing regulatory constraints are more likely to be the stumbling block since they hold down the necessary pilot clinical studies meant to evaluate effectiveness. The key to success is a strong connection between the laboratory and the clinic, along with an eye toward the future. To rapidly evaluate novel vaccine designs and delivery systems for cancer suppression, these three components must all be present simultaneously.

KEYWORDS

- **CD4+**
- **DNA**
- **fusion gene**
- **T cell**
- **vaccines**

REFERENCES

1. Stanley, M. (2007). Prophylactic HPV vaccines. *Journal of Clinical Pathology, 60*(9), 961–965.
2.. Maloney, D. G., Liles, T. M., Czerwinski, D. K., Waldichuk, C., Rosenberg, J., Grillo-Lopez, A., & Levy, R. (1994). Phase I clinical trial using escalating single-dose infusion of chimeric anti-CD20 monoclonal antibody (IDEC-C2B8) in patients with recurrent B-cell lymphoma. *Blood, 84*(8), 2457–2466.
3. Valone, F. H., Kaufman, P. A., Guyre, P. M., Lewis, L. D., Memoli, V., Ernstoff, M. S., Wells, W., Barth, R., Deo, Y., & Fisher, J. (1995). Clinical trials of bispecific antibody MDX-210 in women with advanced breast or ovarian cancer that overexpresses HER-2/neu. *Journal of Hematotherapy, 4*(5), 471–475.
4. Goldman, J. M., Gale, R. P., Horowitz, M. M., Biggs, J. C., Champlin, R. E., Gluckman, E., Hoffmann, R. G., Jacobsen, S. J., Marmont, A. M., McGlave, P. B. (1988). Bone marrow transplantation for chronic myelogenous leukemia in chronic phase. Increased risk for relapse associated with T-cell depletion. *Annals of Internal Medicine, 108*(6), 806–814.
5. Fontaine, P., Roy-Proulx, G., Knafo, L., Baron, C., Roy, D. C., & Perreault, C. (2001). Adoptive transfer of minor histocompatibility antigen-specific T lymphocytes eradicates leukemia cells without causing graft-versushost disease. *Nature Medicine, 7*(7), 789–794.
6. George, A. J. & Stevenson, F. K. (1989). Prospects for the treatment of B cell tumors using idiotypic vaccination. *International Reviews of Immunology, 4*(4), 271–310.
7. Van Der Bruggen, P., Zhang, Y., Chaux, P., Stroobant, V., Panichelli, C., Schultz, E. S., Chapiro, J., Van Den Eynde, B. J., Brasseur, F., & Boon, T. (2002). Tumor-specific shared antigenic peptides recognized by human T cells. *Immunology Reviews, 188*, 51–64.
8. Mantovani, A., Bottazzi, B., Colotta, F., Sozzani, S., & Ruco, L. (1992). The origin and function of tumor-associated macrophages. *Immunology Today, 13*(7), 265–270.
9. Day, S. E., Kettunen, M. I., Gallagher, F. A., Hu, D. E., Lerche, M., Wolber, J., Golman, K., Ardenkjaer-Larsen, J. H., & Brindle, K. M. (2007). Detecting tumor response to treatment using hyperpolarized 13C magnetic resonance imaging and spectroscopy. *Nature Medicine, 13*(11), 1382–1387.
10. Zou, W. (2006). Regulatory T cells, tumour immunity and immunotherapy. *Nature Reviews Immunology, 6*(4), 295–307.
11. Welters, M. J., Piersma, S. J., & van der Burg, S. H. (2008). T-regulatory cells in tumour-specific vaccination strategies. *Expert Opinion on Biological Therapy, 8*(9), 1365–1379.
12. Lutsiak, M. E., Semnani, R. T., De Pascalis, R., Kashmiri, S. V. S., Schlom, J., & Sabzevari, H. (2005). Inhibition of CD4+25+ T regulatory cell function implicated in enhanced immune response by low-dose cyclophosphamide. *Blood, 105*(7), 2862–2868.
13. Phan, G. Q., Yang, J. C., Sherry, R., M., Hwu, P., Topalian, S. L., Schwartzentruber, D. J., Restifo, N. P., Haworth, L. R., Seipp, C. A., Freezer, L. J., Morton, K. E., Mavroukakis, S. A., Duray, P. H., Steinberg, S. M., Allison, J. P., Davis, T. A.,

Rosenberg, S. A. (2003). Cancer regression and autoimmunity induced by cytotoxic T lymphocyte-associated antigen 4 blockade in patients with metastatic melanoma. *Proceedings of the National Academy of Science of the United State of America, 100*(14), 8372–8377.

14. Munn, D. H., & Mellor, A. L. (2007). Indoleamine 2,3- dioxygenase and tumor-induced tolerance. *Journal of Clinical Investigation, 117*(5), 1147–1154.
15. Emens, L. A., Reilly, R. T., & Jaffee, E. M. (2005). Breast cancer vaccines: maximizing cancer treatment by tapping into host immunity. *Endocrine Related Cancer, 12*(1), 1–17.
16. Dell'Agnola, C., & Biragyn, A. (2007). Clinical utilization of chemokines to combat cancer: The double-edged sword. *Expert Review of Vaccines, 6*(2), 267–283.
17. Coscia, M., & Biragyn, A. (2004). Cancer immunotherapy with chemoattractant peptides. *Seminars in Cancer Biology, 14*(3), 209–218.
18. Calarota, S. A., & Weiner, D. B. (2004). Enhancement of human immunodeficiency virus type 1-DNA vaccine potency through incorporation of T-helper 1 molecular adjuvants. *Immunological Reviews, 199*, 84–99.
19. Paparini, D., Gori, S., Grasso, E., Scordo, W., Calo, G., Perez Leiros, C., Ramhorst, R., & Salamone, G. (2015). Acetylcholine contributes to control the physiological inflammatory response during the peri-implantation period. *Acta Physiologica, 214*(2), 237–247.
20. Pomeranz, L. E., Reynolds, A. E., & Hengartner, C. J. (2005). Molecular biology of pseudorabies virus: Impact on neurovirology and veterinary medicine. *Microbiology and Molecular Biology Reviews, 69*(3), 462–500.
21. Immordino, M. L., Dosio, F., & Cattelm, L. (2006). Stealth liposomes: Review of the basic science, rationale, and clinical applications, existing and potential. *International Journal of Nanomedicine, 1*(3), 297–315.
22. Hu, B., Tai, A., & Wang, P. (2011). Immunization delivered by lentiviral vectors for cancer and infectious diseases. *Immunological Reviews, 239*(1), 45–61.
23. McNamara, M. A., Nair, S. K., & Holl, E. K. (2015). RNA-based vaccines in cancer immunotherapy. *Journal of Immunology Research, 2015*, 794528.
24. Brodsky, F. M., & Guagliardi, L. E. (1991). The cell biology of antigen processing and presentation. *Annual Review of Immunology, 9*, 707–744.
25. Loureiro, J., & Ploegh, H. L. (2006). Antigen presentation and the ubiquitin-proteasome system in host-pathogen interactions. *Advances in Immunology*, 92, 225–305.
26. Wong, N. A., & Saier, M. H. (2021). The SARS-coronavirus infection cycle: A survey of viral membrane proteins, their functional interactions and pathogenesis. *International Journal of Molecular Sciences, 22*(3), 1308.
27. Bacik, I. Snyder, H. L., Antón, L. C., Russ, G., Chen, W., Bennink, J. R., Urge, L., Otvos, L., Dudkowska, B., Eisenlohr, L., & Yewdell, J. W. (1997). Introduction of a glycosylation site into a secreted protein provides evidence for an alternative antigen processing pathway: Transport of precursors of major histocompatibility complex class I-restricted peptides from the endoplasmic reticulum to the cytosol. *The Journal of Experimental Medicine, 186*(4), 479–487.
28. Stevenson, F. K., Ottensmeier, C. H., Johnson, P., Zhu, D., Buchan, S. L., McCann, K. J., Roddick, J. S., King, A. T., McNicholl, F., Savelyeva, N., & Rice, J. (2004). DNA

vaccines to attack cancer. *Proceedings of the National Academy of Science of the United State of America*, *101*(2), 14646– 14652.

29. Leifert, J. A., Rodriguez-Carreno, M. P., Rodriguez, F., & Whitton, J. L. (2004). Targeting plasmid-encoded proteins to the antigen presentation pathways. Immunological Reviews, *199*, 40–53.
30. Albert, M. L., Sauter, B., & Bhardwaj, N. (1998). Dendritic cells acquire antigen from apoptotic cells and induce class I-restricted CTLs. *Nature, 392*(6671), 86–89.
31. Hobernik, D., & Bros, M. (2018). DNA vaccines-how far from clinical use? *International Journal of Molecular Sciences*, *19*(11), 3605.
32. Lewis, S. M., Williams, A., & Eisenbarth, S. C. (2019). Structure and function of the immune system in the spleen. *Science Immunology*, *4*(33), eaau6085.
33. Chatterjee, F., & Spranger, S. (2023). MHC-dressing on dendritic cells: Boosting anti-tumor immunity via unconventional tumor antigen presentation. *Seminars in Immunology*, *66*, 101710. Academic Press.
34. Radcliffe, J. N., Roddick, J. S., Friedmann, P. S., Stevenson, F. K., & Thirdborough, S. M. (2006). Prime-boost with alternating DNA vaccines designed to engage different antigen presentation pathways generates high frequencies of peptide-specific CD8+ T cells. *Journal of Immunology*, *177*(10), 6626–6633.
35. Rice, J., Elliott, T., Buchan, S., & Stevenson, F. K. (2001). DNA fusion vaccine designed to induce cytotoxic T cell responses against defined peptide motifs: Implications for cancer vaccines. *Journal of Immunology, 167*(3), 1558–1565.
36. Guermonprez, P., Saveanu, L., Kleijmeer, M., Davoust, J., Van Endert, P., & Amigorena, S. (2003). ER-phagosome fusion defines an MHC class I cross-presentation compartment in dendritic cells. *Nature, 425*(6956), 397–402.
37. Villadangos, J. A., Heath, W. R., & Carbone, F. R. (2007). Outside looking in: the inner workings of the crosspresentation pathway within dendritic cells. *Trends Immunology*, *28*(2), 45–47.
38. Delamarre, L., Pack, M., Chang, H., Mellman, I., & Trombetta, E. S. (2005). Differential lysosomal proteolysis in antigen-presenting cells determines antigen fate. *Science*, *307*(5715), 1630–1634.
39. Luckheeram, R.V., Zhou, R., Verma, A. D., & Xia, B. (2012). CD4$^+$ T cells: Differentiation and functions. *Clinical and Developmental Immunology*, *2012*, 925135.
40. Shedlock, D. J., & Shen, H. (2003). Requirement for CD4 T cell help in generating functional CD8 T-cell memory. *Science, 300*(5617), 337–339.
41. Sun, J. C., & Bevan, M. J. (2003). Defective CD8 T-cell memory following acute infection without CD4 T-cell help. *Science*, *300*(5617), 339–342.
42. Janssen, E. M., Lemmens, E. E., Wolfe, T., Christen, U., von Herrath, M. G., & Schoenberger, S. P. (2003). CD4+ T cells are required for secondary expansion and memory in CD8+ T lymphocytes. *Nature, 421*(6925), 852–856.
43. Melief, C. J., Van Der Burg, S. H., Toes, R. E. M., Ossendorp, F., & Offringa, R. (2002). Effective therapeutic anticancer vaccines based on precision guiding of cytolytic T lymphocytes, *Immunological Reviews, 188*, 177–182.
44. Lu, Z., Yuan, L., Zhou, X., Sotomayor, E., Levitsky, H. I., & Pardoll, D. M. (2000). CD40-independent pathways of T cell help for priming of CD8+ cytotoxic T lymphocytes. *The Journal of Experimental Medicine*, *191*(3), 541–550.

45. Behrens, G. M., Li, M., Davey, G. M., Allison, J., Flavell, R. A., Carbone, F. R., & Heath, W. R. (2004). Helper requirements for generation of effector CTL to islet β cell antigens. *Journal of Immunology*, *172*(9), 5420–5426.
46. Hernandez, J., Aung, S., Marquardt, K., & Sherman, L. A. (2002). Uncoupling of proliferative potential and gain of effector function by CD8+ T cells responding to self-antigens. *The Journal of Experimental Medicine, 196*(3), 323–333.
47. Tan, R., Xu, X., Ogg, G. S., Hansasuta, P., Dong, T., Rostron, T., Luzzi, G., Conlon, C. P., Screaton, G. R., McMichael, A. J., & Rowland-Jones, S. (1999). Rapid death of adoptively transferred T cells in acquired immunodeficiency syndrome. *Blood, 93*(5), 1506–1510.
48. Hamilton, S. E., Wolkers, M. C., Schoenberger, S. P., & Jameson, S. C. (2006). The generation of protective memorylike CD8+ T cells during homeostatic proliferation requires CD4+ T cells. *Nature Immunology, 7*(5), 475–481.
49. Williams, M. A., Tyznik, A. J., & Bevan, M. J. (2006). Interleukin-2 signals during priming are required for secondary expansion of CD8+ memory T cells. *Nature, 441*(7095), 890–893.
50. Janssen, E. M., Droin, N. M., Lemmens, E. E, Pinkoski, M. J., Bensinger, S. J., Ehst, B. D., Griffith, T. S., Green, D. R., & Schoenberger, S. P. (2005). CD4+ T-cell help controls CD8+ T-cell memory via TRAIL-mediated activation-induced cell death. *Nature, 434*(7029), 88–93.
51. Prlic, M., Williams, M. A., & Bevan, M. J. (2007). Requirements for CD8 T-cell priming, memory generation and maintenance. *Current Opinion in Immunology, 19*(3), 315–319.
52. Ebrahimi, N., Akbari, M., Ghanaatian, M., Moghaddam, P. R., Adelian, S., Boroujeni, M. B., Yazdani, E., Ahmadi, A., & Hamblin, M. R. (2022). Development of neoantigens: From identification in cancer cells to application in cancer vaccines. *Expert Review of Vaccines*, *21*(7), 941–955.
53. Savelyeva, N., Munday, R., Spellerberg, M. B., Lomonossoff, G. P., & Stevenson, F. K. (2001). Plant viral genes in DNA idiotypic vaccines activate linked CD4+ T-cell mediated immunity against B-cell malignancies. *Nature Biotechnology*, *19*(8), 760–764.
54. Hung., C. F., Cheng, W. F., Hsu, K. F., Chai, C. Y., He, L., Ling, M., & Wu, T. C. (2001). Cancer immunotherapy using a DNA vaccine encoding the translocation domain of a bacterial toxin linked to a tumor antigen. *Cancer Research*, *61*(9), 3698–3703.
55. Stevenson, F. K., Rice, F., Ottensmeier, C. H., Thirdborough, S. M., & Zhu, D. (2004). DNA fusion gene vaccines against cancer: From the laboratory to the clinic. *Immunological Reviews*, *199*, 156–180.
56. Bergman, P. J., Camps-Palau, M. A., McKnight, J. A., Leibman, N. F., Craft, D. M., Leung, C., Liao, J., Riviere, I., Sadelain, M., Hohenhaus, A. E., Gregor, P., Houghton, A. N., Perales, M. A., & Wolchok, J. D. (2006). Development of a xenogeneic DNA vaccine program for canine malignant melanoma at the Animal Medical Center. *Vaccine*, *24*(21), 4582–4585.
57. Guevara-Patino, J. A., Turk, M. J., Wolchok, J. D., & Houghton, A. N. (2003). Immunity to cancer through immune recognition of altered self: Studies with melanoma. *Advances in Cancer Research*, *90*, 157–177.

58. Bergman, P. J., McKnight, J., Novosad, A., Charney, S., Farrelly, J., Craft, D., Wulderk, M., Jeffers, Y., Sadelain, M., Hohenhaus, A. E., Segal, N., Gregor, P., Engelhorn, M., Riviere, I., Houghton, A. N., & Wolchok, J. D. (2003). Long-term survival of dogs with advanced malignant melanoma after DNA vaccination with xenogeneic human tyrosinase: A phase I trial. *Clinial Cancer Research*, *9*(4), 1284–1290.
59. Garrett, J. T. (2007). *Peptide-based B-cell epitope vaccines targeting HER-2/neu*. The Ohio State University.
60. Wilcox, R. A., Flies, D. A., Wang, H., Tamada, K., Johnson, A. J., Pease, L. R., Rodriguez, M., Guo, Y., & Chen, L. (2002). Impaired infiltration of tumorspecific cytolytic T cells in the absence of interferon-γ despite their normal maturation in lymphoid organs during CD137 monoclonal antibody therapy. *Cancer Research, 62*(15), 4413–4418.
61. Carter, P. J. (2006). Potent antibody therapeutics by design. *Nature Reviews Immunology, 6*(5), 343–357.
62. Hamblin, T. J., Abdul-Ahad, A. K., Gordon, J., Stevenson, F. K., & Stevenson, G. T. (1980). Preliminary experience in treating lymphocytic leukaemia with antibody to immunoglobulin idiotypes on the cell surfaces. *British Journal of Cancer, 42*(4), 495–502.
63. Lowder, J. N., Meeker, T. C., Campbell, M., Garcia, C. F., Gralow, J., Miller, R. A., Warnke, R., & Levy, R. (1987). Studies on B lymphoid tumors treated with monoclonal anti-idiotype antibodies: correlation with clinical responses. *Blood, 69*(1), 199–210.
64. Timmerman, J. M., Singh, G., Hermanson, G., Hobart, P., Czerwinski, D. K., Taidi, B., Rajapaksa, R., Caspar, C. B., Van Beckhoven, A., & Levy, R. (2002). Immunogenicity of a plasmid DNA vaccine encoding chimeric idiotype in patients with B-cell lymphoma. *Cancer Research*, *62*(20), 5845–5852.
65. Stevenson, F., Zhu, K. D., King, C. A., Ashworth, L. J., Kumar, S., Thompsett, A., & Hawkins, R. E. (1995). A genetic approach to idiotypic vaccination for B cell lymphoma. *Annals of the New York Academy of Sciences*, *772*, 212–226.
66. Spellerberg, M. B., Zhu, D., Thompsett, A., King, C. A., Hamblin, T. J., & Stevenson, F. K. (1997). DNA vaccines against lymphoma: promotion of anti-idiotypic antibody responses induced by single chain Fv genes by fusion to tetanus toxin fragment, C. *Journal of Immunology 159*(4), 1885–1892.
67. King, C. A., Spellerberg, M. B., Zhu, D., Rice, J., Sahota, S. S., Thompsett, A. R., Hamblin, T. J., Radl, J., & Stevenson, F. K. (1998). DNA vaccines with single-chain Fv fused to fragment C of tetanus toxin induce protective immunity against lymphoma and myeloma. *Nature Medicine, 4*(11), 1281–1286.
68. Savelyeva, N., King, C. A., Vitetta, E. S., & Stevenson, F. K. (2005). Inhibition of a vaccine-induced anti-tumor B cell response by soluble protein antigen in the absence of continuing T cell help. *Proceedings of the National Academy of Science of the United State of America*, *102*(31), 10987–10992.
69. Padua, R. A., Larghero, J., Robin, M., Pogam, C. L., Schlageter, M. H., Muszlak, S., Fric, J., West, R., Rousselot, P., Phan, T. H., Mudde, L., Teisserenc, H., Carpentier, A. F., Kogan, S., Degos, L., Pla, M., Bishop, J. M., Stevenson, F., Charron, D., & Chomienne, C. (2003). PML-RARA-targeted DNA vaccine induces protective immunity in a mouse model of leukemia. *Nature Medicine, 9*(11), 1413–1417.

70. Smith, C. M., Wilson, N. S., Waithman, J., Villadangos, J. A., Carbone, F. R., Heath, W. R., & Belz, G. T. (2004). Cognate CD4+ T cell licensing of dendritic cells in CD8+ T cell immunity. *Nature Immunology, 5*(11), 1143–1148.
71. Gerloni, M., Castiglioni, P., & Zanetti, M. (2005). The cooperation between two CD4 T cells induces tumor protective immunity in MUC.1 transgenic mice. *Journal of Immunology*, *175*(10), 6551–6559.
72. Mueller, S. N., Jones, C. M., Stock, A. T., Suter, M., Heath, W. R., & Carbone, F. R. (2006). CD4+ T cells can protect APC from CTL-mediated elimination. *Journal of Immunology*, *176*(12), 7379–7384.
73. Yewdell, J. W., & Bennink, J. R. (1999). Immunodominance in major histocompatibility complex class I-restricted T lymphocyte responses. *Annual Reviews of Immunology, 17*, 51–88.
74. Chen, W., & McCluskey, J. (2006). Immunodominance and immunodomination: Critical factors in developing effective CD8+ T-cell-based cancer vaccines. *Advances in Cancer Research*, *95*, 203–247.
75. Le, T. T., Drane, D., Malliaros, J., Cox, J. C., Rothel, L., Pearse, M., Woodberry, T., Gardner, J., & Suhrbier, A. (2001). Cytotoxic T cell polyepitope vaccines delivered by ISCOMs. *Vaccine, 19*(32), 4669–4675.
76. Smith, S. G., Patel, P. M., Porte, J., Selby, P. J., & Jackson, A. M. (2001). Human dendritic cells genetically engineered to express a melanoma polyepitope DNA vaccine induce multiple cytotoxic T-cell responses. *Clinical Cancer Research*, *7*(12), 4253–4261.
77. Rice, J., Buchan, S., & Stevenson, F. K. (2002). Critical components of a DNA fusion vaccine able to induce protective cytotoxic T cells against a single epitope of a tumor antigen. *Journal of Immunology, 169*(7), 3908–3913.
78. Perez-Diez, A., Spiess, P. J., Restifo, N. P., Matzinger, P., & Marincola, F. M. (2002). Intensity of the vaccine-elicited immune response determines tumor clearance. *Journal of Immunology*, *168*(1), 338–347.
79. Snyder, H. L., Bacík, I., Yewdell, J. W., Behrens, T. W., & Bennink, J. R. (1998). Promiscuous liberation of MHC-class I-binding peptides from the C termini of membrane and soluble proteins in the secretory pathway. *European Journal of Immunology, 28*(4), 1339–1346.
80. Rice, J., Buchan, S., Dewchand, H., Simpson, E., & Stevenson, F. K. (2004). DNA fusion vaccines induce targeted epitope-specific CTLs against minor histocompatibility antigens from a normal or tolerized repertoire. *Journal of Immunology, 173*(7), 4492–4499.
81. Rice, J., Dunn, S., Piper, K., Buchan, S. L., Moss, P. A., & Stevenson, F. K. (2006). DNA fusion vaccines induce epitopespecific cytotoxic CD8+ T cells against human leukemia-associated minor histocompatibility antigens. *Cancer Research*, *66*(10), 5436–5442.
82. Li, L., Saade, F., & Petrovsky, N. (2012). The future of human DNA vaccines. *Journal of Biotechnology*, *162*(2–3), 171–182.
83. Shedlock, D. J., & Weiner, D. B. (2000). DNA vaccination: Antigen presentation and the induction of immunity. *Journal of Leukocyte Biology, 68*(6), 793–806.
84. Saade, F., & Petrovsky, N. (2012). Technologies for enhanced efficacy of DNA vaccines. *Expert Review of Vaccines*, *11*(2), 189–209.

85. Bolhassani, A., Safaiyan, S., & Rafati, S. (2011). Improvement of different vaccine delivery systems for cancer therapy. *Molecular Cancer*, *10*, 1–20.
86. McConkey, S. J., Reece, W. H. H., Moorthy, V. S., Webster, D., Dunachie, S., Butcher, G., Vuola, J. M., Blanchard, T. J., Gothard, P., Watkins, K., Hannan, C. M., Everaere, S., Brown, K., Kester, K. E., Cummings, J., Williams, J., Heppner, D. G., Pathan, A., Flanagan, K., Arulanantham, N., Roberts, M. T. M., Roy, M., Smith, G. L., Schneider, J., Peto, T., Sinden, R. E., Gilbert, S. C., & Hill, A. V. S. (2003). Enhanced T-cell immunogenicity of plasmid DNA vaccines boosted by recombinant modified vaccinia virus Ankara in humans. *Nature Medicine, 9*(6), 729–735.
87. Schneider, J., Gilbert, S. C., Blanchard, T. J., Hanke, T., Robson, K. J., Hannan, C. M., Becker, M., Sinden, R., Smith, G. L., & Hill, A. V. (1998). Enhanced immunogenicity for CD8+ T-cell induction and complete protective efficacy of malaria DNA vaccination by boosting with modified vaccinia virus Ankara. *Nature Medicine, 4*(4), 397–402.
88. Moore, A. C., & Hill, A. V. (2004). Progress in DNA-based heterologous prime-boost immunization strategies for malaria. *Immunological Reviews, 199*, 126–143.
89. Ramshaw, I. A., & Ramsay, A. J. (2000). The prime-boost strategy: Exciting prospects for improved vaccination. *Immunology Today, 21*(4), 163–165..
90. Zavala, F., Rodrigues, M., Rodriguez, D., Rodriguez, J. R., Nussenzweig, R. S., & Esteban, M. (2001). A striking property of recombinant poxviruses: Efficient inducers of *in vivo* expansion of primed CD8+ T cells. *Virology*, *280*(2), 155–159.
91. Kundig, T. M., Kalberer, C. P., Hengartner, H., & Zinkernagel, R. M. (1993). Vaccination with two different vaccinia recombinant viruses: Long-term inhibition of secondary vaccination. *Vaccine*, *11*(11), 1154–1158.
92. Cooney, E. L., Collier, A. C., Greenberg, P. D., Coombs, R. W., Zarling, J., Arditti, D. E., Hoffman, M. C., Hu, S. L., & Corey, L. (1991). Safety of and immunological response to a recombinant vaccinia virus vaccine expressing HIV envelope glycoprotein. *Lancet, 337*(8741), 567–572.
93. Rooney, J. F., Wohlenberg, C., Cremer, K. J., Moss, B., & Notkins, A. L. (1988). Immunization with a vaccinia virus recombinant expressing herpes simplex virus type 1 glycoprotein D: Long-term protection and effect of revaccination. *Journal of Virology*, *62*(5), 1530–1534.
94. Kaslow, D. C. (2004). A potential disruptive technology in vaccine development: Gene-based vaccines and their application to infectious diseases. *Transactions of the Royal Society of Tropical Medicine and Hygiene*, *98*(10), 593–601.
95. Alfei, F., Ho, P. C., & Lo, W. L. (2021). DCision-making in tumors governs T cell anti-tumor immunity. *Oncogene, 40*(34), 5253–5261.
96. Greenland, J. R., & Letvin, N. L. (2007). Chemical adjuvants for plasmid DNA vaccines. *Vaccine, 25*(19), 3731–3741.
97. Lofano, G., Mallett, C. P., Bertholet, S., & O'Hagan, D. T. (2020). Technological approaches to streamline vaccination schedules, progressing towards single-dose vaccines. *NPJ Vaccines*, *5*, 88.
98. Mathiesen, I. (1999). Electropermeabilization of skeletal muscle enhances gene transfer *in vivo*. *Gene Therapy*, *6*(4), 508–514.
99. Pollard, A. J., & Bijker, E. M. (2021). A guide to vaccinology: From basic principles to new developments. *Nature Reviews Immunology*, *21*(2), 83–100.

100. Ahlen, G., Söderholm, J., Tjelle, T., Kjeken, R., Frelin, L., Höglund, U., Blomberg, P., Fons, M., Mathiesen, I., & Sällberg, M. (2007). *In vivo* electroporation enhances the immunogenicity of hepatitis C virus nonstructural 3/4A DNA by increased local DNA uptake, protein expression, inflammation, and infiltration of CD3+ T cells. *Journal of Immunology, 179*(7), 4741–4753.
101. Widera, G., Austin, M., Rabussay, D., Goldbeck, C., Barnett, S. W., Chen, M., Leung, L., Otten, G. R., Thudium, K., Selby, M. J., & Ulmer, J. B. (2000). Increased DNA vaccine delivery and immunogenicity by electroporation *in vivo*. *Journal of Immunology, 164*(9), 4635–4640.
102. Babiuk, S., Baca-Estrada, M. E., Foldvari, M., Storms, M., Rabussay, D., Widera, G., & Babiuk, L. A. (2002). Electroporation improves the efficacy of DNA vaccines in large animals. *Vaccine, 20*(27–28), 3399–3408.
103. Tollefsen, S., Tjelle, T., Schneider, J., Harboe, M., Wiker, H., Hewinson, G., Huygen, K., & Mathiesen, I. (2002). Improved cellular and humoral immune responses against Mycobacterium tuberculosis antigens after intramuscular DNA immunisation combined with muscle electroporation. *Vaccine, 20*(27–28), 3370–3378.
104. Buchan, S., Grønevik, E., Mathiesen, I., King, C. A., Stevenson, F. K., & Rice, J. (2005). Electroporation as a "prime/ boost" strategy for naked DNA vaccination against a tumor antigen. *Journal of Immunology, 174*(10), 6292–6298.
105. Smith, H. A., & Klinman, D. M. (2001). The regulation of DNA vaccines. *Current Opinion in Biotechnology*, *12*(3), 299–303.
106. Zahm, C. D., Colluru, V. T., & McNeel, D. G. (2017). DNA vaccines for prostate cancer. *Pharmacology and Therapeutics*, *174*, 27–42.

CHAPTER 8

Utilizing DNA Vaccines and Electroporation to Fight Cancer

ABSTRACT

Due to the invasive nature of standard therapeutic techniques in cancer, the extension of patient survival is typically limited to a few months. An immunization strategy that makes use of naked plasmid DNA has the potential to trigger both cellular and humoral immune responses from the recipient. Recent research has focused on the application of DNA as a means to encode tumor-specific antigens or tumor-associated antigens, revealing a multitude of advantages. Enhancing the effectiveness of vaccines has been a primary objective in the advancement of DNA vaccination as a potential therapeutic for combating tumors. The technique of electroporation (EP) has been employed in fundamental scientific investigations for a considerable duration, facilitating the introduction of DNA into cells in an artificial environment. EP *in vivo* has been found to improve the transmission of DNA vaccines and plasmids to a variety of tissues, including the skin, muscles, tumors, and others. This process leads to significant increases in gene expression, frequently accompanied by positive serological and clinical outcomes. Recent advances in EP technology are a direct result of the growing interest in nonviral gene transfer as a treatment option for a wide variety of diseases and conditions. This chapter has unveiled that EP can be effectively employed in a wide range of species, encompassing the human population.

DNA- and m-RNA-Based Vaccines: An Immunotherapeutic Approach to Cancer.

Sonali Sundram and Rishabha Malviya (Authors)

DOI: 10.1201/9781774919613-8

8.1 INTRODUCTION

Gene transfer-based vaccination methods have been recently introduced. Nonviral vaccination techniques, such as those employing bare DNA molecules, have emerged as a result of advances in our understanding of the basic mechanics of the immune system. Vaccines are widely acknowledged as a comparatively secure and advantageous approach for delivering exogenous antigens into the host organism, thereby eliciting an immune response. There is no replication in DNA vaccines and cellular expression of vaccine products of the host. A subunit vaccine's specificity and safety may be mimicked by making these. DNA vaccines enable the creation and processing of immunogenic proteins within host cells, which means they have the potential to induce immunological responses that are comparable to those triggered by live-attenuated vaccinations. This advantageous characteristic of DNA vaccines allows for the induction of robust immunological reactions without the risk of pathogenic infection in laboratory animals. The antigenic protein is expressed when DNA vaccines are introduced to the host's cells directly to the host. Ag-specific antibodies and cellular responses are both known to be generated as a result of this procedure [1–3]. Evidence suggests that DNA-based immunizations would be long-lasting, cost-effective, and safe in their use.

Studies using DNA vaccines have often focused on administering the vaccine to a muscle or skin tissue for vaccination purposes. Spatial antigen-presenting cells (APCs) and contractile cells take in and express DNA vaccines intramuscularly (IM). Adaptive immune responses are induced when draining lymph nodes become a destination for local APCs [4, 5].

APCs are thought to aid in the cross-presentation of secreted antigens to CD4+ and CD8+ T cells [6, 7], or the direct transfection of DNA vaccine.

APCs can help activate resting T lymphocytes by delivering co-stimulatory signals and cytokines. APCs, non-hematogenous target tissues (such muscle cells), and Ag-specific helper functions all work together to allow B cells to recognize antigenic proteins that are either generated or released (CD4+ T cells when injected intravenously, keratinocytes when injected intradermally (ID)). Langerhans cells and cutaneous dendritic cells provide individualized DNA profiling, which may cause adaptive immune responses in the draining lymph nodes [8]. When it comes to innate immune responses, DNA vaccines manufactured from bacteria include unmethylated CpG patterns, which activate APCs by connecting TLR9 outside the cell. DNA vaccines' ability to stimulate immune responses that are specific to antigens could be limited by the nontargeted activation of APCs. DNA vaccines can be made more effective by combining codon-optimized antigen genes with other DNA sequences encoding immune stimulatory or intracellular antigen-targeting agents. Adjuvants are used in cancer DNA vaccines that enhance the body's natural adaptive immune response. These adjuvants include cytokines and immune response regulators. Increased adaptive immune responses have been demonstrated to be a possible side effect of using the DNA prime-boost method and xenogeneic antigens. DNA vaccines' immunogenicity has been improved by these molecular and biological mechanisms. Because of their high level of self-tolerance, cancer antigens are often regarded as having low immunogenicity. Immunological tolerance to cancer antigens must be broken down before cancer DNA vaccination may produce strong adaptive immune responses [9]. On top of that, the antigens that are specific to cancer may be found in healthy tissues. As a result, immune cells that are hypersensitive to cancer might target healthy tissues, resulting in autoimmune disorders. Many cancer antigens have been discovered to date. However, further effort is required to uncover other malignancy-derived antigens that might serve as cancer antigens in the future. Cancer immunotherapy relies heavily on CTLs, which specifically target and kill neoplastic cells. When it comes to the apoptosis of cancer-reactive CTLs, the Fas/Fas ligand route and the perforin/granzyme B pathway are both extremely important [10, 11]. However, even if CTL activity is induced and enhanced against cancer Ag, the cancer cells themselves may develop immunological resistance and stop responding to CTL recognition and attack. Resistance to immunotherapy and immune selection often develops in cancer cells throughout treatment. Cancer cells have been found to employ a wide variety of mechanisms that act as defenses against the host immune system. Due to their ineffectiveness against cancer-reactive CTLs, cancer DNA vaccines are not a viable option for cancer treatment. As a result, probably, preventing cancer and preventing cancerous cells from hiding from the body's immune system is crucial for effective treatment [12].

DNA vaccines and common medical practices such as operations, x-rays, and drugs, all of which have distinct mechanisms for killing cancer cells, might be used in combination to stop cancer cells from developing immunological resistance and so improve cancer control. Pre-clinical and clinical testing of DNA vaccines coding for research on a plethora of cancer-related antigens and antigens not previously linked to cancer has been carried out. This chapter will cover how to administer DNA vaccines, how to manipulate antigens and how to employ xenogeneic antigens, how to boost the cancer antigens that are most immunogenic for DNA vaccines, and how cancer cells use immune evasion mechanisms.

In recent years, EP has gained significant traction in the fields of biotechnology and medicine. EP was first used to increase the permeability of the cellular membrane, allowing substances like genes and drugs to cross over when they normally couldn't [13]. Following its success in delivering genes and drugs into specific cells, this method was used in a wide variety of additional contexts [14]. The utilization of EP is widely recognized as a highly efficient strategy for the delivery of genes into various animal tissues and organs [15]. This technique functions as a potent mechanism for gene replacement and can furthermore be employed as a physical approach for immunization against various illnesses. Additionally, electrochemotherapy, which is now recognized as a potent method for delivering drugs in cancer treatment, was introduced [16].

8.2 VARIOUS TYPES OF CANCER ANTIGENS

A lot of cancer antigens have been discovered thus far. As a general rule, cancer antigens may be divided into mutated self-antigens, testis cancer antigens, overexpressed cancer antigens, and differentiated cancer antigens, including those unique to various cancers. The antigens linked to prostate, breast, and testicular cancers consist of a diverse set of proteins, including Survivin, carcinoembryonic antigen (CEA), telomerase reverse transcriptase (hTERT), alpha-fetoprotein (AFP), HER2/neu, prostatic acid phosphatase (PAP), prostate-specific antigen (PSA), Wilm's tumor (WT1) antigens, prostate-specific membrane antigen (PSMA), and melanoma-associated antigen (PRAME). These body-derived cancer antigens tend to be rather feeble.

8.3 ANTIGENS OVEREXPRESSED BY CANCER

Overexpression of apoptosis-inhibiting proteins such as survivin and hTERT is common in initial tumors [17–20]. A mouse model of melanoma was used to study the effects of priming with IL-2 CDNA and survivin

DNA vaccines, followed by reactivation with rAd, on antitumor responses. Antitumor responses to Ag-expressing tumor cells may also be induced by hTERT DNA vaccines [21, 22]. To eradicate cancers that express survivin and hTERT, these animal studies suggest that Agspecific CTL responses may be induced by using survivin and hTERT.

Cancers of the colon (CEA) and breasts (HER2/neu) both overexpress CEA [23, 24]. CD8+ T lymphocytes and perforin-dependent antitumor immunity were bolstered by the injection of IL-12 cDNA along with a DNA vaccination against CEA [25]. This study used a combination of antitumor protective responses against CEA-expressing malignancies that may benefit from priming with CEA DNA and boosting with adenovirus [26]. The tumor growth of mice, which was transgenic for both CEA and HER2, as well as mice that were transgenic for either NOD or SCID, was observed to be reduced upon administration of cancer antigen (CEA) and HER2 nucleic acid (DNA) vaccinations [27]. In light of the failure of prime-boost vaccination strategies, these results highlight the importance of overcoming immunological tolerization before generating antigen-specific immune responses in people employing genetically engineered vaccines and an adenovirus that expresses HER2/CEA. Many hepatocellular cancers over-express AFP, an oncofetal protein. Antitumor protective responses in mice were elicited by DNA encoding for adenovirus (producing AFP) primed with GM-CSF vaccinations [28, 29]. Patients with hepatocellular carcinoma were vaccinated with AFP DNA primed by adenovirus, and one of them had stronger Ag-specific T cell responses and improved PFS [30] suggesting that AFP could be a promising antigen for immunotherapy of hepatocellular carcinoma. Leukaemia cells, as well as specific solid tumors, including lung and colon cancer, have an elevated expression of the WT1 antigen, which functions as a transcription factor [31, 32]. WT1-derived epitope DNA vaccines, in particular WT137–45, elicited Ag-specific CTL responses in humanized transgenic mice, which identified leukemia cells [33]. WT1 has the potential to be utilized in therapeutic immunization strategies for the treatment of leukemia and other cancers that express WT1. This is because of the observed efficacy of expanded human cytotoxic T lymphocytes *in vitro* against human target cells expressing the antigen [34, 35] Men with suspected or confirmed prostate cancer often have PSA levels measured as part of routine screening procedures. There is also evidence that PSMA and PAP are elevated in prostate cancer [36, 37]. PSA DNA vaccines injected ID led to robust antibody and cell-based responses to Ag and antitumor resistance in a mouse model of Ag-expressing tumors [38]. Immune responses to both PSA and PSMA were strongly elicited in mice by immunization with DNA vaccines that expressed both antigens [39]. Ag-specific humoral and cellular men with advanced prostate cancer were given intravenous and intradermal PSA DNA vaccinations in addition to subcutaneous GM-CSF and IL-2 injections [40]. Prostate cancer patients treated with PAP DNA vaccines and GM-CSF cDNA ID injections experienced a decrease in PSA doubling time and an increase in CD4+ and CD8+ T-cell proliferative responses in 41% of cases [41]. Patients who were vaccinated against PAP using DNA and then given GM-CSF cDNA as a booster demonstrated instances of cytolytic T-cell responses. Individuals with recurrent prostate cancer elicited anti-DOM IgG and CD4+ T cell responses after receiving DNA vaccines encoding PSMA CTL epitopes associated with the tetanus toxin DOMmain [42]. This occurred alongside the induction of PSMA-specific CD8+ T cell responses. Although no partial or complete response was observed, 63 patients with Ag-positive solid tumors were given intranasal melanoma vaccines consisting of a DNA prime and then a peptide boost (PRAME + PSMA). Patients developed antigen-specific T-cell responses after receiving these vaccinations. Several people who took part in the study had much lower than average PSA values. These encouraging results highlight the need for further investigation into the treatment of prostate cancer with IM-EP and the intranasal injection of PSMA, PSA, and PAP DNA vaccines.

8.4 CANCER-RELATED AND TESTICULAR TUMOR-ASSOCIATED ANTIGENS

Both MAGE and NY-ESO-1, two different types of cancer cells, express cancer/testis antigens that are found nowhere else in the body except in the testes [43]. Using a mouse model, researchers found that HSP70/MAGE-3 fusion proteins were immunogenic and evoked a potent anticancer response against MAGE-3-expressing tumors. In 16 patients with advanced malignancy, DNA vaccines against NY-ESO-1 delivered via particle-mediated ID elicited CD4 and/or CD8 T cell responses [45]. The great majority of those tested had reactions that were not clinically relevant. Antibodies that target NY-ESO-1 have not yet been linked to clinical outcomes, according to this study.

8.5 ANTIGENS INVOLVED IN TUMOR DIFFERENTIATION

Melanoma cells and normal melanocytes exhibit antigens for racial and ethnic differences, including gp100, Trp2, and MART-1 (or Melan-A) [46–48]. Evidence suggests that a xenogeneic antigen can stimulate cross-reactive anticancer reactions toward cancerous cells that produce self-antigens [49], as demonstrated by the success of DNA vaccines encoding human gp100 and Trp2. Human Trp2-encoding DNA-vaccinated mice produce CD8(+) T cells and antibodies against B16 melanoma cross-reactive antigens. Patients with melanoma who got gp100 injections IM or IM showed no clinical or immunological responses [50–51]. After being delivered by particle-mediated epidermal means to unaffected skin from melanoma patients, moderate activation of anti-melanoma responses demonstrated the method's safety and tolerability [52]. DNA vaccines that target tyrosinases have shown that 42% of patients without any clinical reactions will still have a specific immune response, and those patients will have a better chance of survival in the long run if they do. Ag-specific immune responses were observed following intranasal DNA vaccination in patients having stage IV malignancy expressing MART-1 [53]. However, these responses did not translate into any clinical benefit for the patients.

Cancer recurrence may be prevented by establishing immunological responses with long-term memory during treatment for hematological malignancies. Furthermore, B cell immunoglobulin variable regions and idiotype immunoglobulin variable regions have different protein sequences [54, 55]. A tumor-specific antigen (TSA) may be present in malignant B-idiotype cells. Mice are protected from cancer by a T cell-dependent immune response after being vaccinated with DNA vaccines comprising of just the light and heavy chain antigenic changeable regions [56]. Follicular B-cell lymphoma patients who had received intramuscular injections of a DNA vaccine were shown to have developed immunity to the vaccination, which included chimeric idiotypes.

When it comes to managing hematological malignancies, differentiation antigens provide a prospective target for sustained tumor-specific CTL immunity.

8.6 P53, A MUTATED ANTIGEN,

Cell cycle progression, genomic stability, angiogenesis, and apoptosis are all controlled by the p53 protein [57, 58]. The *p53* gene, which is frequently altered in cancer, has been suggested as a target for immunotherapy. Animal studies using an IM-EP DNA vaccine encoding mutant human p53 demonstrated that CD8+ T cell responses are critical for antitumor protection and treatment [59], and p53 mutations may be an attractive immunotherapeutic target for cancer.

8.7 DNA VACCINES AGAINST MALIGNANT TUMORS

TSAs and tumor-associated antigens (TAA) found on cancer cells provide motivation for the pursuit of cancer vaccines. Tumor-immune system connections are intricate and difficult to understand. The term "cancer immunoediting" refers to a complex chain of events involving neoplastic growths and the immune system. The aforementioned interactions can be broken down into three distinct phases, which are collectively known as the three Es that comprise cancer immunoediting [60]. These phases are known as Elimination, Equilibrium, and Escape. During the Elimination phase, the intrinsic part of the immune system holds the power to destroy cells that have undergone a modification or change. Throughout the progression of cancer, specific tumor cells undergo a biological phenomenon in which the immune system triggers a specialized immune response that specifically targets tumor antigens (TAs). The immune system engages in a response against cancer growth by means of targeted T and B lymphocytes, which serve to safeguard the host from the load imposed by the tumor. Certain changes in cancer cells are induced by the immune system's selective pressure. Therefore, decreased TA expression levels or a changed TA repertoire can be related to the decreased immunogenicity of malignant cells. Major histocompatibility complexes I (MHC-I) and II (MHC-II) are downregulated on the cell surface of these malignant cells [61–64], leading to the production of mutant antigens.

The dynamic balance between tumor elimination and cancer migration is a major focus during the equilibrium phase. The outcome observed is a conspicuous state of tumor dormancy and a deficiency in immune reactions [65]. The immune system's ability to keep a dynamic balance with the expanding cancer diminishes in the final phase, called the Escape phase. When it comes to boosting cancer growth, the equilibrium between antitumor and tumor-promoting immunity is of utmost importance. In addition, cancer cells contribute to an impaired immune response by secreting cytokines with immunosuppressive properties [66].

While it is true that cancer cells use a wide variety of strategies to avoid being detected by the immune system, researchers have still been able to identify a number of consistent TAAs and TSAs that have been used to advance therapeutic vaccination approaches across a range of tumor types.

As an alternative to conventional subunit immunizations, cancer vaccines that use plasmid DNA encoding for TAAs have proven effective. DNA-based vaccines have exciting potential in cancer immunotherapy since they do not rely on refined or crude antigens like recombinant proteins and peptides. Understanding the immune system's role in the development of malignant tumors has drawn the attention of the scientific community in testing the efficacy of DNA vaccines in cancer treatment.

Both the antibody-mediated response, which is reliant on the function of B lymphocytes, and the cellular immunological response, which is carried out by CTLs, are used by the human immune system to combat cancer. Upon activation against TAAs, these T cells acquire the capability to identify and eliminate cancer cells that express the antigens. While both immune responses are critical, it is important to remember that stopping cancer's progression just through the body's own creation of antibodies against TAs is not enough. Therefore, in order to successfully destroy malignant cells, it is crucial to elicit a tailored cytolytic immune response against specific epitopes.

In this specific context, the DNA molecule that codes for TA has shown great promise as a means of creating vaccinations. DNA vaccines possess the capacity to deliver specific target antigens (TAs) to certain processing pathways. Furthermore, additional activation elements can be incorporated with little changes to improve the immune response. Antigens are produced, taken up by antigen presentation cells (APCs), and presented along with major histocompatibility complex class I (MHC-I) and class II (MHC-II) molecules when the DNA vaccine is injected into muscle or the skin [67]. Since DNA vaccines may directly carry heterologous antigens to the antigen-processing pathways required for the stimulation of MHC-I-restricted CTL responses, they provide a significant advantage over other sub-unit vaccines [68]. The major goal is to induce a comprehensive immune system reaction by the activation of B and T cells, which will selectively target antigenic epitopes that are typically prevalent in particular types of tumors. The primary aim is to develop a vaccine that can be used effectively against a wide range of cancers.

8.8 THE UTILIZATION OF EP TO TRANSMIT DNA AS A CANCER VACCINE

In 1998, Aihara and Miyazaki undertook an experiment to demonstrate the feasibility of utilizing electroporation (EP) as a method for transferring genes into a specific organ. The study used electrical pulses to inject plasmid DNA encoding interleukin 5 (IL-5) into mouse tibialis anterior muscles. Other scientists also had achievements in the same field simultaneously [69–71].

The utilization of electric pulses as a secure mechanism for the administration of therapeutic compounds to tissues and organs has experienced significant growth during the past decade. *In vivo*, gene transfer aided by EP has been studied extensively in a variety of animal models, with a primary emphasis on mice. The researchers in these studies are primarily interested in this method's applicability to therapeutic interventions for a variety of diseases [72–75].

EP has been effectively utilized in DNA vaccination to avoid viral infections and cancer treatment. EP in conjunction with intramuscular administration of plasmid DNA vaccines has demonstrated significant promise. This event not only accelerates the procedure of antigen absorption and synthesis within the skeletal muscle but also causes an adjuvant effect by triggering an immune system response [76].

When electrical pulses are applied to certain tissues, like skeletal muscle, the cell surfaces are momentarily exposed to high-intensity electrical fields. The cell membrane becomes temporarily and locally unstable as a result of this process. One of the many complex steps in the uptake of DNA by cells is the electrophoretically generated interaction between the DNA molecule and the destabilized cell membrane during the administration of an electric pulse. The DNA molecule then translocates across the cell membrane, entering the cell successfully [77–79].

8.8.1 *ELECTROPORATION THROUGH SKELETAL MUSCLE*

Skeletal muscle is frequently selected as the principal tissue for EP treatment because of its extensive application and several advantages. In mammalian organisms, the skeletal muscle is extensively dispersed, constituting around 30% of the total body mass. The structure consists of several cylindrical muscle fibers that are distinguished by stable and large syncytial cells with many nuclei. These cells are interconnected by connective tissue, which facilitates the passage of profuse blood vessels. Muscle fibers, being postmitotic in nature, possess the advantageous characteristic of enabling an extended lifespan and sustained expression of injected plasmid DNA over an extended period.

Muscle fibers are regarded as an optimal choice for DNA transfection due to their convenient accessibility and well-developed blood supply. These properties render them appropriate for the systemic injection of proteins such as Apolipoprotein [80, 81], Erythropoietin [82], Kallikrein [83], VEGF [84], and for the transportation of DNA vaccines. Moreover, the skeletal muscle's active involvement in immune responses further supports its suitability for this purpose. DNA-based vaccination has been shown to activate all three arms of adaptive immunity, including antibodies, helper T cells, and CTLs, leading to a strong immunological response. Furthermore, this approach allows for the prompt and efficient generation of innate immune responses, while ensuring the preservation of immunological elements crucial for pathogen recognition, while simultaneously avoiding the activation of unwanted proteins or immune reactions [85].

Brief electric pulses on muscle tissue have been offered as a possible technique for optimizing DNA immunization protocols. LV electric pulses alone or in combination with electric pulses are just one of many approaches documented. When EP-induced injury is a possibility, the phenomenon of myoblast fusion is generally recognized as a process for the rapid recovery and regrowth of muscle fibers. By taking up the transfected DNA, satellite cells help kickstart the regeneration process. Electrotransfer of bare DNA, as described above, has the potential to have a lasting effect on gene expression in skeletal muscle. This is evident as the regenerated myofibers demonstrate the expression of the transfected DNA. Several investigations have been carried out to determine the optimal circumstances that ensure efficient DNA uptake and optimal levels of expression, while additionally taking into account the proper settings that minimize the possibility of tissue damage related to this method.

Transgenic expression in mouse skeletal muscle can be short- or long-lived depending on a number of circumstances. Plasmid DNA dose, electric pulse parameters, and the time elapsed between DNA injection and electric pulse application are all variables. Hence, it is imperative to exercise caution in the selection of electrotransfection techniques that effectively regulate transgene expression in muscle, taking into account the potential toxicity associated with this procedure.

There are several variables that contribute to DNA electrotransfer and the initiation of muscle damage. Electrotransfer toxicity has been linked to cell permeabilization, which has been well studied [86]. Research findings have shown that the occurrence of cell necrosis significantly escalates during an extended period of exposure to a higher quantity and longer duration of pulses directed toward the tissue. Exposure of muscle cells to high electric fields has been shown to cause cellular necrosis and a consequent decrease in gene expression [87].

The potential toxicity associated with DNA electrotransfer may be influenced by the quantity of DNA administered throughout the process. Research findings indicate that electrotransfer leads to the development of muscle lesions that are dependent on the presence of plasmids and are characterized by necrotic myofibers. However, no discernible differences are observed between electrotransferred muscles and untreated control muscles. The predominant factor contributing to muscle injury seems to be the intracellular existence and manifestation of plasmid DNA. It has been observed that necrotic fibers do not demonstrate transgenic expression. Moreover, it is worth noting that the afflicted region exhibits a restricted presence of positive muscle cells, whereas the neighboring intact cells exhibit a strong expression of the transgene [88].

Therefore, it may not be too detrimental to utilize electrotransfer techniques in cases when an immunological response is required [89]. The presence of muscular inflammation, together with a degree of muscle injury and necrosis, is expected to enhance immune responses by creating suitable inflammatory surroundings and increasing the likelihood of antigen cross-presentation. In a study, researchers have presented evidence about the induction of specific local damage by EP leads to temporary alterations in the structure of skeletal muscle. This process triggers the immediate release of endogenous cytokines, which play a crucial role in signaling local distress. As a result, the signaling cascade induces the mobilization of dendritic cells, macrophages, and T lymphocytes, without any observable effect on the general physiological state. To mitigate any potential adverse impact of EP on the experimental subjects, the researchers proceeded by collecting spleens and blood samples subsequent to EP treatment. The aforementioned samples were later evaluated for the existence of signal danger compounds.

The available findings indicate that EP have the capacity to attract and stimulate cells engaged in antigen presentation and immune response, albeit just within a localized context. The present discovery confirms the safety and high tolerance of electrotransfer as a viable approach for administering genetic vaccination protocols. The adjuvant-like characteristics of electrotransfer do not exert any influence on the general physiological state of the animals subjected to this treatment [90]. Using a sequential approach with a short-duration high-voltage (HV) pulse following a longer-duration LV pulse in order to accomplish successful DNA electrotransfer into the skeletal muscle of mice and rats provides additional support for the limited interference with cellular physiology and function observed [91]. The researchers conducted an analysis of gene expression profiling subsequent to the transfer of skeletal muscle DNA using HVand LV EP techniques. The expression levels of both structural proteins like sarcospan and catalytic enzymes were lowered as a result of this therapeutic intervention. The temporary nature of the effects on muscle fibers was seen, as evidenced by the close similarity in expression profiles between the treated muscles and the control group three weeks post-treatment. Significantly, the study demonstrated the absence of any detrimental impacts on muscle functionality or modifications in the gene expression patterns of proteins related to cellular apoptosis, inflammatory response, or muscle repair subsequent to both brief and extended therapeutic interventions. The histological investigation demonstrated the presence of cells exhibiting morphological alterations at both the 4-h and 48-h time points. Additionally, a small number of cells were observed to possess central nuclei after a three-week period [92]. The conclusion derived from the aforementioned facts is that methods employing high and low voltage are seen to be safe, as they effectively facilitate DNA electrotransfer while minimizing muscle injury, hence maintaining optimal efficiency. The aforementioned findings hold significant importance for the prospective implementation of DNA EP in clinical settings. Preclinical research has revealed that EP is effective, and Phase I clinical trials are currently examining its safety and tolerability. EP is also used to transport plasmid DNA directly into tumors in these experiments [93 -95]. The examination of potential harmful effects associated with the administration process is currently underway, yielding positive outcomes.

8.8.2 ELECTROPORATION THROUGH INTRADERMAL

Numerous preclinical investigations documented in scholarly literature have commonly employed intramuscular DNA transfer and EP as methods for gene vaccination against cancer. However, it should be noted that the skeletal muscle is not the only tissue that can be targeted for vaccine administration. Vaccination is also important at the skin level.

A very attractive DNA delivery technique for possible therapeutic uses is the Skin EP of genetic vaccines, which has shown substantial effectiveness in immune responses across both small [96–98] as well as big animal models [99, 100]. The skin is considered a very accessible region for the administration of DNA vaccines due to its favorable characteristics. The tissue is home to a sizeable population of APCs, including dermal dendritic cells and Langerhans' cells, for example. Additionally, it facilitates convenient surveillance of the immunization site. The Skin EP allows for the application of a local anesthetic through topical means, as well as the utilization of short electrode needles that have a minimal level of invasiveness [101]. It is anticipated that the utilization of intradermal EP will yield notable enhancements in the acceptability of vaccine administration in comparison to intramuscular EP, as the electrodes exert a lesser impact on muscle contraction.

Previous comparative investigations conducted on big animals have indicated that intramuscular administration of DNA via EP appears to be advantageous for the development of cellular immunity. On the other hand, intradermal EP delivery may be more conducive to the generation of humoral immunity. Nevertheless, numerous investigations have provided evidence indicating that intradermal EP can also elicit immune responses mediated by antibody-dependent cytotoxicity [102].

The effects of intradermal EP on gene expression, DNA persistence, and the local tissue microenvironment have been the subject of a vast number of studies [103, 104]. Transgenic expression was rapidly initiated, antigen production was boosted, and genes involved in local inflammatory and immune reactions were activated, as demonstrated by the study. EP was incorporated into the intradermal delivery of DNA. At the same time, there was no difference in the number of stable plasmid copies in the skin between the two methods of distribution (plasmid injection alone and skin EP).

In a subsequent investigation, the researchers examined a novel pulse protocol characterized by exceedingly brief intervals. Using an enhanced gene delivery technology, they demonstrated that a single immunization can induce robust and sustained *in vivo* protein expression and cytotoxic antigen-specific T cells that are marked by IFN and CD107a (lysosomal-associated membrane protein 1). Researchers suggest that intradermal EP may be linked to a less unpleasant sensation due to the utilization of shorter needles and a decrease in the frequency and intensity of muscle contractions. Furthermore, the researchers of the study provided evidence of the clinical advantages of intradermal EP, including enhanced tolerability and safety. Antigen-specific T cell production and functioning were not significantly affected by pre-vaccination use of a topical anesthetic cream. Based on these findings, local anesthetics may be a useful adjunct in reducing patients' awareness of pulse delivery [105].

At present, needle electrodes are placed into the muscle to administer electrical stimulation for electrically mediated DNA vaccinations. Intradermal EP may have advantages over traditional skin penetration because less invasive electroporators can make contact with the skin's surface without penetrating the skin. The skin is much thinner than skeletal muscle, therefore the possibility exists. Researchers [106] advocated for the use of a non-invasive electrode design called a multi-electrode array (MEA). This electrode is placed on the skin's surface in a flat orientation, without penetrating deeper into the body. The MEA (microneedle array) device was utilized to administer intradermal immunization of guinea pigs using a plasmid containing the genetic information for Hepatitis B surface antigen (HBsAg). The MEA EP intradermal delivery approach exhibited superior protein expression compared to the exclusive use of DNA plasmid injection. Animals subjected to intradermal EP exhibited the initiation of a cellular infiltration within a span of 48 h post-treatment. When compared to the DNA vaccination alone, the humoral immune response was significantly longer lasting and stronger. In conclusion, the results of this work illustrate the captivating capabilities of microelectrode array (MEA) technology in enhancing intradermal DNA vaccination by the use of electrical stimulation.

8.9 THE TECHNIQUES FOR ENHANCING IMMUNOGENICITY

Cancer antigens, as previously said, are often immunogenic in a weak way and need particular approaches to improve their immunogenicity. A variety of tactics have been used to date, including DNA editing and DNA prime-boost immunization systems, alternative DNA delivery methods, and the injection of cytokines and other compounds together are all examples of this. Researchers have used the following strategies to boost the immune response of cancer DNA vaccines:

8.9.1 INFESTATION WITH FOREIGN ANTIGENS AND THE USE OF SYNTHETIC DNA

Generating and modifying DNA has never been simpler because of advances in molecular biological technology. The codon-optimized antigen genes used in most recent DNA vaccines enable greater antigenic protein synthesis. Additional research has looked at the method of combining genetic sequences outside of the genes encoding antigens whose products are involved in antigen recognition and presentation or immunological stimulation and cell antigen targeting. When exposed to tumor cells (TC-1) that express both E6 and E7, those whose codon use was optimized for E7 elicited stronger Ag-specific CTL and antitumor responses [107].

E7 DNA vaccination efficacy against TC-1 cells was further increased by conjugating temperature-shock protein for human papillomavirus type 16 E7 antigens [108]. The anticancer effectiveness against TC-1 cell challenges was considerably improved by combining the first few bases of the IgE molecule, including the codon-optimized *E6* and *E7* genes [109].

Humans have been exposed to combinations of the combination of CTL epitope sequences with Epitope regions for CD4+ T helper cells to detect whether this enhances CTL responses.

In CTL and antitumor responses have been increased by Identifying the genes that code for E7 DNA sequences the proteins that target the endolysosomal membrane protein 1-targeting peptide, bacterial toxin, endoplasmic reticulum, viral protein 22, and tubulin [110, 111]. It is possible that approaches such as improvements in the targeting of antigens to specific subcellular locations within cells employing fine-tuning their CD4+ T helper cell epitope domain fusion, antigen codon use, and subcellular localization can enhance antigen-specific CTL responses and anticancer efficacy in preclinical trials.

In the context of invariant self-antigens, an alternative approach to addressing immunological tolerance toward self-antigens involves the administration of an exogenous antigen. These antigens may be identified by T cells and immune systems are prepared to mount immunological because xenogeneic antigens are just modified self-proteins with an amino acid alteration in one or more epitopes, immune responses to them are similar to those to native antigens. Identical proteins found in different species referred to as xenogeneic antigens have been found to trigger an immune response in humans gp100 and tyrosinase may be used as immunogens [112, 113]. CD8+ T cell responses against melanoma and cross-reactivity were elicited in a mouse model by Human gp100-expressing DNA vaccines, but not murine gp100-expressing DNA vaccines [114].

8.9.2 DNA VACCINATION BASED ON XENOGENIC TYROSINASE

Extensive research has been conducted on the proteins affiliated with the tyrosinase family, namely as differentiation antigens. These antigens have demonstrated excellent recognition by antibodies and T cells in individuals who have been diagnosed with melanoma. Preclinical research in murine models demonstrated that xenogeneic DNA vaccination, using genes encoding members of the tyrosinase family, can elicit immunological responses, including antibody formation and cytotoxic T-cell activation. These immune responses subsequently result in the removal of malignancies [115, 116]. Mice that were given a plasmid containing an autologous construct of melanocyte antigen tyrosinase-related protein-2 through EP saw significant increases in CD8+ T lymphocyte numbers and significant slowing of tumor growth after being exposed to the generate [117]. The findings of this work prompted further investigation into the long-term viability of DNA vaccination with xenogeneic human tyrosinase in dogs with advanced spontaneous malignant melanoma [118, 119]. The Biojector2000, a needle-free delivery device, was used to inject human tyrosinase plasmid DNA IM into nine dogs. The results of the trial demonstrated the efficacy and safety of the vaccination. The median survival period observed in vaccinated dogs was somewhat more than one year, in contrast to dogs treated with conventional therapy utilizing historical controls, which exhibited survival durations ranging from one to five months. A subsequent paper reported the antibody responses, revealing that three out of the nine dogs exhibited a reaction [120].

In light of these promising findings, a clinical study was carried out to evaluate the immunogenicity and safety of TYR DNA vaccines in a group of 18 patients with stage III/IV melanoma. The phase I experiment encompassed the injection of TYR DNA vaccines in both mouse and human subjects, employing the Biojector2000 equipment [121]. T-cell responses were detected in seven out of ten people who were given the vaccine via the needle-free injection method. The study did not provide information regarding the determination of median survival time beyond a follow-up period of more than 42 months. A deeper investigation into alternative DNA delivery methods has been inspired by the findings of this study and the development of efficient EP devices. To learn more about the topic at hand, researchers launched a phase I clinical trial to test the efficacy and immunogenicity of a xenogeneic tyrosinase DNA vaccine. EP made it possible for people with stage IIB, IIC, III, or IV melanoma to get the vaccination IM. This clinical trial is registered under the identifier NCT00471133 on ClinicalTrials.gov. Th safety and efficacy of EP-enhanced intramuscular injection, as well as the amplitude and frequency of immune responses targeting tyrosinase in immunized patients, will be the primary outcome measures. Patients with observable tumors following vaccination will be used for the study of anticancer responses. Increasing immunological responses, inducing anticancer effects, and maybe extending overall survival are all possibilities when the xenogeneic tyrosinase DNA vaccine is combined with EP. This holds promise for surpassing the outcomes observed when the vaccine is used as an alone intervention.

8.9.3 MODULATING IMMUNE REACTIONS WITH A NOVEL DRUG

T-cell destiny is determined by two classes of molecules that are surface-expressed. These substances regulate immune responses.

CD27 and CD30 are cell surface markers that are commonly used in immunology research. Inducible T cell co-stimulator (ICOS), programmed death (PD), and cytotoxic T lymphocyte-associated antigen-4 (CTLA-4) make up the repertoire of co-stimulatory molecules, whereas programmed death (PD), CTLA-4, and B and T lymphocyte attenuator make up the repertoire of co-inhibitory molecules [122, 123]. The capacity of these molecules to modulate cancer treatment has been subjected to several clinical and animal trials. Combining agonistic anti-4-1BB antibodies with tumor vaccinations has been demonstrated to significantly improve the success of cancer treatment. Increased antigen-specific CTL activity is responsible for this improvement, as seen in two different animal cancer models [124, 125].

In a HER2/neu transgenic animal model, anti-OX-40 and anti-4-1BB antibodies showed improved antitumor effectiveness [126]. Mice received greater protection from a potentially fatal B16 melanoma treatment when anti-GITR antibodies were added to DNA vaccines encoding for gp100 and Trp2 [127]. Mice with tumors have better anticancer T-cell responses when CTLA-4 is suppressed by antagonistic anti-CTLA-4 Abs [128, 129]. Together, an anti-CTLA-4 antibody and DNA vaccines encoding for Trp2- and gp100-encoding proteins increased the relationship between anti-melanoma activity and T-cell responses to antigen [130]. Anti-CTLA-4 antibodies have been found to extend the lives of patients with metastatic melanoma in clinical trials. These results suggest that anti-CTLA-4 antibodies activate Ag-specific T cells in a more direct fashion than was previously thought [131, 132]. Animal studies and preliminary human clinical trials have demonstrated that cancer DNA vaccines are more immunogenic when combined with immune response regulators. Patients in the US with metastatic melanoma (skin cancer) now have access to ipilimumab, an anti-CTLA-4 blocking Ab.

8.9.4 CO-INJECTION OF CYTOKINES AND OTHER SUBSTANCES

One promising strategy in the fight against cancer is the use of recombinant cytokines. However, unpleasant responses and toxicity are common when large doses are consistently administered, limiting the safe dosage [133]. Therefore, there exists a substantial need for innovative therapeutic alternatives. Interleukin (IL)-2 and IL-12 have been proven to have favorable anticancer effects in a number of preclinical investigations, where they were found to augment immune responses. The precise mechanism of these effects, however, remains unclear [134–136].

Previous research has investigated the efficacy of treating murine ovarian teratocarcinoma in mice by administering IL plasmid DNA in combination with a cationic lipid [137]. When plasmid DNA (pDNA) encoding IL-2 was given, the concentration of the cytokine produced locally went up. Furthermore, it was observed that by using plasmid DNA, the expression time could be increased from 24 h (as demonstrated with the recombinant form) to a maximum of 10 days. Furthermore, the data demonstrated a considerable anti-cancer impact together with an important increase in overall survival. In a mouse model of melanoma, prolonged remission without disease recurrence was obtained by giving bleomycin in combination with IL-2 plasmid utilizing EP [138].

The IL-2 transgene was tested for local expression and systemic distribution in mice as part of the preclinical research for an investigational new medication application. The application also sought to assess whether or not this therapy could slow the progression of preexisting malignancies [139]. According to the findings of the study, IL-2 levels within the tumor significantly increased after EP-assisted administration was implemented. Specifically, the size of this increase ranged from 3 to 7 times higher compared to the delivery strategy that did not use EP. The study observed the presence of continuous amounts of IL-2 inside the tumor microenvironment, while relatively low and transient levels of IL-2 were found in the bloodstream. The study observed a reduction in tumor size when IL-2plus EP was administered, in comparison to the administration of IL-2 alone. Subcutaneous infusions of VCL-IM01, a plasmid DNA encoding human IL-2 (VCL-1102), dissolved in phosphate-buffered saline (PBS), and provided in conjunction with EP, were studied further to evaluate safety in a rat model. No deaths occurred, there was no indication of drug-induced toxicity, no injection-related redness or adverse reactions, and the treatment was generally well received. Based on these results, as well as those from the safety study with VCL-1102 Pdna [140], a phase I clinical trial of VCL-IM01 with EP has begun (ClinicalTrials.gov ID NCT00223899). Thirty patients were chosen to take part in an investigation in which they will receive VCL-IM01 therapy for their metastatic melanoma. The Medpulser EPT System will be used to perform EP after this treatment is injected immediately into the tumor at varied concentrations. The major purpose of this research is to evaluate the treatment's safety. Secondary outcomes, such as response rate, examination of injected tumors for induration, inflammation, and erythema, and examination of IL-2 blood levels, will also be assessed. Furthermore, the assessment will involve the measurement of tumor burden, evaluation of response rate, and monitoring of disease progression.

Since plasmid IL-2 treatment was so successful in a mouse melanoma tumor model, researchers have begun looking into the feasibility of using IL-12 in conjunction with EP. Results showed a reduction in systemic cytokine levels in addition to a local antitumor effect. When EP was used in conjunction with plasmids encoding murine interleukin-2 (IL-2) or interleukin-12 (IL-12), growth was significantly slowed by 5–15 days compared to when either plasmid was used alone or with a control plasmid [141]. Subsequent investigations have provided additional evidence indicating that the administration of plasmid IL-12 via intratumoral injection, together with EP, in mice with B16.F10 melanoma tumors, led to a remarkable outcome where 80% of the subjects remained free of tumors for a period exceeding 100 days. Furthermore, these animals exhibited resistance when subsequently exposed to B16 cells, indicating a robust and enduring response [142, 143]. The B16.F10 melanoma model was used for toxicity testing in order to bring this technique closer to clinical use. The study demonstrated a notable upregulation in the expression levels of IL-12 when administered alongside EP, leading to total tumor regression. Furthermore, the administration of plasmid IL-12 with EP exhibited low to no observed harmful effects, as indicated by the data [144].

In patients with a suspicion of Stage IIIB/c or IV malignant melanoma, the primary goal of the phase I clinical investigation (ClinicalTrials.gov ID NCT00323206) was to assess the safety, tolerability, optimum dosage, and efficacy of intratumoral pIL-12 EP treatment. Twenty-four participants were included in the study. The Medpulser EPT System was used to conduct the EP. Local and systemic response, as well as local and systemic expression of IL-12 and IFN-, were among the key outcome measures, along with toxicity profile, maximum-tolerated dose, the suggested dose for a phase II investigation, and others. The study found that while IL-12 and IFN- expression increased within the treated tumors, there was no corresponding increase in circulation. The biopsies that were performed on the treated lesions revealed a notable presence of necrotic tissue and infiltration of lymphocytes. Furthermore, out of the total sample size of 24 patients, it was discovered that 8 individuals exhibited stable condition. Notably, two of these patients demonstrated a full response, indicating the absence of either treated or untreated lesions. The first clinical trial to examine *IL-12* gene transfer in patients with metastatic melanoma using *in vivo* DNA EP. The trial provided evidence to support the assertion that this particular strategy is both safe and efficacious, yielding consistent outcomes that can be modified as required [145].

The results of the preclinical studies show that the therapeutic potential of cytokines can be increased by administering them singly or in combination with EP. The anticipated outcome of the clinical studies is to provide evidence supporting the efficacy of combining EP with cytokine-expressing plasmids as a potential treatment for individuals afflicted with melanoma.

8.9.5 IMMUNIZATION STRATEGIES UTILIZING DNA PRIME-BOOST PROTOCOLS

DNA prime-boost vaccination is an approach that shows great promise for DNA-based vaccinations. When compared to solely using DNA immunization, the immune response achieved by employing the prime-boost strategy was stronger and more long-lasting. The administration of CEA DNA vaccines in a prime-boost manner has demonstrated potential efficacy in circumventing self-tolerance and inducing robust immune responses. This is evidenced by the sequential application of intramuscular electroporation (IM-EP) following the administration of the vaccinations, leading to subsequent expression of the CEA antigen. Previous studies have demonstrated that the prime-boost approach elicits Ag-specific CD8+ T cell responses in CEA transgenic mice, which are comparable to those observed in wild-type mice [146]. To boost immunity, it is possible to use either a DNA vaccination consisting of CEA fused with Adenoviruses that express the fused CEA/toxin C or toxin fragment C [147].

The present study investigates the immunogenicity and safety of adenovirus prime-boost regimens in monkeys for the CEA DNA vaccine. The clinical trials employing the HER2/CEA DNA vaccine/adenovirus prime-boosting technique have demonstrated a lack of T cell response activation for both tested antigens [148].

8.9.6 MULTIPLE DNA-DELIVERY METHADOLOGIES

In addition to the previously mentioned gene gun delivery and EP techniques, extensive investigations have been undertaken to explore many additional cancer medicine delivery systems. The primary goal of these studies has been to find ways to make DNA vaccines more effective. It has been shown that gene guns provide superior tumor protection via antigen-specific CTL responses as compared to jet injectors when administering HER2/neu DNA vaccines. DNA vaccines that contain a portion of the tetanus toxin conjugated to MART-1 have also proven highly immunogenic in humans when delivered through tattooing. The effectiveness of direct intranodal DNA vaccine administration was also evaluated. Tests on the effectiveness of these vaccinations were also carried out with the use of chemical components (such as polymers or nanoparticles). In other terms, the utilization of a liposome DNA vaccination combination yielded superior outcomes compared to the use of DNA vaccination alone [149]. This approach demonstrated enhanced efficacy in augmenting the population of CD8+ T lymphocytes and inhibiting tumor growth by boosting the production of interferon-gamma (IFN-γ) by natural killer (NK) cells. Similarly, DNA vaccines formulated with nanoparticles induced greater anti-melanoma immune responses than DNA vaccines alone [150]. Cancer DNA vaccines may benefit from the use of these formulations and improved ways of delivering them.

8.10 CONCLUSION

In this chapter, we take a close look at the promising use of EP for the transfer of cancer vaccines in the treatment and prevention of the disease. Further investigation into this methodology will facilitate the broader application of this technology to a multitude of illnesses that currently lack efficacious treatments. EP has been shown in recent research to attract and activate cells important for antigen presentation and immune response, and this effect is independent of the mechanism employed to deliver the DNA. Hence, it may be inferred that EP exhibits characteristics similar to adjuvants, thereby augmenting the ongoing progress and efficacy of DNA vaccines and immunotherapeutics. EP has many benefits, including the enhancement of humoral and cellular immune responses, the reduction of injection volume, the minimization of administration frequency, and the extension of the period of vaccination or treatment efficacy. The influence of the route of administration is anticipated to exert a substantial influence on the effective delivery of EP to human subjects. The latest advancements in the field of electrophysiology mostly focus on therapeutic applications. The success of DNA vaccinations and the widespread adoption of DNA-based immunotherapies and other therapeutic techniques hinges on the continued study and development of EP.

KEYWORDS

- **cancer antigens**
- **DNA**
- **electroporation**
- **immunogenicity**
- **malignant**
- **tumor**

REFERENCES

1. Kuhober, A., Pudollek, H. P., Reifenberg, K., Chisari, F. V., Schlicht, H. J., Reimann, J., & Schirmbeck, R. (1996). DNA immunization induces antibody and cytotoxic T cell responses to hepatitis B core antigen in H-2b mice. *Journal of Immunology*, *156*(10), 3687–3695.
2. Wang, B., Ugen, K. E., Srikantan, V., Agadjanyan, M. G., Dang, K., Refaeli, Y., Sato, A., Boyer, J. D., Williams, W. V., & Weiner, D. B. (1993). Gene inoculation generates immune responses against human immunodeficiency virus type 1. *Proceedings of the National Academy of Science of the United State of America*, *90*(9), 4156–4160.
3. Corr, M., Lee, D. J., Carson, D. A., & Tighe, H. (1996). Gene vaccination with naked plasmid DNA: Mechanism of CTL priming. *The Journal of Experimental Medicine*, *184*(4),1555–1560.
4. Casares, S., Inaba, K., Brumeanu, T. D., Steinman, R. M., & Bona, C. A. (1997). Anitigen presentation by dendritic cells after immunization with DNA encoding a major histocompatibility complex class II-restricted viral epitope. *The Journal of Experimental Medicine*, *186*(9), 1481–1486.
5. Chattergoon, M. A., Robinson, T. M., Boyer, J. D., & Weiner, D. B. (1998). Specific immune induction following DNA-based immunization through *in vivo* transfection and activation of macrophages. *Journal of Immunology*, *160*(12), 5707–5718.
6. Fu, T., Ulmer, J. B., Caulfield, M. J., Deck, R. R., Friedman, A., Wang, S., Liu, X., Donnelly, J. J., & Liu, M. A. (1997). Priming of cytotoxic T lymphocytes by DNA vaccines: requirement for professional antigen presenting cells and evidence for antigen transfer from myocytes. *Molecular Medicine*, *3*(6), 362–371.
7. Iwasaki, A., Torres, C. A., Ohashi, P. S., Robinson, H. L., & Barber, B. H. (1997). The dominant role of bone marrow-derived cells in CTL induction following plasmid DNA immunization at different sites. *Journal of Immunology*, *159*(1), 11–14.
8. Condon, C., Watkins, S. C., Celluzzi, C. M., Thompson, K., & Falo, L. D. (1996). DNA-based immunization by *in vivo* transfection of dendritic cells. *Nature Medicine*, *2*(10), 1122–1128.

9. Liu, M., & Ulmer, J. B. (2005). Human clinical trials of plasmid DNA vaccines. *Advances in Genetics*, *55*, 25–40.
10. Atkinson, E. A., & Bleackley, R. C. (1995). Mechanisms of lysis by cytotoxic T cells. *Critical Reviews in Immunology*, *15*(3–4), 359–384.
11. Groscurth, P., & Filgueira, L. (1998). Killing mechanisms of cytotoxic T lymphocytes. *News in Physiological Sciences*, *13*, 17–21.
12. Rajput, S., Sharma, P. K., & Malviya, R. (2023). Herbal drugs inducing autophagy for the management of cancer: Mechanism and utilization. *Current Pharmaceutical Biotechnology*.
13. Neumann, E., Schaefer-Ridder, M., Wang, Y., & Hofschneider, P. (1982). Gene transfer into mouse lyoma cells by electroporation in high electric fields. *The EMBO Journal*, *1*(7), 841–845.
14. Okino, M., & Mohri, H. (1987). Effects of a high-voltage electrical impulse and an anticancer drug on *in vivo* growing tumors. *Japanese Journal of Cancer Research: GANN*, *78*(12), 1319–1321.
15. Mir, L. M. (2009). Nucleic acids electrotransfer-based gene therapy (electrogenetherapy): Past, current, and future. *Molecular Biotechnology*, *43*(2), 167–176.
16. Cemazar, M., Tamzali, Y., Sersa, G., Tozon, N., Mir, L. M., Miklavcic, D., Lowe, R., & Teissie, J. (2008). Electrochemotherapy in veterinary oncology. *Journal of Veterinary Internal Medicine*, *22*(4), 826–831.
17. Altieri, D. C. (2008). Survivin, cancer networks and pathway-directed drug discovery. *Nature Reviews Cancer*, *8*(1), 61–70.
18. Kim, N. W, Piatyszek, M. A., Prowse, K. R., Harley, C. B., West, M. D., Ho, P. L., Coviello, G. M., Wright, W. E., Weinrich, S. L., & Shay, J. W. (1994). Specific association of human telomerase activity with immortal cells and cancer. *Science*, *266*(5193), 2011–2015.
19. Hiyama, E., & Hiyama, K. (2003). Telomerase as tumor marker. *Cancer Letters*, *194*(4), 221–233.
20. Zhang, H., Wang, Y., Liu, C., Zhang, L., Xia, Q., Zhang, Y., Wu, J., Jiang, C., Chen, Y., Wu, Y., & Zha, X. (2012). DNA and adenovirus tumor vaccine expressing truncated survivin generates specific immune responses and anti-tumor effects in a murine melanoma model. *Cancer Immunology, Immunotherapy*, *61*(10), 1857–18567.
21. Yan, J., Pankhong, P., Shin, T. H., Obeng-Adjei, N., Morrow, M. P., Walters, J. N., Khan, A. S., Sardesai, N. Y., & Weiner, D. B. (2013). Highly optimized DNA vaccine targeting human telomerase reverse transcriptase stimulates potent antitumor immunity. *Cancer Immunology Research*, *1*(3), 179–189.
22. Tsuboi, A., Oka, Y., Ogawa, H., Elisseeva, O. A., Li, H., Kawasaki, K., Aozasa, K., Kishimoto, T., Udaka, K., & Sugiyama, H. (2000). Cytotoxic T-lymphocyte responses elicited to Wilms' tumor gene WT1 product by DNA vaccination. *Journal of Clinical Immunology*, *20*(3), 195–202.
23. Thompson, J., & Zimmermann, W. (1988). The carcinoembryonic antigen gene family: Structure, expression and evolution. *Tumor Biology*, *9*(2–3), 63–83.
24. Thompson, J. A., Grunert, F., & Zimmermann, W. (1991). Carcinoembryonic antigen gene family: Molecular biology and clinical perspectives. *Journal of Clinical Laboratory Analysis*, *5*(5), 344–366.

25. Slamon, D. J., Godolphin, W., Jones, L. A., Holt, J. A., Wong, S. G., Keith, D. E., Levin, W. J., Stuart, S. G., Udove, J., Ullrich, A., et al. (1989). Studies of the HER-2/neu proto-oncogene in human breast and ovarian cancer. *Science, 244*(4905), 707–712.
26. Song, K., Chang, Y., & Prud'homme, G. J. (2000). Regulation of T-helper-1 versus T-helper-2 activity and enhancement of tumor immunity by combined DNA-based vaccination and nonviral cytokine gene transfer. *Gene Therapy*, *7*(6), 481–492.
27. Aurisicchio, L., Peruzzi, D., Koo, G., Wei, W. Z., La Monica, N., & Ciliberto, G. (2014). Immunogenicity and therapeutic efficacy of a dual-component genetic cancer vaccine cotargeting carcinoembryonic antigen and HER2/neu in preclinical models. *Human Gene Therapy*, *25*(2), 121–131.
28. Ruoslahti, E., & Seppälä, M. (1979). α-Fetoprotein in cancer and fetal development. *Advances in Cancer Research*, *29*, 275–346.
29. Meng, W., Butterfield, L. H., Ribas, A., Dissette, V. B., Heller, J. B., Miranda, G. A., Glaspy, J. A., McBride, W. H., & Economou, J. S. (2001). Alpha-fetoprotein-specific tumor immunity induced by plasmid prime-adenovirus boost genetic vaccination. *Cancer Research*, *61*(24), 8782–8786.
30. Butterfield, L., Economou, J. S., Gamblin, T. C., & Geller, D. A. (2014). Alpha fetoprotein DNA prime and adenovirus boost immunization of two hepatocellular cancer patients. *Journal of Translational Medicine, 12*, 86.
31. Oji, Y., Miyoshi, S., Maeda, H., Hayashi, S., Tamaki, H., Nakatsuka, S., Yao, M., Takahashi, E., Nakano, Y., Hirabayashi, H., Shintani, Y., Oka, Y., Tsuboi, A., Hosen, N., Asada, M., Fujioka, T., Murakami, M., Kanato, K., Motomura, M., Kim, E. H., Kawakami, M., Ikegame, K., Ogawa, H., Aozasa, K., Kawase, I., & Sugiyama, H. (2002). Overexpression of the Wilms' tumor gene WT1 in de novo lung cancers. *International Journal of Cancer*, *100*(3), 297–303.
32. Koesters, R., Linnebacher, M., Coy, J. F., Germann, A., Schwitalle, Y., Findeisen, P., & von Knebel Doeberitz, M. (2004). WT1 is a tumor-associated antigen in colon cancer that can be recognized by *in vitro* stimulated cytotoxic T cells. *International Journal of Cancer*, *109*(3), 385–392.
33. Chaise, C., Buchan, S. L., Rice, J., Marquet, J., Rouard, H., Kuentz, M., Vittes, G. E., Molinier-Frenkel, V., Farcet, J. P., Stauss, H. J., & Delfau-Larue, M. H. (2008). DNA vaccination induces WT1-specific T-cell responses with potential clinical relevance. *Blood*, *112*(7), 2956–2964.
34. Wang, M., Kuriyama, M., Papsidero, L., Loor, R., Valenzyela, L., Murphy, G., & Chu, T. (1982). Prostate antigen of human cancer patients. *Methods Cancer Research*, *19*, 179–197.
35. Moul, J. W. (2000). Prostate specific antigen only progression of prostate cancer. *The Journal of Urology*, *163*(6), 1632–1642.
36. Schmittgen, T. D., Teske, S., Vessella, R. L., True, L. D., & Zakrajsek, B. A. (2003). Expression of prostate specific membrane antigen and three alternatively spliced variants of PSMA in prostate cancer patients. *International Journal of Cancer*, *107*(2), 323–329.
37. Gutman, A. B., & Gutman, E. B. (1938). An "acid" phosphatase occurring in the serum of patients with metastasizing carcinoma of the prostate gland. *The Journal of Clinical Investigation*, *17*(4), 478–478.

38. Marshall, D., San Mateo, L. R., Rudnick, K. A., McCarthy, S. G., Harris, M. C., McCauley, C., Schantz, A., Geng, D., Cawood, P., & Snyder, L. A. (2005). Induction of Th1-type immunity and tumor protection with a prostate-specific antigen DNA vaccine. *Cancer Immunology, Immunotherapy*, *54*(11), 1082–1094.
39. Ferraro, B., Cisper, N. J., Talbott, K. T., Philipson-Weiner, L., Lucke, C. E., Khan, A. S., Sardesai, N. Y., & Weiner, D. B. (2011). Co-delivery of PSA and PSMA DNA vaccines with electroporation induces potent immune responses. *Human Vaccines*, *7*, 120–127.
40. Pavlenko, M., Roos, A. K., Lundqvist, A., Palmborg, A., Miller, A. M., Ozenci, V., Bergman, B., Egevad, L., Hellström, M., Kiessling, R., Masucci, G., Wersäll, P., Nilsson, S., & Pisa, P. (2004). A phase I trial of DNA vaccination with a plasmid expressing prostate-specific antigen in patients with hormone-refractory prostate cancer. *British Journal of Cancer*, *91*(4), 688–694.
41. McNeel, D. G., Dunphy, E. J., Davies, J. G., Frye, T. P., Johnson, L. E., Staab, M. J., Horvath, D. L., Straus, J., Alberti, D., Marnocha, R., & Liu, G. (2009). Safety and immunological efficacy of a DNA vaccine encoding prostatic acid phosphatase in patients with stage D0 prostate cancer. *Journal of Clinical Oncology*, *27*(25), 4047–4054.
42. Becker, J. T., Olson, B. M., Johnson, L. E., Davies, J. G., Dunphy, E. J., & McNeel, D. G. (2010). DNA vaccine encoding prostatic acid phosphatase (PAP) elicits long-term T-cell responses in patients with recurrent prostate cancer. *Journal of Immunotherapy*, *33*(6), 639–647.
43. Yoshida, N., Abe, H., Ohkuri, T., Wakita, D., Sato, M., Noguchi, D., Miyamoto, M., Morikawa, T., Kondo, S., Ikeda, H., & Nishimura, T. (2006). Expression of the MAGE-A4 and NYESO-1 cancer-testis antigens and T cell infiltration in non-small cell lung carcinoma and their prognostic significance. *International Journal of Oncology*, *28*(5), 1089–1098.
44. Ma, J., Sui, Y. F., Ye, J., Huang, Y. Y., Li, Z. S., Chen, G. S., Qu, P., Song, H. P., & Zhang, X. M. (2005). Heat shock protein 70/MAGE-3 fusion protein vaccine can enhance cellular and humoral immune responses to MAGE-3 *in vivo*. *Cancer Immunology, Immunotherapy*, *54*(9), 907–914.
45. Gnjatic, S., Altorki, N. K., Tang, D. N., Tu, S. M., Kundra, V., Ritter, G., Old, L. J., Logothetis, C. J., & Sharma, P. (2009). NY-ESO-1 DNA vaccine induces T-cell responses that are suppressed by regulatory T cells. *Clinical Cancer Research*, *15*(6), 2130–2139.
46. Kawakami, Y., Eliyahu, S., Delgado, C. H., Robbins, P. F., Rivoltini, L., Topalian, S. L., Miki, T., & Rosenberg, S. A. (1994). Cloning of the gene coding for a shared human melanoma antigen recognized by autologous T cells infiltrating into tumor. *Proceedings of the National Academy of Science of the United State of America*, *91*(9), 3515–3519.
47. Kawakami, Y., Eliyahu, S., Delgado, C. H., Robbins, P. F., Sakaguchi, K., Appella, E., Yannelli, J. R., Adema, G. J., Miki, T., & Rosenberg, S. A. (1994). Identification of a human melanoma antigen recognized by tumor-infiltrating lymphocytes associated with *in vivo* tumor rejection. *Proceedings of the National Academy of Science of the United State of America*, *91*(14), 6458–6462.

48. Brichard, V., Van Pel, A., Wölfel, T., Wölfel, C., De Plaen, E., Lethé, B., Coulie, P., & Boon, T. (1993). The tyrosinase gene codes for an antigen recognized by autologous cytolytic T lymphocytes on HLA-A2 melanomas. *Journal of Experimental Medicine*, *178*(2), 489–495.
49. Tanaka, M., Kaneda, Y., Fujii, S., Yamano, T., Hashimoto, K., Huang, S. K., & Hoon, D. S. (2002). Induction of a systemic immune response by a polyvalent melanoma-associated antigen DNA vaccine for prevention and treatment of malignant melanoma. *Molecular Therapy*, *5*(3), 291–299.
50. Steitz, J., Brück, J., Steinbrink, K., Enk, A., Knop, J., & Tüting, T. (2000). Genetic immunization of mice with human tyrosinase-related protein 2: Implications for the immunotherapy of melanoma. *International Journal of Cancer*, *86*(1), 89–94.
51. Rosenberg, S., Yang, J. C., Sherry, R. M., Hwu, P., Topalian, S. L., Schwartzentruber, D. J., Restifo, N. P., Haworth, L. R., Seipp, C. A., Freezer, L. J., Morton, K. E., Mavroukakis, S. A., & White, D. E. (2003). Inability to immunize patients with metastatic melanoma using plasmid DNA encoding the gp100 melanoma-melanocyte antigen. *Human Gene Therapy*, *14*(8), 709–714.
52. Cassaday, R., Sondel, P. M., King, D. M., Macklin, M. D., Gan, J., Warner, T. F., Zuleger, C. L., Bridges, A. J., Schalch, H. G., Kim, K. M., Hank, J. A., Mahvi, D. M., & Albertini, M. R. (2007). A phase I study of immunization using particle–mediated epidermal delivery of genes for gp100 and GM-CSF into uninvolved skin of melanoma patients. *Clinical Cancer Research*, *13*(2 Pt 1), 540–549.
53. Tagawa, S., Lee, P., Snively, J., Boswell, W., Ounpraseuth, S., Lee, S., Hickingbottom, B., Smith, J., Johnson, D., & Weber, J. S. (2003). Phase I study of intranodal delivery of a plasmid DNA vaccine for patients with Stage IV melanoma. *Cancer*, *98*(1), 144–154.
54. Sirisinha, S., & Eisen, H. N. (1971). Autoimmune-like antibodies to the ligand-binding sites of myeloma proteins. *Proceedings of the National Academy of Sciences*, *68*(12), 3130–3135.
55. Lynch, R. G., Graff, R. J., Sirisinha, S., Simms, E. S., & Eisen, H. N. (1972). Myeloma proteins as tumorspecific transplantation antigens. *Proceedings of the National Academy of Sciences*, *69*(6), 1540–1544.
56. Qin, H., Cha, S. C., Neelapu, S. S., Lou, Y., Wei, J., Liu, Y. J., & Kwak, L. W. (2009). Vaccine site inflammation potentiates idiotype DNA vaccine-induced therapeutic T cell-, and not B cell-, dependent antilymphoma immunity. *Blood*, *114*(19), 4142–4149.
57. Levine, A. J. (1997). p53, the cellular gatekeeper for growth and division. *Cell*, *88*(3), 323–331.
58. Oren, M. (1999). Regulation of the p53 tumor suppressor protein. *Journal of Biological Chemistry*, *274*(51), 36031–36034.
59. Soong, R. S., Trieu, J., Lee, S. Y., He, L., Tsai, Y. C., Wu, T. C., & Hung, C. F. (2013). Xenogeneic human p53 DNA vaccination by electroporation breaks immune tolerance to control murine tumors expressing mouse p53. *PLoS One*, *8*(2), e56912.
60. Dunn, G. P., Old, L. J., & Schreiber, R. D. (2004). The three Es of cancer immunoediting. *Annual Review of Immunology*, *22*, 329–360.
61. List, A. F., Spier, C. M., Miller, T. P., & Grogan, T. M. (1993). Deficient tumor-infiltrating T-lymphocyte response in malignant lymphoma: Relationship to HLA expression and host immunocompetence. *Leukemia*, *7*(3), 398–403.

62. Stopeck, A. T., Gessner, A., Miller, T. P., Hersh, E. M., Johnson, C. S., Cui, H., Frutiger, Y., & Grogan, T. M. (2000). Loss of B7. 2 (CD86) and intracellular adhesion molecule 1 (CD54) expression is associated with decreased tumor-infiltrating T lymphocytes in diffuse B-cell large-cell lymphoma. *Clinical Cancer Research*, *6*(10), 3904–3909.
63. Bushway, M., Cycon, K. A., Mulvaney, K., & Murphy, S. P. (2010). Coordinate loss of MHC class II expression in the diffuse large B cell lymphoma cell line OCI-Ly2 is due to a novel mutation in RFX–AP. *Immunogenetics*, *62*(2), 109–116.
64. Khanna, R. (1998). Tumour surveillance: Missing peptides and MHC molecules. *Immunology and Cell Biology*, *76*(1), 20–26.
65. Rajput, S., Sharma, P. K., & Malviya, R. (2023). Fluid, mechanics in circulating tumour cells: Role in metastasis and treatment strategies. *Medicine in Drug Discovery*, *18*(6382), 100158.
66. Zou, W. (2005). Immunosuppressive networks in the tumour environment and their therapeutic relevance. *Nature Reviews Cancer*, *5*(4), 263–274.
67. Van den Berg, J. H., Oosterhuis, K., Beijnen, J. H, Nuijen, B., & Haanen, J. B. A. G. (2010). DNA vaccination in oncology: Current status, opportunities and perspectives. *Current Clinical Pharmacology*, *5*(3), 218–225.
68. Liu, M. A. (2010). Gene-based vaccines: Recent developments. *Current Opinion in Molecular Therapeutics, 12*(1), 86–93.
69. Aihara, H., & Miyazaki, J, I. (1998). Gene transfer into muscle by electroporation *in vivo*. *Nature Biotechnology*, *16*(9), 867–870.
70. Suzuki, T., Shin, B. C., Fujikura, K., Matsuzaki, T., & Takata, K. (1998). Direct gene transfer into rat liver cells by *in vivo* electroporation. *FEBS Letters*, *425*(3), 436–440.
71. Mir, L. M., Bureau, M. F., Gehl, J., Rangara, R., Rouy, D., Caillaud, J. M., Delaere, P., Branellec, D., Schwartz, B., & Scherman, D. (1999). High-efficiency gene transfer into skeletal muscle mediated by electric pulses. *Proceedings of the National Academy of Sciences*, *96*(8), 4262–4267.
72. Ayuni, E. L., Gazdhar, A., Giraud, M. N., Kadner, A., Gugger, M., Cecchini, M., Caus, T., Carrel, T. P., Schmid, R. A., & Tevaearai, H. T. (2010). *In vivo* electroporation mediated gene delivery to the beating heart. *Plos One*, *5*(12), e14467.
73. Blair-Parks, K., Weston, B. C., & Dean, D. A. (2002). High-level gene transfer to the cornea using electroporation. *The Journal of Gene Medicine*, *4*(1), 92–100.
74. Heller, R., Jaroszeski, M., Atkin, A., Moradpour, D., Gilbert, R., Wands, J., & Nicolau, C. (1996). *In vivo* gene electroinjection and expression in rat liver. *FEBS Letters*, *389*(3), 225–228.
75. Martin, J. B., Young, J. L., Benoit, J. N., & Dean, D. A. (2000). Gene transfer to intact mesenteric arteries by electroporation. *Journal of Vascular Research*, *37*(5), 372–380.
76. Chiarella, P., Massi, E., De Robertis, M., Sibilio, A., Parrella, P., Fazio, V. M., & Signori, E. (2008). Electroporation of skeletal muscle induces danger signal release and antigen-presenting cell recruitment independently of DNA vaccine administration. *Expert Opinion on Biological Therapy*, *8*(11), 1645–1657.
77. Escoffre, J. M., Portet, T., Wasungu, L., Teissié, J., Dean, D., & Rols, M. P. (2009). What is (still not) known of the mechanism by which electroporation mediates

gene transfer and expression in cells and tissues. *Molecular Biotechnology*, *41*(3), 286–295.

78. Bureau, M. F., Gehl, J., Deleuze, V., Mir, L. M., & Scherman, D. (2000). Importance of association between permeabilization and electrophoretic forces for intramuscular DNA electrotransfer. *Biochimica et Biophysica Acta (BBA)*, *1474*(3), 353–359.
79. Gehl, J., Sørensen, T. H., Nielsen, K., Raskmark, P., Nielsen, S. L., Skovsgaard, T., & Mir, L. M. (1999). *In vivo* electroporation of skeletal muscle: threshold, efficacy and relation to electric field distribution. *Biochimica et Biophysica Acta (BBA)*, *1428*(2–3), 233–240.
80. Rinaldi, M., Catapano, A. L., Parrella, P., Ciafre, S. A., Signori, E., Seripa, D., Uboldi, P., Antonini, R., Ricci, G., Farace, M. G., & Fazio, V. M. (2000). Treatment of severe hypercholesterolemia in apolipoprotein E-deficient mice by intramuscular injection of plasmid DNA. *Gene Therapy*, *7*(21), 1795–1801.
81. Signori, E., Rinaldi, M., Fioretti, D., Iurescia, S., Seripa, D., Perrone, G., Norata, G. D., Catapano, A. L., & Fazio, V. M. (2007). ApoE gene delivery inhibits severe hypercholesterolemia in newborn ApoE-KO mice. *Biochemical and Biophysical Research Communications*, *361*(2), 543–548.
82. Tripathy, S. K., Svensson, E. C., Black, H. B., Goldwasser, E., Margalith, M., Hobart, P. M., & Leiden, J. M. (1996). Long-term expression of erythropoietin in the systemic circulation of mice after intramuscular injection of a plasmid DNA vector. *Proceedings of the National Academy of Sciences*, *93*(20), 10876–10880.
83. Ma, J. X., Yang, Z., Chao, J., & Chao, L. (1995). Intramuscular delivery of rat kallikrein-binding protein gene reverses hypotension in transgenic mice expressing human tissue kallikrein. *Journal of Biological Chemistry*, *270*(1), 451–455.
84. Tsurumi, Y., Takeshita, S., Chen, D., Kearney, M., Rossow, S. T., Passeri, J., Horowitz, J. R., Symes, J. F., & Isner, J. M. (1996). Direct intramuscular gene transfer of naked DNA encoding vascular endothelial growth factor augments collateral development and tissue perfusion. *Circulation*, *94*(12), 3281–3290.
85. Liu, M. A. (2011). DNA vaccines: An historical perspective and view to the future. *Immunological Reviews*, *239*(1), 62–84.
86. Gehl, J., & Mir, L. M. (1999). Determination of optimal parameters for *in vivo* gene transfer by electroporation, using a rapid *in vivo* test for cell permeabilization. *Biochemical and Biophysical Research Communications*, *261*(2), 377–380.
87. Mathiesen, I. (1999). Electropermeabilization of skeletal muscle enhances gene transfer *in vivo*. *Gene Therapy*, *6*(4), 508–514.
88. Trollet, C., Scherman, D., & Bigey, P. (2008). Delivery of DNA into muscle for treating systemic diseases: Advantages and challenges. *Methods in Molecular Biology*, *423*, 199–214.
89. McMahon, J. M., Signori, E., Wells, K. E., Fazio, V. M., & Wells, D. J. (2001). Optimisation of electrotransfer of plasmid into skeletal muscle by pretreatment with hyaluronidase–increased expression with reduced muscle damage. *Gene Therapy*, *8*(16), 1264–1270.
90. Chiarella, P., Massi, E., De Robertis, M., Sibilio, A., Parrella, P., Fazio, V. M., & Signori, E. (2008). Electroporation of skeletal muscle induces danger signal release and antigen-presenting cell recruitment independently of DNA vaccine administration. *Expert Opinion on Biological Therapy*, *8*(11), 1645–1657.

91. Hojman, P., Gissel, H., Andre, F. M., Cournil-Henrionnet, C., Eriksen, J., Gehl, J., & Mir, L. M. (2008). Physiological effects of high-and low-voltage pulse combinations for gene electrotransfer in muscle. *Human Gene Therapy*, *19*(11), 1249–1260.
92. Hojman, P., Zibert, J. R., Gissel, H., Eriksen, J., & Gehl, J. (2007). Gene expression profiles in skeletal muscle after gene electrotransfer. *BMC Molecular Biology*, *8*, 56.
93. Radkevich-Brown, O., Piechocki, M. P., Back, J. B., Weise, A. M., Pilon-Thomas, S., & Wei, W. Z. (2010). Intratumoral DNA electroporation induces anti-tumor immunity and tumor regression. *Cancer Immunology, Immunotherapy*, *59*(3), 409–417.
94. Mahvi, D. M., Henry, M. B., Albertini, M. R., Weber, S., Meredith, K., Schalch, H., Rakhmilevich, A., Hank, J., & Sondel, P. (2007). Intratumoral injection of IL-12 plasmid DNA-results of a phase I/IB clinical trial. *Cancer Gene Therapy*, *14*(8), 717–723.
95. Prud'homme, G. J., Glinka, Y., Khan, A. S., & Draghia-Akli, R. (2006). Electroporation-enhanced nonviral gene transfer for the prevention or treatment of immunological, endocrine and neoplastic diseases. *Current Gene Therapy*, *6*(2), 243–273.
96. Roos, A. K., Moreno, S., Leder, C., Pavlenko, M., King, A., & Pisa, P. (2006). Enhancement of cellular immune response to a prostate cancer DNA vaccine by intradermal electroporation. *Molecular Therapy*, *13*(2), 320–327.
97. Drabick, J. J., Glasspool-Malone, J., Somiari, S., King, A., & Malone, R. W. (2001). Cutaneous transfection and immune responses to intradermal nucleic acid vaccination are significantly enhanced by *in vivo* electropermeabilization. *Molecular Therapy*, *3*(2), 249–255.
98. Hooper, J. W., Golden, J. W., Ferro, A. M., & King, A. D. (2007). Smallpox DNA vaccine delivered by novel skin electroporation device protects mice against intranasal poxvirus challenge. *Vaccine*, *25*(10), 1814–1823.
99. Babiuk, S., Baca-Estrada, M. E., Foldvari, M., Baizer, L., Stout, R., Storms, M., Rabussay, D., Widera, G., & Babiuk, L. (2003). Needle-free topical electroporation improves gene expression from plasmids administered in porcine skin. *Molecular Therapy*, *8*(6), 992–998.
100. Hirao, L. A., Wu, L., Khan, A. S., Satishchandran, A., Draghia-Akli, R., & Weiner, D. B. (2008). Intradermal/subcutaneous immunization by electroporation improves plasmid vaccine delivery and potency in pigs and rhesus macaques. *Vaccine*, *26*(3), 440–448.
101. Gothelf, A., Mahmood, F., Dagnaes-Hansen, F., & Gehl, J. (2011). Efficacy of transgene expression in porcine skin as a function of electrode choice. *Bioelectrochemistry*, *82*(2), 95–102.
102. Hirao, L. A., Draghia-Akli, R., Prigge, J. T., Yang, M., Satishchandran, A., Wu, L., Hammarlund, E., Khan, A. S., Babas, T., Rhodes, L., & Silvera, P. (2011). Multivalent smallpox DNA vaccine delivered by intradermal electroporation drives protective immunity in nonhuman primates against lethal monkeypox challenge. *Journal of Infectious Diseases*, *203*(1), 95–102.
103. Gothelf, A., Eriksen, J., Hojman, P., & Gehl, J. (2010). Duration and level of transgene expression after gene electrotransfer to skin in mice. *Gene Therapy*, *17*(7), 839–845.
104. Roos, A. K., Eriksson, F., Timmons, J. A., Gerhardt, J., Nyman, U., Gudmundsdotter, L., Bråve, A., Wahren, B., & Pisa, P. (2009). Skin electroporation: Effects on transgene expression, DNA persistence and local tissue environment. *Plos One*, *4*(9), e7226.

105. Roos, A. K., Eriksson, F., Walters, D. C., Pisa, P., & King, A. D. (2009). Optimization of skin electroporation in mice to increase tolerability of DNA vaccine delivery to patients. *Molecular Therapy*, *17*(9), 1637–1642.
106. Donate, A., Coppola, D., Cruz, Y., & Heller, R. (2011). Evaluation of a novel non-penetrating electrode for use in DNA vaccination. *PLoS One*, *6*(4), e19181.
107. Kim, M. S., & Sin, J. I. (2005). Both antigen optimization and lysosomal targeting are required for enhanced anti-tumour protective immunity in a human papillomavirus E7-expressing animal tumour model. *Immunology*, *116*(2), 255–266.
108. Hsu, K. F., Hung, C. F., Cheng, W. F., He, L., Slater, L. A., Ling, M., & Wu, T. C. (2001). Enhancement of suicidal DNA vaccine potency by linking mycobacterium tuberculosis heat shock protein 70 to an antigen. *Gene Therapy*, *8*(5), 376–383.
109. Yan, J., Reichenbach, D. K., Corbitt, N., Hokey, D. A., Ramanathan, M. P., McKinney, K. A., Weiner, D. B., & Sewell, D. (2009). Induction of antitumor immunity *in vivo* following delivery of a novel HPV-16 DNA vaccine encoding an E6/E7 fusion antigen. *Vaccine*, *27*(3), 431–440.
110. Low, L., Mander, A., McCann, K., Dearnaley, D., Tjelle, T., Mathiesen, I., Stevenson, F., & Ottensmeier, C. H. (2009). DNA vaccination with electroporation induces increased antibody responses in patients with prostate cancer. *Human Gene Therapy*, *20*(11), 1269–1278.
111. Chudley, L., McCann, K., Mander, A., Tjelle, T., Campos-Perez, J., Godeseth, R., Creak, A., Dobbyn, J., Johnson, B., Bass, P., Heath, C., Kerr, P., Mathiesen, I., Dearnaley, D., Stevenson, F., & Ottensmeier, C. (2012). DNA fusion-gene vaccination in patients with prostate cancer induces high-frequency CD8(+) T-cell responses and increases PSA doubling time. *Cancer Immunology Immunotherapy*, *61*(11), 2161–2170.
112. Bergman, P. J., Camps-Palau, M. A., McKnight, J. A., Leibman, N. F., Craft, D. M., Leung, C., Liao, J., Riviere, I., Sadelain, M., Hohenhaus, A. E., Gregor, P., Houghton, A. N., Perales, M. A., & Wolchok, J. D. (2006). Development of a xenogeneic DNA vaccine program for canine malignant melanoma at the Animal Medical Center. *Vaccine*, *24*(21), 4582–4585.
113. Liao, J., Gregor, P., Wolchok, J. D., Orlandi, F., Craft, D., Leung, C., Houghton, A. N., & Bergman, P. J. (2006). Vaccination with human tyrosinase DNA induces antibody responses in dogs with advanced melanoma. *Cancer Immunity*, *6*, 8.
114. Gold, J. S., Ferrone, C. R., Guevara-Patiño, J. A., Hawkins, W. G., Dyall, R., Engelhorn, M. E., Wolchok, J. D., Lewis, J. J., & Houghton, A. N. (2003). A single heteroclitic epitope determines cancer immunity after xenogeneic DNA immunization against a tumor differentiation antigen. *Journal of Immunology*, *170*(10), 5188–5194.
115. Hollstein, M., Shomer, B., Greenblatt, M., Soussi, T., Hovig, E., Montesano, R., & Harris, C. C. (1996). Somatic point mutations in the p53 gene of human tumors and cell lines: updated compilation. *Nucleic Acids Research*, *24*(1), 141–146.
116. Bowne, W. B., Srinivasan, R., Wolchok, J. D., Hawkins, W. G., Blachere, N. E., Dyall, R., Lewis, J. J., & Houghton, A. N. (1999). Coupling and uncoupling of tumor immunity and autoimmunity. *The Journal of Experimental Medicine*, *190*(11), 1717–1722.
117. Kalat, M., Küpcü, Z., Schüller, S., Zalusky, D., Zehetner, M., Paster, W., & Schweighoffer, T. (2002). *In vivo* plasmid electroporation induces tumor

antigen-specific CD8+ T-cell responses and delays tumor growth in a syngeneic mouse melanoma model. *Cancer Research*, *62*(19), 5489–5494.

118. Bergman, P. J., McKnight, J., Novosad, A., Charney, S., Farrelly, J., Craft, D., Wulderk, M., Jeffers, Y., Sadelain, M., Hohenhaus, A. E., & Segal, N. (2003). Long-term survival of dogs with advanced malignant melanoma after DNA vaccination with xenogeneic human tyrosinase: a phase I trial. *Clinical Cancer Research*, *9*(4), 1284–1290.
119. Bergman, P. J., Camps-Palau, M. A., McKnight, J. A., Leibman, N. F., Craft, D. M., Leung, C., Liao, J., Riviere, I., Sadelain, M., Hohenhaus, A. E., & Gregor, P. (2006). Development of a xenogeneic DNA vaccine program for canine malignant melanoma at the Animal Medical Center. *Vaccine*, *24*(21), 4582–4585.
120. Liao, J. C. F., Gregor, P., Wolchok, J. D., Orlandi, F., Craft, D., Leung, C., Houghton, A. N., & Bergman, P. J. (2006). Vaccination with human tyrosinase DNA induces antibody responses in dogs with advanced melanoma. *Cancer Immunity*, *6*, 8.
121. Wolchok, J. D., Yuan, J., Houghton, A. N., Gallardo, H. F., Rasalan, T. S., Wang, J., Zhang, Y., Ranganathan, R., Chapman, P. B., Krown, S. E., & Livingston, P. O. (2007). Safety and immunogenicity of tyrosinase DNA vaccines in patients with melanoma. *Molecular Therapy*, *15*(11), 2044–2050.
122. Peggs, K. S., Quezada, S. A., & Allison, J. P. (2009). Cancer immunotherapy: Co-stimulatory agonists and co-inhibitory antagonists. *Clinical and Experimental Immunology*, *157*(1), 9–19.
123. Pentcheva-Hoang, T., Corse, E., & Allison, J. P. (2009). Negative regulators of T-cell activation: potential targets for therapeutic intervention in cancer, autoimmune disease, and persistent infections. *Immunological Reviews*, *229*(1), 67–87.
124. Sin, J. I., Kim, H., Ahn, E., Jeon, Y. H., Park, W. S., Lee, S. Y., & Kwon, B. (2013). Combined stimulation of TLR9 and 4.1BB augments Trp2 peptide vaccine-mediated melanoma rejection by increasing Ag-specific CTLs and their infiltration into tumor sites. *Cancer Letters*, *330*(2), 190–199.
125. Kim, H., Kwon, B., & Sin, J. I. (2013). Combined stimulation of IL-2 and 4-1BB receptors augments the antitumor activity of E7 DNA vaccines by increasing Ag-specific CTL responses. *PLoS One*, *8*(12), e83765.
126. Cuadros, C., Dominguez, A. L., Lollini, P. L., Croft, M., Mittler, R. S., Borgström, P., & Lustgarten, J. (2005). Vaccination with dendritic cells pulsed with apoptotic tumors in combination with anti-OX40 and anti-4-1BB monoclonal antibodies induces T cellmediated protective immunity in Her-2/neu transgenic mice. *International Journal of Cancer*, *116*(6), 934–943.
127. Cohen, A. D., Diab, A., Perales, M. A., Wolchok, J. D., Rizzuto, G., Merghoub, T., Huggins, D., Liu, C., Turk, M. J., Restifo, N. P., Sakaguchi, S., & Houghton, A. N. (2006). Agonist anti-GITR antibody enhances vaccine-induced CD8(+) T-cell responses and tumor immunity. *Cancer Research*, *66*(9), 4904–4912.
128. Van Elsas, A., Hurwitz, A. A., & Allison, J. P. (1999). Combination immunotherapy of B16 melanoma using anti-cytotoxic T lymphocyte–associated antigen 4 (CTLA-4) and granulocyte/macrophage colony-stimulating factor (GM-CSF)-producing vaccines induces rejection of subcutaneous and metastatic tumors accompanied by autoimmune depigmentation. *The Journal of Experimental Medicine*, *190*(3), 355–366.

129. Quezada, S. A., Peggs, K. S., Curran, M. A., & Allison, J. P. (2006). CTLA4 blockade and GM-CSF combination immunotherapy alters the intratumor balance of effector and regulatory T cells. *Journal of Clinical Investigation*, *116*(7), 1935–1945.
130. Gregor, P. D., Wolchok, J. D., Ferrone, C. R., Buchinshky, H., Guevara-Patiño, J. A., Perales, M. A., Mortazavi, F., Bacich, D., Heston, W., Latouche, J. B., Sadelain, M., Allison, J. P., Scher, H. I., & Houghton, A. N. (2004). CTLA-4 blockade in combination with xenogeneic DNA vaccines enhances T-cell responses, tumor immunity and autoimmunity to self antigens in animal and cellular model systems. *Vaccine*, *22*(13–14), 1700–1708.
131. Hodi, F. S., O'Day, S. J., McDermott, D. F., Weber, R. W., Sosman, J. A., Haanen, J. B., Gonzalez, R., Robert, C., Schadendorf, D., Hassel, J. C., Akerley, W., Van den Eertwegh, A. J., Lutzky, J., Lorigan, P., Vaubel, J. M., Linette, G. P., Hogg, D., Ottensmeier, C. H., Lebbé, C., Peschel, C., Quirt, I., Clark, J. I., Wolchok, J. D., Weber, J. S., Tian, J., Yellin, M. J., Nichol, G. M., Hoos, A., & Urba, W. J. (2010). Improved survival with ipilimumab in patients with metastatic melanoma. *The New England Journal of Medicine*, *363*(8), 711–723.
132. Kvistborg, P., Philips, D., Kelderman, S., Hageman, L., Ottensmeier, C., Joseph-Pietras, D., Welters, M. J., Van der Burg, S., Kapiteijn, E., Michielin, O., Romano, E., Linnemann, C., Speiser, D., Blank, C., Haanen, J. B., & Schumacher, T. N. (2014). Anti-CTLA-4 therapy broadens the melanoma-reactive CD8+ T cell response. *Science Translational Medicine*, *6*(254), 254ra128.
133. Chada, S., Ramesh, R., & Mhashilkar, A. M. (2003). Cytokine-and chemokine-based gene therapy for cancer. *Current Opinion in Molecular Therapeutics*, *5*(5), 463–474.
134. Lotze, M. T., Shurin, M., Esche, C., Tahara, H., Storkus, W., Kirkwood, J. M., Whiteside, T. L., Elder, E. M., Okada, H., & Robbins, P. (2000). Interleukin-2: Developing additional cytokine gene therapies using fibroblasts or dendritic cells to enhance tumor immunity. *The Cancer Journal from Scientific American*, *6*(Suppl 1), S61–S66.
135. Shimizu, K., Fields, R. C., Redman, B. G., Giedlin, M., & Mulé, J. J. (2000). Potentiation of immunologic responsiveness to dendritic cell-based tumor vaccines by recombinant interleukin-2. *The Cancer Journal from Scientific American*, *6*(Suppl 1), S67–S75.
136. Weiss, J. M., Subleski, J. J., Wigginton, J. M., & Wiltrout, R. H. (2007). Immunotherapy of cancer by IL-12-based cytokine combinations. *Expert Opinion on Biological Therapy*, *7*(11), 1705–1721.
137. Horton, H. M., Dorigo, O., Hernandez, P., Anderson, D., Berek, J. S., & Parker, S. E. (1999). IL-2 plasmid therapy of murine ovarian carcinoma inhibits the growth of tumor ascites and alters its cytokine profile. *The Journal of Immunology*, *163*(12), 6378–6385.
138. Heller, L., Pottinger, C., Jaroszeski, M. J., Gilbert, R., & Heller, R. (2000). *In vivo* electroporation of plasmids encoding GM-CSF or interleukin-2 into existing B16 melanomas combined with electrochemotherapy induces long-term antitumour immunity. *Melanoma Research*, *10*(6), 577–583.
139. Horton, H. M., Lalor, P. A., & Rolland, A. P. (2008). IL-2 plasmid electroporation: from preclinical studies to phase I clinical trial. *Methods in Molecular Biology*, *423*, 361–372.

140. Parker, S. E., Vahlsing, H. L., Lew, D., Martin, T., Hall, B., Kornbrust, D., & Norman, J. (1999). Cancer gene therapy using plasmid DNA-Pharmacokinetics and safety evaluation of an IL-2 plasmid DNA expression vector in rodents and nonhuman primates. *Biopharm-The Applied Technologies of Biopharmaceutical Development*, *12*, 18–24.
141. Lohr, F., Lo, D. Y., Zaharoff, D. A., Hu, K., Zhang, X., Li, Y., Zhao, Y., Dewhirst, M. W., Yuan, F., & Li, C. Y. (2001). Effective tumor therapy with plasmid-encoded cytokines combined with *in vivo* electroporation. *Cancer Research*, *61*(8), 3281–3284.
142. Lucas, M. L., Heller, L., Coppola, D., & Heller, R. (2002). IL-12 plasmid delivery by *in vivo* electroporation for the successful treatment of established subcutaneous B16. F10 melanoma. *Molecular Therapy*, *5*(6), 668–675.
143. Lucas, M. L., & Heller, R. (2003). IL-12 gene therapy using an electrically mediated nonviral approach reduces metastatic growth of melanoma. *DNA and Cell Biology*, *22*(12), 755–763.
144. Heller, L., Merkler, K., Westover, J., Cruz, Y., Coppola, D., Benson, K., Daud, A., & Heller, R. (2006). Evaluation of toxicity following electrically mediated interleukin-12 gene delivery in a B16 mouse melanoma model. *Clinical Cancer Research*, *12*(10), 3177–3183.
145. Daud, A. I., DeConti, R. C., Andrews, S., Urbas, P., Riker, A. I., Sondak, V. K., Munster, P. N., Sullivan, D. M., Ugen, K. E., Messina, J. L., & Heller, R. (2008). Phase I trial of interleukin-12 plasmid electroporation in patients with metastatic melanoma. *Journal of Clinical Oncology*, *26*(36), 5896 –5903.
146. Mennuni, C., Calvaruso, F., Facciabene, A., Aurisicchio, L., Storto, M., Scarselli, E., Ciliberto, G., & La Monica, N. (2005). Efficient induction of T-cell responses to carcinoembryonic antigen by a heterologous prime-boost regimen using DNA and adenovirus vectors carrying a codon usage optimized cDNA. *International Journal of Cancer*, *117*(3), 444–455.
147. Facciabene, A., Aurisicchio, L., Elia, L., Palombo, F., Mennuni, C., Ciliberto, G., & La Monica, N. (2006). DNA and adenoviral vectors encoding carcinoembryonic antigen fused to immunoenhancing sequences augment antigen-specific immune response and confer tumor protection. *Human Gene Therapy*, *17*(1), 81–92.
148. Diaz-Montero, C. M., Chiappori, A., Aurisicchio, L., Bagchi, A., Clark, J., Dubey, S., Fridman, A., Fabregas, J. C., Marshall, J., Scarselli, E., La Monica, N., Ciliberto, G., & Montero, A. J. (2013). Phase 1 studies of the safety and immunogenicity of electroporated HER2/CEA DNA vaccine followed by adenoviral boost immunization in patients with solid tumors. *Journal of Translational Medicine*, *11*, 62.
149. U'Ren, L., Kedl, R., & Dow, S. (2006). Vaccination with liposome-DNA complexes elicits enhanced antitumor immunity. *Cancer Gene Therapy*, *13*(11), 1033–1044.
150. Li, A., Qin, L., Wang, W., Zhu, R., Yu, Y., Liu, H., & Wang, S. (2011). The use of layered double hydroxides as DNA vaccine delivery vector for enhancement of anti-melanoma immune response. *Biomaterials*, *32*(2), 469–477.
151. Inoue, K., Ogawa, H., Sonoda, Y., Kimura, T., Sakabe, H., Oka, Y., Miyake, S., Tamaki, H., Oji, Y., Yamagami, T., Tatekawa, T., Soma, T., Kishimoto, T., & Sugiyama, H. (1997). Aberrant overexpression of the Wilms tumor gene (WT1) in human leukemia. *Blood*, *89*(4), 1405–1412.

152. Weber, L. W., Bowne, W. B., Wolchok, J. D., Srinivasan, R., Qin, J., Moroi, Y., Clynes, R., Song, P., Lewis, J. J., & Houghton, A. N. (1998). Tumor immunity and autoimmunity induced by immunization with homologous DNA. *The Journal of Clinical Investigation*, *102*(6), 1258–1264.

CHAPTER 9

Promoting DNA-Based Cancer Vaccine Research

ABSTRACT

Cancer immunotherapy has emerged as a highly influential and transformative strategy in the ongoing fight against cancer, exhibiting significant accomplishments and successes in recent times. Among these, DNA-based cancer vaccines present a promising area of research, as they utilize the immune system of the body to selectively target and eradicate cancerous cells. This chapter examines the present state of research and development of DNA-based cancer vaccines, with a focus on their potential to significantly transform the landscape of cancer therapy. Immune responses innate immune suppression tumor-derived immunosuppressive networks and evasion mechanisms are among the numerous challenges facing cancer immunotherapy. For cancer prevention, plasmid DNA provides a unique vaccination method that may boost the body's immunological system to create antibodies and cells while also being delivered safely and made inexpensively. Although DNA vaccines have had encouraging outcomes their widespread use in human clinical trials, as seen in animal studies, has so far had little effect on cancer regression in the field. This chapter also discusses the possible advantages and limitations of DNA-based cancer vaccines when compared to other immunotherapeutic methods, such as checkpoint inhibitors and adoptive T-cell therapies. Furthermore, it explores the potential of personalized cancer vaccines, which are specifically designed for each patient, and their significance within the context of precision medicine. This chapter delivers a complete analysis of the present state of DNA-based cancer vaccine research, explaining its potential to significantly transform

DNA- and m-RNA-Based Vaccines: An Immunotherapeutic Approach to Cancer.
Sonali Sundram and Rishabha Malviya (Authors)

DOI: 10.1201/9781774919613-9

cancer immunotherapy and make significant contributions to the ongoing fight against this challenging disease.

9.1 INTRODUCTION

Tumor growth has been shown to spontaneously regress after exposure to bacteria, fungi, viruses, and protozoa. Intratumoral infections can cause tumor regression by reactivating defensive functions. These phenomena prompted the creation of several basic immunotherapies for cancer, starting with methods that do not target specific cells, first employed by William Coley [1] and culminating in the idea of cancer vaccination. For large-scale manufacturing of vaccines, using plasmid DNA rather than recombinant protein or entire tumor cells offers many practical advantages that are not available when using alternative vaccine delivery systems [2]. They may encode a variety of immune components and can be manufactured utilizing bacterial expression systems to administer them. The present standard of treatment procedures, such as surgery, radiation, and chemotherapy, has not had a significant impact on the dissemination and reoccurrence of progressive cancers [3]. Previously, Wolff et al. [4] demonstrated that continuous gene regulation in mice skeletal muscles could be achieved by directly administering plasmid DNA into the muscle. Initially, Wolff and associates showed sustaining gene expression by direct intramuscular injections of plasmid DNA mouse muscle for extended periods [4]. Because of these and other early research showing the viability of genetic vaccines, plasmid DNA was initially used to test vaccines against influenza and HIV-1 [5, 6]. Immunotherapy is gaining popularity as a cancer treatment strategy, and numerous methodologies are now being developed to enhance the clinical results seen in individuals diagnosed with cancer [7]. Plasmid-borne gene constructs are typically expressed in the host cell after vaccination using a bare DNA vector. The protein may travel through the proper channels for immunological presentation, where it may elicit immune responses from cells and antibodies, aiding in the fight against illness. Immunization with recombinant soluble protein, which enters exogenous presentation routes and primarily causes humoral immunity [1], has the opposite effect on the immune system.

One significant illustration of a contemporary genetic vaccination is the DNA vaccine, which involves the application of unencapsulated plasmid DNA as an immunization immune system activation approach response against various illnesses and offers several practical advantages for the production of vaccines on a large scale. These benefits are not as simply controllable when using additional vaccinations, such as recombinant protein or whole tumor cells [8, 9]. The rapid screening of antigens and the ability to design specific expression constructs have contributed to the significance of studying DNA vaccines in cancer immunotherapy. The development of new technologies, such as gene-expression profiling, has expanded the range of potential tumor antigens. Researchers have directed their attention toward specific targets in their investigations, such as tumor-specific antigens (TSAs) like idiotypic antigens found in B-cell tumors [10], as well as tumor-associated antigens (TAAs) [11]. These TAAs are also shown by the healthy cells that cancer emerged [12], and they encompass a collection of antigens identified together as cancer antigens found in the testis [13]. DNA vaccines allow for the incorporation of other gene-producing molecules to overcome tumor antigen immunogenicity and the patients' tolerized immune assortment. DNA vaccination signifies a potentially effective approach to manipulating the immune system. DNA vaccines are plasmid-specific engineered to transport genes that encode TAAs. These vaccines aim to stimulate or enhance the adaptive immune response against tumor cells that express these TAs. Cancer DNA vaccines work as "danger signals" to activate numerous DNA-sensing pathways in transfected cells' cytosol, triggering the innate immune response. This activation is due to CpG motifs and DNA double-stranding [14].

9.2 TUMOR ANTIGENS (TAS)

Numerous carcinoma-associated antigens have been discovered by scientists, and many of these are currently being used in both basic and clinical research to create cancer treatment vaccines. The regular expansion of tumor antigens is primarily attributable to the development of genetic methods, including monitoring the expression of genes and sequencing the human genome. Antigens found in tumors have been divided into two primary groups: common antigens and unique proteins that are only found in tumors [15]. Unique TAAs are specific to each tumor since they are the result of mutations generated by chemical or physical carcinogens. To achieve positive clinical outcomes, cancer vaccines should incorporate optimal immunotherapy drugs and administration methods along with the optimal selection of tumor antigens. However, a challenge inefficient immunity against the intended target may be induced without inducing deleterious autoimmunity by immunizing against overemphasized TAAs. DNA vaccines offer precise targeting of selected antigens, but careful selection of targets is necessary to prevent autoimmunity as their potency increases [16–19]. Since the initial identification of the first tumor antigen, specifically the tumor antigen (MAGE), in 1991 [20], there has been a continuous rise in tumor antigens that have been discovered. TAs can be categorized into two primary types, as indicated in Table 9.1.

TABLE 9.1 Types of Tumor Antigens.

Types of Tumor Antigen	Subtypes	Illustrations
Mutation antigens	The outcomes of mutated gene oncogenes (TSA)	Ras, P53, and Bcr-Abl
	Neoantigens	Case-dependent mutations
TAAs or tumor-associated antigens	Genes with inactive products	Antigens for cancer and the testis (a-fetoprotein, MAGE-1, and NY-ESO1)
	Type-specific antigens	Tyrosinase, Melan-A, MART-1, TRP-1/ 2, Gp100, and Melan-A
	Antigens prevalent in tumors	Her2/neu, telomerase, and surviving

9.2.1 MUTATION-SPECIFIC ANTIGENS

Mutation-specific antigens (MSAs) comprise a subset of tumor antigens that have garnered a lot of interest in cancer immunotherapy. The presence of these antigens on individual cancer cells is attributed to genetic mutations in their DNA, thereby establishing a distinctive characteristic that differentiates them from normal, healthy cells. MSAs present a promising avenue for precision cancer treatment due to their ability to be selectively recognized and targeted by the immune system. These are produced when self-proteins undergo mutations; they are not expected to be found in healthy cells. Oncogenes and tumor suppressor genes, including Ras and Bcr-Abl, may have a direct association with the growth of cancer [21]. These antigens are often referred to as "TSAs." Their specificity is relative, as they might be present in many cancers or aberrant noncancerous cells [22]. While some unique TAs may or may not be linked to tumor growth, they are a subgroup of tumor antigens this is because cancer cells' genes are not stable. Initially, these are referred to as "neoantigens." The capacity to recognize and capitalize on MSAs has facilitated the advancement of individualized cancer vaccines and immunotherapies, customized to correspond with the genetic characteristics of each patient's malignancy. By focusing on these MSAs, investigators hope to enhance the precision and efficiency of cancer treatment. This could change the way a wide range of cancers are treated while causing the least amount of harm to healthy tissues.

9.2.2 TUMOR-ASSOCIATED ANTIGENS (TAAS)

TAAs, which are a heterogeneous collection of molecules that are ubiquitously found on melanoma cell membranes, are crucial in the field of cancer immunotherapy. TAAs are attractive targets for immune-based therapies because they are widely shared among cancer cells, in contrast to MSAs, specific to particular tumors. These antigens are overexpressed or improperly generated by cancerous cells [22, 23]. These involve silent gene products like oncofetal or cancer/testis antigens, differentiating antigens, and universal tumor antigens, which show low expression in healthy tissues but are high in tumors [22]. Oncoviral TAAs are a type of TAA that is made up of nonhuman TAs and proteins that are only found in cancer cells that have been infected with an oncogenic virus [24]. Some examples of oncogenic viruses include the human papillomavirus, which has been linked to cervical cancer, which has been linked to nasopharyngeal carcinoma. Cancer cells differentiate from normal tissues by a variety of antigens, such as proteins, glycoproteins, and other molecules. Utilizing the immune system's capacity to identify and target TAAs, researchers have created a variety of immunotherapeutic strategies that target cancer with precision while sparing healthy cells. These strategies include adoptive cell therapies, cancer vaccines, and monoclonal antibodies. TAAs have helped develop targeted immunotherapies that could treat a variety of cancers and improve cancer patient outcomes.

9.3 THE CONCEPT OF ONE'S OWN IDENTITY

Extrinsic genetic defects, such as contracting a virus or being exposed to a carcinogen, can also initiate cancer-causing cell processes [25].

Epstein-Barr and human papillomaviruses are carcinogenic viruses linked to many forms of cancer [26]. Cells that generate tumors by secreting proteins from other viruses are good candidates for vaccine development after viral infections. Other identified variables that do not have an obvious immunogenic profile in the host's central tolerance system form the bulk of tumors throughout many different cancers. Self-antigen tolerance is the product of early immunological mechanisms that remove lymphocytes in the bone marrow and thymus that attack their own body generated by the host may be developed. Despite this, self-reacting lymphocytes survive the host's central tolerance systems and may be found in the periphery, giving the possibility of breaking self-tolerance [27, 28]. As an example, positive selection lymphocytes that respond weakly to either a self-antigen or an exogenous antigen that reacts with proteins found in the body, are included in these populations [29].

Selecting an appropriate DNA vaccine to attack a specific subset of cancer cells presents several challenges. Vaccine candidacy is heavily influenced by factors such as the antigen's molecular makeup and the tissues in which it is expressed. Antigens are both prevalent in protein targets whose expression is restricted to a single tumor type and which are identified by the immune system [30–32]. Due to the high similarity between tumor cells and healthy cell expression of self-antigens, these preferences are not always possible. Since DNA vaccines have to deal with breaking self-tolerance and not triggering medically uncontrolled autoimmune responses in the body, it is important to look at the whole picture.

An ever-growing collection of tumor self-antigens has been developed by researchers, which gives prospective vaccination targets for certain human tumors. Table 9.2 lists several of the most prevalent self-antigens, and they are categorized by antigen type. Many genes encode T lymphocyte-recognizable human tumor antigens, such as MAGE-A1 [33]. In cancer cells and germline organs, this antigen class is identified (e.g., testis, placenta, ovary). Since lacking appropriate antigen-presenting receptors in immune systems, mature cells, and reproductive organs cannot mount an effective defense against pathogens, CT antigens are suitable candidates for vaccine application [34]. Patients with cancer have been discovered to have CT antigen-specific antibodies and T lymphocytes, including those that target NY-ESO-1 [35]. A possible explanation for NY-heightened ESO-1's immunogenicity, despite its origin in the host, is that the protein is only found in immune-privileged cells in locations such as the testis, which sidesteps the body's primary toleration centers. In contrast to the normal cell equivalent, cells' proteins, called self-proteins, including HER-2/neu are overproduced and overexpressed in cancers. Differentiated antigens like MART-1/Melan-A, on the other hand, are unique to tumors in addition to typical cells descended from a given precursor. When alterations to TSAs drive cells toward a transformed state, this is called oncogenesis; they serve as targets against cancerous cells. This type of antigen is more representative of viral oncoproteins. Several of the aforementioned tumor antigens have been extensively studied into DNA vaccines in mouse trials. A protective immunological reaction may occur in response to cancer exposure if DNA vaccines are developed and given correctly. The outcomes of these animal models have already been described in great depth [36].

TABLE 9.2 T Cells Frequently Detect Self-Antigens From Tumors.

Category of Antigen	Antigen	Cancer in Its Various Manifestations
Disease-specific chemotherapy	CDK-4	Melanoma
	b-catenin	Melanoma
	Caspase-8	Head/neck
Differences	CEA	Colon
	Gp100	Melanoma
	MART-1/ Melan-A	Melanoma
	Tyrosinase	Melanoma
	PSA	Prostrate
High expression	MUC1	Breast
	HER-2/neu	Melanoma
	PSMA	Ovarian prostate

9.4 BENEFITS AND DRAWBACKS OF CANCER DNA VACCINATIONS

The use of DNA-mediated immunization was first employed throughout the 1990s, whereby a plasmid containing DNA that encodes the influenza A nucleoprotein was shown to induce a targeted and protective cytotoxic T lymphocyte (CTL) response [37]. Since then, DNA-mediated immunization has been widely used. Subsequently, DNA vaccines have been developed to combat a wide range of diseases and conditions, from allergens to cancer. Bacterial plasmids encoding antigens and immunostimulatory molecules (IL-2, GM-CSF, etc.) form the basis of DNA vaccines. They are administered intramuscularly (IM), topically, subcutaneously (SC), or orally. Various physical techniques have been used in genetic research, including electroporation (EP) [38], sonoporation [39, 40], DNA tattooing [41], and gene guns [42], which are widely used because they can successfully transport DNA into the nucleus despite the presence of both extracellular and intracellular barriers. To activate T cells, the DNA vaccine's encoded antigen must first be produced and expressed on the molecules of the MHC after entering the nucleus. DNA vaccines have the potential to stimulate CD4 and CD8 T cells and, indirectly, humoral immunity because the encoded antigen can be delivered by MHC class I and class II [43]. DNA vectors are a significant tool for clinical applications, particularly in cases where producing vaccines on a large scale is challenging using other vaccine forms such as recombinant protein, whole cancer cells, or viral vectors [44]. The use of genetically altered lentiviruses, adenoviruses, and retroviruses for viral-mediated gene transfer is advantageous due to their stable, efficient transfection [45]. However, a major challenge in utilizing viral vectors is the need to address the immunogenicity associated with viruses' packaging proteins. Viral approaches are also expensive, toxic, transgenic size-restrictive, and prone to insertional mutagenesis [46].

Nonviral vectors provide benefits, including greater flexibility, the ability to encode multiple immunological components, reduced cytotoxicity, relative stability, and potential cost savings during production and storage (Table 9.1). The security of injection-related side effects was established in both clinical trials and trials on animal models [47, 48]. The initial clinical trial, which was conducted to assess the security and effectiveness of a DNA vaccine targeting HIV-1 infection, provided evidence that DNA plasmid vaccinations were secure and elicited immune cell and antibody reactions [49]. Activation of innate immunity can also occur as a result of cytosolic sensors recognizing the double-stranded DNA structure [50, 51]. In murine models, the successful elicitation of a targeted and defensive immunological response is currently being observed within a range of antigens, such as surface and core antigens for hepatitis B, HIV Env, Gag, and TAAs in various cancer models [52, 53]. Cancer DNA vaccines offer certain advantages over nonspecific and non-targeted therapies in terms of antigen specificity and safety. Unlike therapies that lack specificity, vaccinations have been developed to specifically target certain antigens associated with cancer cells. This targeted approach reduces the risk of side effects and minimizes damage to healthy tissues [54]. Cancer DNA vaccines can induce a comprehensive immune response throughout the body, making them a viable treatment option for metastatic cancer, which poses challenges for surgical removal. Furthermore, in contrast to antibodies and other types of inhibitory small molecules, DNA vaccines have been shown to enhance the development of immunological memory [55, 56]. Incorporating genes into plasmids and using gene manipulation technology enables *in vivo* expression in cells.

While the efficiency of the transfection process is limited and can differ depending on the target tissue and method of administration, it typically achieves adequate DNA uptake to stimulate the immune response [52]. DNA vaccines offer numerous benefits over recombinant protein vaccines, as they are not burdened by the issues typically associated with their production. Additionally, DNA vaccines are considered safer than live vaccines with attenuation, which have the potential to induce pathogenic infections within the host organism. Furthermore, research conducted on DNA vaccination causes the development of anti-DNA antibodies. It does not occur even after repeated immunizations [57]. The unique characteristic of DNA vaccines lies in their capacity to introduce antigens to the immune system of the host, thereby facilitating the generation of robust Th1-type CD4+ T cells and CD8+ cytotoxic T cells. This sets them apart from conventional protein or peptide vaccines [58]. Plasmid-mediated gene transfer can introduce oligonucleotides into cells, thereby modifying gene splicing or gene expression. An example of such oligonucleotides is siRNA. Human studies of DNA vaccines showed very modest immunogenicity due to their delivery methods despite advancements in this area [59, 60]. Various molecular techniques have been examined to enhance their effectiveness, including the utilization of codon optimization. The utilization of increased production of proteins and plasmids immunity may be achieved with this gene engineering method by replacing synonymous codons [56]. Cancer DNA vaccines have shown promising results in several preclinical experiments, especially preventive ones, and have a generally encouraging safety profile in humans. Despite promising results in animal trials, medicinal vaccination has yet to fully realize its potential [61]. The primary factor contributing to this limitation is the diverse array of resistance mechanisms that arise during tumor development. These immune-suppressive cells produce cytokines such as TGF-β and IL-10, which further hinder immune responses. Additionally, the tumor microenvironment can deprive immune cells of essential nutrients and oxygen [62, 63].

9.5 THE AUGMENTATION OF IMMUNOGENICITY IN DNA VACCINES

Immunogenicity of DNA vaccines may be improved in several ways to stimulate a stronger immune response to the foreign DNA. Antigen expression may be improved by adjusting the vaccination plasmid's design, immunological activation can be increased by adding adjuvants or cytokines, and cellular absorption of the DNA can be increased by using delivery techniques like EP. A DNA vaccination followed by a protein-based or viral vector-based booster may further improve the immune response in a prime-boost strategy. Increasing immunogenicity also relies heavily on selecting the right target antigens and epitopes for a certain pathogen. All of these strategies are aimed at stimulating an immune response that will continue for an extended period, something that is essential for DNA vaccines to do their job of protecting against infectious illnesses.

9.5.1 DESIGNING PLASMIDS

During the initial stages of DNA vaccine research, it was evident that the optimization of antigen expression was crucial for the effective stimulation of immune responses. CMV-intA, a type of viral promoter known for its substantial activity, is typically the preferred promoter that is overactive or found naturally in eukaryotic cells [64]. Additionally, the incorporation of a nuclear targeting sequence (NTS) is a method that has been suggested to enhance the effectiveness of intramuscular injection in inducing nuclear plasmid uptake [65, 66].

The implementation of alternative coding sequences that have been codon-optimized is a widely applicable and effective approach for enhancing the efficacy of vaccination. The determination of an optimal coding sequence involves the utilization of algorithms that consider the expected structure of the messenger RNA (mRNA) and the quantity of certain transfer RNAs (tRNAs) in the cytoplasm of human cells. This coding sequence is derived in a reverse manner from the amino acid sequence of the antigen. Subsequently, the chosen genetic sequence is synthesized in a laboratory setting through the utilization of artificial oligonucleotides. Efforts are made to prevent the occurrence of unfavorable rare codons, while also minimizing mRNA secondary structures. Thus, the synthetic gene exhibits optimal characteristics for efficient expression and subsequently, the induction of an immune response [67]. Plasmid design flexibility and gene manipulation technology enable "gene enhancement [68]." Technical DNA vaccine development improves immunity to particular epitopes through sequence modifications. New strategies for enhancing immune responses are emerging from molecular recognition of the immune system's reaction. T cells selective for effective epitopes may be deleted due to self-tolerance, retaining only low-avidity T cells [69, 70]. Hence, it may be inferred that not all combinations possess the desirable characteristics of antigenic epitopes. The phenomenon of epitope enhancement has the potential to increase the immunogenicity of cancer epitope sequences [71].

9.5.2 THE ADMINISTERING METHOD

There seems to be a strong correlation between the route of administration and the immunogenicity of DNA vaccines [72]. Antiangiogenic plasmids expressing angiostatin and endostatin were intratumorally delivered in a melanoma mouse model with DNA immunization. The combined melanoma immunization increased tumor-free survival from baseline by 57% at 90 days postexposure [73]. Intratumoral DNA injection resulted in tumor regression at distant locations in a small percentage of individuals with malignant illness [74], Compared to alternative delivery techniques that inject DNA into different chemical solutions, current investigations have proven that physical approaches are preferable [75, 76]. Using a high-pressure tool, bare DNA is attached to gold beads for a biolistic gene gun delivery. This approach is a very effective method for delivering DNA to skin and Langerhans cells. Tumor immunity may be achieved with less vaccine and a higher CD8+ T cell response after gene gun vaccination [77].

To overcome the challenge of transferring the efficacy of transplanting DNA vaccines from rodents used in preclinical studies to larger animals and eventually humans via EP is a promising technique that boosts both the amount and breadth of response in primates [78, 79]. The absorption of DNA vaccines by cells is greatly improved by the use of EP-based DNA delivery technology. EP acts as an additive to boost electroporating experimental mouse DNA vaccines into bigger animals and humans may pick up on them. Significant immunological responses, including antibody and T-cell responses, are triggered by the inflammation and attracting DCs, macrophages, and lymphocytes to injection sites that EP produces [80, 81]. And since it is well tolerated without anesthesia and does not provoke the immune system to attack the delivery system, it may be used again. The tattoo technique is an innovative method of intradermal DNA delivery. The tattoo technology uses a cartridge with nine small metal-puncturing needles oscillating at high frequencies to pierce the skin and transfer genes to epidermal-associated cells. Strong T-cell responses are triggered by the expression of reporter genes [82].

9.5.3 PRIME-BOOST METHODS

It seems that the DNA vaccine platform has successfully improved with heterologous prime-boost immunization techniques employing several vectors for antigen delivery. Prime-boost regimens have shown the potential to involve a more robust immune response in people when compared to the use of DNA vaccine alone [83]. The DNA-prime-boosted-viral vector strategy prioritizes the stimulation of T-cell-mediated immune responses. In this particular methodology, the homologous boost vaccination entails the administration of an antigen that is comparable to the one used in the preceding immunization. Adenovirus and vaccinia virus are among the viral vectors that have been subjected to assessment for their potential as booster vaccines [84, 85], along with the virus of vesicular stomatitis that has been recombined [86]. The DNA-prime-protein-boost method uses regenerated protein antigens that match those employed in DNA prime immunization [87–89]. The objective of this method is to cultivate an immunological response that is equally effective via humoral and cell-mediated means, emphasizing the generation of robust and effective protective antibody responses. The use of distinct priming and boosting vectors enables a more extensive proliferation of T-cell populations that are specific to the illness antigen [90]. Currently, heterologous prime-boost regimens are considered to be one of the most effective techniques for eliciting cellular immune responses. When comparing the homologous prime-boost strategy to the use of a heterologous vector for boosting a primary response with the identical DNA vaccine, the latter strategy has been found to result in T cells that are 4–10 times greater [91–93].

9.5.4 MOLECULAR IMMUNOMODULATORS AND IMMUNOENHANCING AGENTS

Although naked DNA vaccinations have been proven to produce specific antibody and CTL responses in clinical studies, it was found that substantial amounts of DNA were needed to measure immunological responses when administered via the parenteral or intradermal route [94, 95]. Significant amounts, ranging from 5 to 10 mg, are necessary to elicit only moderate immunogenicity.

Enhancing DNA vaccine immunogenicity may be increased by modifying the vaccinated microenvironment location by the simultaneous delivery of genetic elements, such as DNA plasmids encoding immunostimulatory molecules, proteins, or chemical adjuvants. Significant advancements have been achieved in the enhancement of methods for enclosing plasmid DNA, utilizing liposomes, polymers, and microparticles. However, only a limited number of these formulations have demonstrated immune responses that surpass the effectiveness of basic intramuscular plasmid DNA administration. Regrettably, this outcome has persisted in human clinical studies [96]. To make defense reactions against tumor proteins more effective and have low immunogenicity, supplementary approaches include the use of vaccines that use DNA fusion genes to get T cells to help fight tumors. The CD4+ T helper cell (Th cells) is an important part of the defense system by promoting strong immunological responses and sustaining the response and has been thoroughly investigated by Stevenson et al. [97]. The need for foreign sequences to elicit T-helper cell activation in the B-cell response and facilitate CTL response has been well established in the scientific literature for a considerable period [98, 99]. Given that Th cells are very important for controlling immunity reactions to vaccination, it is evident that self-antigens lacking epitopes that can be identified by existing Th cells are unable to elicit an immune response.

9.6 DNA VACCINE-INDUCED IMMUNE RESPONSES

One significant benefit DNA vaccines may induce cellular (CD4+ and CD8+ T cells) and humoral immune responses. This is achieved by processing the encoded antigen through both endogenous and exogenous pathways, resulting in the presentation of peptide epitopes by both MHC Class I and Class II complexes (Figure 9.1) [100].

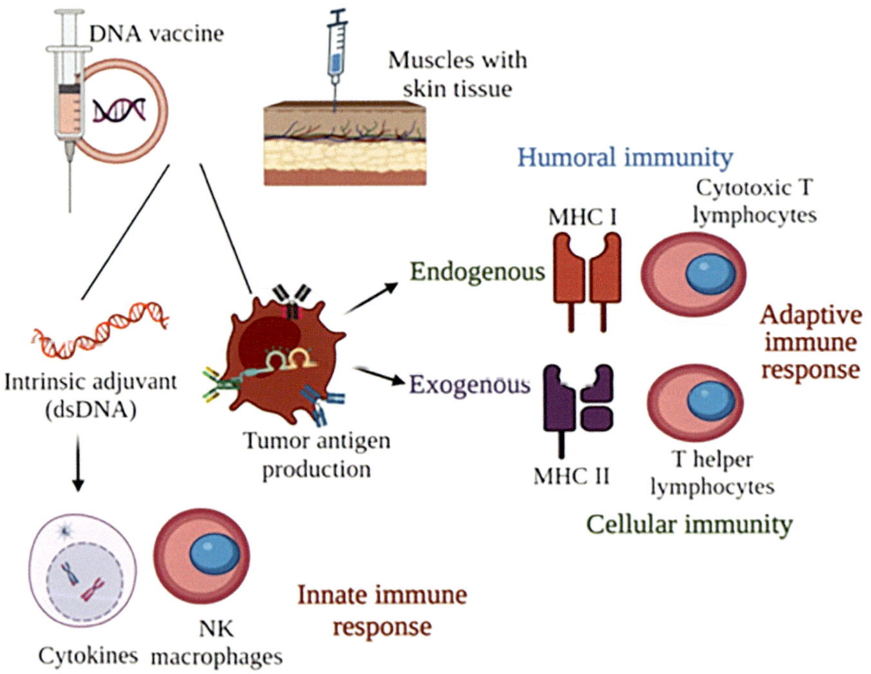

FIGURE 9.1 Antigen processing occurs through both endogenous and exogenous pathways, leading to the presentation of peptide epitopes by MHC Class I and Class II complexes.

9.6.1 CELLULAR IMMUNE RESPONSE

Intradermal injection of the target antigen may be produced by directly transfected cells (DC, Langerhans cells, and other APC). The proteasome is responsible for breaking down naturally occurring proteins into smaller pieces called peptides. Antigenic peptides are transported into the endoplasmic reticulum to be presented on major histocompatibility complex (MHC) class I molecules by peptide transporters that are attached to membranes that are antigenic (TAP). The induction of CD8+ T-cell response may be facilitated by the presence of co-stimulatory molecules. Intramuscular injection of transfected myocytes results in protein release upon lysis. The proteins are then internalized, digested, and presented by dendritic cells (DCs) via cross-priming, therefore inducing the activation of CD4+ T cells. Previous studies have shown that foreign proteins can be internalized by specialized DCs and subsequently presented via the MHC class I route [101, 102].

The studies used a DNA vaccine to generate tumor immunity specific to HER2, and it was shown that the antitumor response was dependent on the presence of both CD4+ and CD8+ T cells. Among the cytokines studied, IFN-c and, to a lesser degree, IL-4 were shown to play pivotal roles in tumor rejection [103]. The significance of IFN-c in tumor rejection provides support for the utilization of DNA vaccines, which seem to induce IFN-c-based Th1-type responses with greater reproducibility. DNA immunization was shown by Amici et al. [104] to bias the phenotype of transgenic FVB/neu mice toward a Th1 response. Previous studies have shown that CTL+ and Th1-associated tumor immunity need IL-4 during the priming phase, which may explain the requirement for IL-4 in Her-2/neu tumor rejection [105]. The specific function of CD4+ assistance in CD8+ CTL production remains unclear. As an example, the administration of anti-HIV vaccinations to CD4-/- mice resulted in a significant decrease in CTL memory and a notable reduction in the efficacy of the vaccine. Simultaneously, it has been shown that animals deficient in CD4+ T cells have mostly intact initial CTL responses [106]. In a separate investigation, CTL activity was shown to be correlated with an increased antibody response after DNA vaccination [107]. The C57BL/6 mice exhibited a more robust antibody response to OVA DNA vaccination than the congenic bm1 animals, whereby the immunodominant CTL epitope of OVA was not further expressed. In addition, preexisting OVA-specific CTL enhanced the immune response in terms of antibody production when a second antigen, b-galactosidase, was delivered concurrently with OVA. One proposed method is that CTL may release antigens from cells transfected with DNA by causing their death or damage. This released antigen may then be accessed by DC and B cells [108].

9.6.2 *HUMORAL IMMUNE RESPONSE*

DNA vaccines frequently demonstrate lower efficacy compared to protein vaccinations in terms of stimulating antibody responses. The modest quantities of antigen generated might be one reason, along with the propensity to promote a Th1 dominant reaction. To induce antibodies, complete protein must be released and absorbed. When muscle cells transfected with the target gene are administered IM, CTL is likely to recognize and lyse them to liberate soluble antigens for B-cell recognition. The detection of muscle fiber destruction has been seen after DNA vaccination; however, the precise contribution of muscle cells in eliciting antibody responses remains uncertain [109]. Several physical approaches, including EP and DNA delivery on small particles, have been utilized to boost antigen levels by improving transfection efficiency.

Several animals, including nonhuman primates, showed potent humoral and cellular reactions to *in vivo* EP [110]. To increase the efficacy of an HIV DNA vaccination in rhesus macaques, Otten et al. [111] utilized *in vivo* EP. The findings indicated a significant enhancement in the initiation, intensity, and longevity of both defense system cells and antibody reactions, hence highlighting the effectiveness of EP technology in the context of big animal applications. Microparticle administration is used as a means to augment humoral responses triggered by DNA vaccines, particularly when administered via mucosal immunization pathways. The study demonstrated that plasmid DNA attached to cationic microparticles caused higher antibody titers than when DNA was released from the particles [112]. DNA vaccines are potential cancer therapeutic methods.

9.7 INCREASING THE EFFICACY OF DNA VACCINES

The optimization of immunotherapeutic capability is a multidimensional activity in the attempt to enhance DNA effectiveness in vaccinations. At the core of this endeavor lies the enhancement of delivery mechanisms, whereby techniques such as EP and nanoparticle-mediated carriers are used to enhance the intracellular absorption of DNA. Furthermore, it is essential to customize the design of DNA vaccine constructions, which entails the careful selection and optimization of antigens, integration of immune-stimulating adjuvants, and employment of sophisticated synthetic biology methodologies to augment antigen expression. Many factors may be at play, including the failure of DNA vaccinations to produce strong, individualized immune responses across patients, the presence of self-antigens in the DNA vaccine, and the overall patient immunodeficiency. Plasmid DNA's lack of immunogenicity in cancer patients can be circumvented in many other ways in addition to combinatorial procedures that impede tumor cells' evasive tactics. As a result of elevated amounts immature myeloid cells may be drawn at the tumor growth site, where they may develop into immature DCs and stay in the presence of VEGF, TGF-b, and IL-10 [113]. A lack of immune infiltration and activation has been connected to immature DCs at the cancer site. When T cells connect to them, these cells behave as suppressors, producing lymphocyte energy and activating regulatory T cells (Tregs). As a result, blocking the processes that define suppressor DC activity might have an influence on tumor growth in conjunction with VEGF decrease. Several receptors that define dendritic cells (DCs) generated by tumors, such as B7-H1 and B7-H, enhance their suppressive capabilities and serve as promising targets for immunotherapeutic intervention [114]. The deliberate use of powerful adjuvants serves to enhance immune responses, effectively balancing the desired outcome of effectiveness with the need for safety. Furthermore, the exploration of personalized DNA vaccines, which are customized to the distinct genetic profiles of individual patients, has the potential for increased precision and effectiveness in the selective targeting of cancer cells. The convergence of many methodologies contributes to the ongoing development of DNA vaccines as a potent tool in the field of cancer immunotherapy, presenting a possibility for enhanced and individualized therapeutic approaches.

9.8 IMPROVING THE IMMUNE RESPONSE

Plasmid DNA expression may be directed to particular locations to modify the body's immunological response to DNA immunization. DNA vaccines may induce systemic immunity if they are injected into the skin or muscles of animals in the majority of experiments. The main development and proliferation of certain cancer types might be prevented, however, by using alternate DNA injection pathways. For example, intranasal and oral distribution of plasmid DNA might be used to limit the spread of malignant development that originates in the mucosa. There has been a lot of work done on mucosal-based DNA vaccines to prevent infectious illness since many viruses initially invade the mucosal channels of the gastrointestinal, vaginal, and nasal tracts [115]. There have been some successes with DNA vaccines aimed specifically at the mucosal epithelium [116–118]. It is advantageous to use mucosal priming because it allows CTLs to be activated in both mucosal-associated lymphoid tissues and systemic lymphoid locations. Parenteral immunization, on the other hand, primarily promotes CTL activity systemically and does not prepare mucosal locations [119]. Attenuated *Salmonella typhimurium* is a typical tiny intestinal bacterium that transports plasmid DNA, where it may be transfected into M cells by oral treatment. DNA delivery vehicles, including microparticles and liposomes, have been developed for use in the mucosal epithelium; however, these vehicles have been tested on animals [120]. DNA vaccinations and the progression of mucosa cancer are an intriguing topic that needs more study. Alternate injection methods, biological adjuvants, and prime-boost tactics can all augment the uptake and immunogenicity of a DNA vaccine. Plasmid DNA vaccines may be more successful if these changes complement the current applications of plasmid DNA. It is possible to use a biolistic gene pistol to transfer plasmid DNA instead of injecting it. This technique includes attaching DNA to gold beads and firing them via a high-pressure device. Langerhans cells and other immunological-based components [121] help prime the immune system via this system's DNA delivery to the skin and Langerhans cells. Gene cannon delivery of DNA vectors to cells is a very effective method of genetic expression. When compared to alternative plasmid injection techniques, increased CD8+ T cell response after immunization uses gene gun [122] and needs less vaccine to establish tumor immunity [123]. DNA vaccines may also be made more immunogenic by the use of an extra technique called EP. To improve plasmid DNA uptake by cells and, by extension, gene expression, an electrical current is applied to a specific area of the body. Cancer vaccine delivery by plasmid DNA EP has shown early promise by inhibiting the growth of B16 melanoma tumors [124]. Numerous studies have examined the benefits of plasmid DNA transfection versus direct intramuscular injection in skeletal muscle. Quaglino et al. [125] tested a DNA vaccination therapy HER-2/neu overexpression in a transgenic mouse model of breast cancer. After detecting *in situ* carcinomas in mice, researchers injected or electroporated animals using plasmid DNA that recognizes the HER-2/neu extracellular and transmembrane domains. It was found that mice given a DNA vaccine directly had little success in halting the development of mammary lesions; however, EP protected against tumor formation. Unmethylated DNA sequences called CpG oligodeoxynucleotides (ODNs) naturally occur in bacterially derived plasmid DNA and promote innate immunity. Pro-inflammatory cytokines and chemokines are released when CpG ODNs bind to specialist APCs and secrete a protein called Toll-like receptor 9 (TLR9). Additionally, CpG-neutralizing sequences may be included inside the backbone of the plasmid, which can inhibit DNA-absorbing APC activity [126]. CpG ODNs may be used as both a preventive and a therapeutic therapy to prevent malignant development, according to many studies [127]. When administered in cancer treatment, it has been found to boost immune responses that provide protective tumor immunity in combination with DNA plasmid vaccination as an adjuvant. Plasmid vectors with optimal CpG sequences may be useful because they can direct the growth of specific types of immune cells while suppressing local inhibitory patterns. Adjuvants such as CpG ODNs, which are injected together with particular DNA vaccines, may help activate the immune system.

Historically, bioadjuvants include cytokines and costimulatory substances in DNA vaccines [128]. Th1 differentiation and CTL activity can be stimulated by cytokines like IL-12 and IFN-g, while a Th2 bias and B-cell activation can be generated by IL-4. DNA immunization has been proposed as a means to enhance antigen presentation by inducing the synthesis of chemokines such as RANTES and MIP1a. To recruit and activate DCs, the cytokine GM-CSF is commonly used in plasmid DNA research. Improved CD4+ and CD8+ T-cell activation has been achieved by using DNA vaccines in combination with the costimulatory molecules B7-1 and B7-2. Plasmid DNA is easily produced, allowing for the encoding of biological adjuvants like cytokines, chemokines, and costimulatory molecules inside the same DNA vector used to target a specific tumor. A preferred immune response that promotes tumor cell lysis may be activated at the location of DNA transfection by delivering an adjuvant at the time of DNA transfection. Adjuvants in their natural protein form would no doubt be less expensive and time-consuming to produce if this technique was implemented. In conclusion, several vaccine moieties may be employed to make up for DNA vaccines' lackluster immune response. After priming the immune system using plasmid DNA, the target antigen can be carried as a recombinant protein or vaccine viral vector. An impressive immune response to tumorigenic challenge was induced in mice trials using this approach, which lasted for a long time and was more potent than injections of the prime-boost regime's components [129]. Studies on humans have also included vaccination against infectious diseases using vaccines made from recombinant proteins or modified viral vectors. DNA vaccines were given to patients first as a sort of "primer" before they were given the whole vaccination. McConkey et al. [130] used a vaccinia virus vector with the malaria antigen expressed in it to stimulate and increase the immune response of malaria patients. IFN-g CD8+-specific T cells increased much more dramatically in those who were given either plasmid DNA or a viral vector alone according to the study's findings, and this rise lasted for many months after vaccination. However, although studies like these and others have shown that prime-boost may raise the amount when it comes to cancer patients and their levels of immune response to vaccination, prime-boost approaches have not been conclusively shown to be successful.

9.9 INNOVATIVE APPROACHES TO ADVANCING DNA VACCINE DEVELOPMENT

The progression of DNA vaccine development entails the investigation of novel strategies to address current challenges and optimize their effectiveness. To improve the transport of DNA into target cells and provide the best possible gene expression and immune response, researchers are currently exploring innovative delivery technologies such as viral vectors and lipid nanoparticles. The use of cutting-edge adjuvants such as TLR agonists attempts to increase the immunogenicity of the vaccine, stimulating a strong and prolonged immune response. Identifying and incorporating highly immunogenic antigens, optimizing codon use, and synthetic biology approaches help build more effective and personalized DNA vaccines. The benefit of microarray technology is that it may help investigators to characterize and comprehend the expression profile of a particular genotype linked to illness, as well as recognize or estimate immunological responses to certain antigens. The use of microarray-based DNA sequencing has facilitated the thorough examination of several mutations in genes and expressed sequences. The provided knowledge is beneficial in promoting the creation of innovative medication designs, enhancing our comprehension of host–pathogen relations, and aiding in the formulation of innovative vaccines. By comparing gene expression across many pathophysiological conditions, virulence factors (such as malignancy factors in tumors) may be identified for vaccine creation [131].

Villaret et al. [132] used cDNA subtractive methods and microarray methods to recognize head-and-neck squamous cell cancer genes in 2000. A library using a subtractive approach was constructed using two samples of squamous cell cancers in the head and neck and six samples of normal tissues. Out of the total number of genes investigated, a total of 107 genes exhibited differential expression patterns when comparing tumor tissues to normal tissues. Among the identified genes, a total of 13 independent genes were shown to exhibit overexpression in tumor tissues. Out of the total of 13 genes examined, 9 were already documented in earlier studies, whereas the other 4 genes had not been found before this investigation. The genes that were previously found consist of Keratins K6 and K16, and tumor antigen CaN19. It is possible to use these genes as tumor indicators, therapeutic targets, or in cancer vaccines, and the four newly discovered ones have the same potential.

Combining computer methods with DNA microarrays, Sturniolo et al. [133] were the first to find possible tumor antigens in an organized manner. Virtual HLA-DR arrays were made that show most of the HLA-DR peptide-binding affinity in humans. The incorporation of matrices into computer software (TEPITOPE) enabled the prediction of promiscuous HLA Class II ligands, totaling 126. DNA microarrays were used to identify genes that exhibit particular expression or increased activity in colon cancer. A compilation of 130 T-cell epitopes unique to colon cancer, which were promiscuous, was created using a database consisting of around 20,000 genes. Antibodies targeting certain candidate antigens identified by microarray analysis were shown to be present in patients, providing evidence that supports further investigation into the properties and potential applications of these molecules. Having access to their whole DNA sequences makes them more viable DNA vaccine candidates. Alizadeh and Staudt [134] developed a specialized microarray known as a "lymphoid" to investigate particular genes within both healthy and cancerous lymphocyte environments. The cDNA microarray known as the "lymphoid" offers two comprehensive perspectives on both normal and malignant lymphocytes at a genetic level. This technology facilitates the generation of valuable insights and hypotheses that are relevant to established cellular pathways. This also offers a wide range of possible targets that might be included in DNA vaccines for the treatment of lymphoid malignancies. The use of antibody microarray technology has also been employed for screening and identifying potential biomarkers. In their study, Miller et al. [135] devised an effective approach for conducting serum protein profiling via the use of antibody microarrays. They then employed this technique to identify possible biomarkers in blood samples from individuals with prostate cancer.

The use of advanced technologies, such as CRISPR/Cas9, enables the precise manipulation of genomes to promote antigen expression and vaccinations' effectiveness should be increased. By using these pioneering methodologies, the domain of DNA vaccine creation is positioned to open novel possibilities, hence facilitating the advancement of more efficient and focused methodologies in the prevention of infectious illnesses and the reduction of different health obstacles. DNA microarrays are a relatively newly developed and very effective instrument that enables the simultaneous examination of many important genes that exhibit differential expression. This technology offers a speedy and efficient means of conducting such analyses.

9.10 CONCLUSION

DNA vaccines have substantial immunotherapeutic potential for use in the fight against cancer in humans. Among its many benefits as a vaccine delivery system are its high levels of safety, simplicity, low cost, mass manufacturing, and the capacity to elicit antibody defense and CTL immunological responses. Despite the disappointing results of plasmid DNA-based research in shrinking human tumors in clinical trials, this approach is far from being written off as hopeless. A new generation of DNA vaccinations must integrate a variety of immunogenicity-enhancing and immunosuppression-targeting techniques to achieve success. There is little question that DNA vaccine creation and treatment optimization will need extra time and research and may incorporate methods such as surgery, chemotherapy, or radiation that are not currently used in cancer treatments. Cancer vaccines are designed to induce antigen-specific immunity, hence potentially inhibiting the progression of cancer or curing it at early stages, therefore inhibiting its progression or recurrence. For cancer vaccines to be operative, they must include a strong immune response, including both cellular and humoral components, as well as establish a durable immunological memory. Furthermore, cancer vaccines must possess both affordability and practicality to facilitate their widespread administration to the vast population of cancer patients. In the pursuit of this objective, DNA vaccines have been proven to stimulate immunological responses at many levels, while also exhibiting ease of production and distribution. DNA vaccines have recently emerged as a promising novel tool in the battle against tumors, thanks to the development of innovative technologies.

KEYWORDS

- **cancer**
- **DNA**
- **immunization**
- **immunotherapy**
- **T cells**
- **tumor antigen**

REFERENCES

1. Hoption Cann, S. A., Van Netten, J. P., & Van Netten, C. (2003). Dr William Coley and tumour regression: A place in history or in the future. *Postgraduate Medical Journal, 79*(938), 672–680.
2. Yannelli, J. R., & Wroblewski, J. M. (2004). On the road to a tumor cell vaccine: 20 years of cellular immunotherapy. *Vaccine, 23*(1), 97–113.
3. Varmus, H. (2006). The new era in cancer research. *Science, 312*(5777), 1162–1165.
4. Wolff, J. A., Malone, R. W., Williams, P., Chong, W., Acsadi, G., Jani, A., & Felgner, P. L. (1990). Direct gene transfer into mouse muscle in vivo. *Science, 247*(4949), 1465–1468.
5. Ulmer, J. B., Donnelly, J. J., Parker, S. E., Rhodes, G. H., Felgner, P. L., Dwarki, V. J., Gromkowski, S. H., Deck, R. R., DeWitt, C. M., Friedman, A., & Hawe, L. A. (1993). Heterologous protection against influenza by injection of DNA encoding a viral protein. *Science, 259*(5102), 1745–1749.

6. Wang, B., Ugen, K. E., Srikantan, V., Agadjanyan, M. G., Dang, K., Refaeli, Y., Sato, A. I., Boyer, J., Williams, W. V., & Weiner, D. B. (1993). Gene inoculation generates immune responses against human immunodeficiency virus type 1. *Proceedings of the National Academy of Sciences, 90*(9), 4156–4160.
7. Fry, T. J., & Mackall, C. L. (2013). T-cell adoptive immunotherapy for acute lymphoblastic leukemia. In *Hematology the American society of hematology education program book* (Vol. *2013*(1), pp. 348–353).
8. Haupt, K., Roggendorf, M., & Mann, K. (2002). The potential of DNA vaccination against tumor-associated antigens for antitumor therapy. *Experimental Biology and Medicine, 227*(4), 227–237.
9. Ribas, A., Butterfield, L. H., Glaspy, J. A., & Economou, J. S. (2003). Current developments in cancer vaccines and cellular immunotherapy. *Journal of Clinical Oncology, 21*(12), 2415–2432.
10. George, A. J., & Stevenson, F. K. (1989). Prospects for the treatment of B cell tumors using idiotypic vaccination. *International Reviews of Immunology, 4*(4), 271–310.
11. Van Der Bruggen, P., Zhang, Y., Chaux, P., Stroobant, V., Panichelli, C., Schultz, E. S., Chapiro, J., Van den Eynde, B. J., Brasseur, F., & Boon, T. (2002). Tumor-specific shared antigenic peptides recognized by human T cells. *Immunological Reviews, 188*(1), 51–64.
12. Stevenson, F. K., Rice, J., & Zhu, D. (2004). Tumor vaccines. *Advances in Immunology, 82*, 49–104.
13. Caballero, O. L., & Chen, Y. T. (2012). Cancer/testis antigens: Potential targets for immunotherapy. *Innate Immune Regulation and Cancer Immunotherapy*, 347–369.
14. Herrada, A. A., Rojas-Colonelli, N., González-Figueroa, P., Roco, J., Oyarce, C., Ligtenberg, M. A., & Lladser, A. (2012). Harnessing DNA-induced immune responses for improving cancer vaccines. *Human Vaccines & Immunotherapeutics, 8*(11), 1682–1693.
15. Wang, R. F., & Rosenberg, S. A. (1999). Human tumor antigens for cancer vaccine development. *Immunological Reviews, 170*(1), 85–100.
16. Robbins, P. F., El-Gamil, M., Kawakami, Y., & Rosenberg, S. A. (1994). Recognition of tyrosinase by tumor-infiltrating lymphocytes from a patient responding to immunotherapy. *Cancer Research, 54*(12), 3124–3126.
17. Kawakami, Y., Eliyahu, S., Delgado, C. H., Robbins, P. F., Rivoltini, L., Topalian, S. L., Miki, T., & Rosenberg, S. A. (1994). Cloning of the gene coding for a shared human melanoma antigen recognized by autologous T cells infiltrating into tumor. *Proceedings of the National Academy of Sciences, 91*(9), 3515–3519.
18. Kawakami, Y., Eliyahu, S., Delgado, C. H., Robbins, P. F., Sakaguchi, K., Appella, E., Yannelli, J. R., Adema, G. J., Miki, T., & Rosenberg, S. A. (1994). Identification of a human melanoma antigen recognized by tumor-infiltrating lymphocytes associated with in vivo tumor rejection. *Proceedings of the National Academy of Sciences, 91*(14), 6458–6462.
19. Doehn, C., Böhmer, T., Kausch, I., Sommerauer, M., & Jocham, D. (2008). Prostate cancer vaccines: Current status and future potential. *BioDrugs, 22*, 71–84.
20. Boon, T., & van der Bruggen, P. (1996). Human tumor antigens recognized by T lymphocytes. *The Journal of Experimental Medicine, 183*(3), 725–729.

21. Finn, O. J. (2017). Human tumor antigens yesterday, today, and tomorrow. *Cancer Immunology Research, 5*(5), 347–354.
22. Strioga, M. M., Darinskas, A., Pasukoniene, V., Mlynska, A., Ostapenko, V., & Schijns, V. (2014). Xenogeneic therapeutic cancer vaccines as breakers of immune tolerance for clinical application: To use or not to use?. *Vaccine, 32*(32), 4015–4024.
23. Li, L., Goedegebuure, S. P., & Gillanders, W. E. (2017). Preclinical and clinical development of neoantigen vaccines. *Annals of Oncology, 28*, xii11-7.
24. Alibek, K., Baiken, Y., Kakpenova, A., Mussabekova, A., Zhussupbekova, S., Akan, M., & Sultankulov, B. (2014). Implication of human herpesviruses in oncogenesis through immune evasion and supression. *Infectious Agents and Cancer, 9*(1), 1–8.
25. Hanahan, D., & Weinberg, R. A. (2000). The hallmarks of cancer. *Cell, 100*(1), 57–70.
26. Damania, B. (2007). DNA tumor viruses and human cancer. *Trends in Microbiology, 15*(1), 38–44.
27. Hogquist, K. A., Baldwin, T. A., & Jameson, S. C. (2005). Central tolerance: Learning self-control in the thymus. *Nature Reviews Immunology, 5*(10), 772–782.
28. Gallegos, A. M., & Bevan, M. J. (2006). Central tolerance: good but imperfect. *Immunological Reviews, 209*(1), 290–296.
29. Kreuwel, H. T., & Sherman, L. A. (2001). The T-cell repertoire available for recognition of self-antigens. *Current Opinion in Immunology, 13*(6), 639–643.
30. Renkvist, N., Castelli, C., Robbins, P. F., & Parmiani, G. (2001). A listing of human tumor antigens recognized by T cells. *Cancer Immunology Immunotherapy, 50*(1), 3–15.
31. Lewis, J. D., Reilly, B. D., & Bright, R. K. (2003). Tumor-associated antigens: From discovery to immunity. *International Reviews of Immunology, 22*(2), 81–112.
32. Novellino, L., Castelli, C., & Parmiani, G. (2005). A listing of human tumor antigens recognized by T cells: March 2004 update. *Cancer Immunology, Immunotherapy, 54*, 187–207.
33. van der Bruggen, P., Traversari, C., Chomez, P., Lurquin, C., De Plaen, E., Van den Eynde, B., Knuth, A., & Boon, T. (1991). A gene encoding an antigen recognized by cytolytic T lymphocytes on a human melanoma. *Science, 254*(5038), 1643–1647.
34. Van Der Bruggen, P., Zhang, Y., Chaux, P., Stroobant, V., Panichelli, C., Schultz, E. S., Chapiro, J., Van den Eynde, B. J., Brasseur, F., & Boon, T. (2002). Tumor-specific shared antigenic peptides recognized by human T cells. *Immunological Reviews, 188*(1), 51–64.
35. Simpson, A. J., Caballero, O. L., Jungbluth, A., Chen, Y. T., & Old, L. J. (2005). Cancer/testis antigens, gametogenesis and cancer. *Nature Reviews Cancer, 5*(8), 615–625.
36. Yu, M., & Finn, O. J. (2006). DNA vaccines for cancer too. *Cancer Immunology, Immunotherapy, 55*, 119–30.
37. Yankauckas, M. A., Morrow, J. E., Parker, S. E., Abai, A., Rhodes, G. H., Dwarki, V. J., & Gromkowski, S. H. (1993). Long-term anti-nucleoprotein cellular and humoral immunity is induced by intramuscular injection of plasmid DNA containing NP gene. *DNA and Cell Biology, 12*(9), 771–776.

38. Lambricht, L., Lopes, A., Kos, S., Sersa, G., Préat, V., & Vandermeulen, G. (2016). Clinical potential of electroporation for gene therapy and DNA vaccine delivery. *Expert Opinion on Drug Delivery, 13*(2), 295–310.
39. Liu, Y., Yan, J., Santangelo, P. J., & Prausnitz, M. R. (2016). DNA uptake, intracellular trafficking and gene transfection after ultrasound exposure. *Journal of Controlled Release, 234*, 1–9.
40. Miller, D. L., Pislaru, S. V., & Greenleaf, J. F. (2002). Sonoporation: Mechanical DNA delivery by ultrasonic cavitation. *Somatic Cell and Molecular Genetics, 27*(1-6), 115–134.
41. Qiu, Y., Luo, Y., Zhang, Y., Cui, W., Zhang, D., Wu, J., Zhang, J., & Tu, J. (2010). The correlation between acoustic cavitation and sonoporation involved in ultrasound-mediated DNA transfection with polyethylenimine (PEI) in vitro. *Journal of Controlled Release, 145*(1), 40–48.
42. Bergmann-Leitner, E. S., & Leitner, W. W. (2015). Vaccination using Gene-gun technology. In A. Vaughan (Ed.), *Malaria vaccines: Methods and protocols* (pp. 289–302). Springer New York
43. Li, L., & Petrovsky, N. (2016). Molecular mechanisms for enhanced DNA vaccine immunogenicity. *Expert Review of Vaccines, 15*(3), 313–329.
44. Lowe, D. B., Shearer, M. H., Jumper, C. A, & Kennedy, R. C. (2007). Towards progress on DNA vaccines for cancer. *Cellular and Molecular Life Sciences, 64*, 2391–2403.
45. Gregorevic, P., Blankinship, M. J., & Chamberlain, J. S. (2004). Viral vectors for gene transfer to striated muscle. *Current Opinion in Molecular Therapeutics, 6*(5), 491–498.
46. Hacein-Bey-Abina, S., Von Kalle, C., Schmidt, M., McCormack, M. P., Wulffraat, N., Leboulch, P. A., Lim, A., Osborne, C. S., Pawliuk, R., Morillon, E., & Sorensen, R. (2003). LMO2-associated clonal T cell proliferation in two patients after gene therapy for SCID-X1. *Science, 302*(5644), 415–419.
47. Fazio, V. M., Ria, F., Franco, E., Rosati, P., Cannelli, G., Signori, E., Parrella, P., Zaratti, L., Iannace, E., Monego, G., & Blogna, S. (2004). Immune response at birth, long-term immune memory and 2 years follow-up after in-utero anti-HBV DNA immunization. *Gene Therapy, 11*(6), 544–551.
48. Rinaldi, M., Signori, E., Rosati, P., Cannelli, G., Parrella, P., Iannace, E., Monego, G., Ciafrè, S. A., Farace, M. G., Iurescia, S., & Fioretti, D. (2006). Feasibilty of in utero DNA vaccination following naked gene transfer into pig fetal muscle: Transgene expression, immunity and safety. *Vaccine, 24*(21), 4586–4591.
49. MacGregor, R. R., Boyer, J.D., Ugen, K. E., Lacy, K. E., Gluckman, S. J., Bagarazzi, M. L., Chattergoon, M. A., Baine, Y., Higgins, T. J., Ciccarelli, R. B., & Coney, L. R. (1998). First human trial of a DNA-based vaccine for treatment of human immunodeficiency virus type 1 infection: Safety and host response. *Journal of Infectious Diseases, 178*(1), 92–100.
50. Ori, D., Murase, M., & Kawai, T. (2017). Cytosolic nucleic acid sensors and innate immune regulation. *International Reviews of Immunology, 36*(2), 74–88.
51. Tang, C. K., & Pietersz, G. A. (2009). Intracellular detection and immune signaling pathways of DNA vaccines. *Expert Review of Vaccines, 8*(9), 1161–1170.

52. Boyer, J., Ugen, K., Wang, B., Chattergoon, M., Tsai, A., Merva, M., & et al. (1998). Induction of a TH1 type cellular immune response to the human immunodeficiency type 1 virus by in vivo DNA inoculation. *Developments in Biological Standardization, 92*, 169–174.
53. Schirmbeck, R., Bohm, W., Ando, K., Chisari, F. V., & Reimann, J. (1995). Nucleic acid vaccination primes hepatitis B virus surface antigen-specific cytotoxic T lymphocytes in nonresponder mice. *Journal of Virology, 69*(10), 5929–5934.
54. Amara, S., & Tiriveedhi, V. (2017). The five immune forces impacting DNA-based cancer immunotherapeutic strategy. *International Journal of Molecular Sciences, 18*, 650. https://doi.org/10. 3390/ijms18030650.
55. Denies, S., Cicchelero, L., Polis, I., & Sanders, N. N. (2016). Immunogenicity and safety of xenogeneic vascular endothelial growth factor receptor-2 DNA vaccination in mice and dogs. *Oncotarget, 7*(10), 10905–10916.
56. Lopes, A., Vanvarenberg, K., Preat, V., & Vandermeulen, G. (2017). Codon-optimized P1Aencoding DNA vaccine: Toward a therapeutic vaccination against P815 Mastocytoma. *Molecular Therapy Nucleic Acids, 8*, 404–415.
57. Smith, H. A. (2000). Regulation and review of DNA vaccine products. *Developments in Biologicals, 104*, 57–62.
58. Cui, Z. (2005). DNA vaccine. *Advances in Genetics, 54*, 257–289.
59. Suschak, J. J., Williams, J. A., Schmaljohn, C. S. (2017). Advancements in DNA vaccine vectors, non-mechanical delivery methods, and molecular adjuvants to increase immunogenicity. *Human Vaccines & Immunotherapeutics, 13*(12), 2837–2848.
60. Jorritsma, S. H. T., Gowans, E. J., Grubor-Bauk, B., & Wijesundara, D. K. (2016). Delivery methods to increase cellular uptake and immunogenicity of DNA vaccines. *Vaccine, 34*(46), 5488–5494.
61. Lambricht, L., Vanvarenberg, K., De Beuckelaer, A., Van Hoecke, L., Grooten, J., Ucakar, B., & et al. (2016). Coadministration of a plasmid encoding HIV-1 gag enhances the efficacy of Cancer DNA vaccines. *Molecular Therapy: The Journal of the American Society of Gene Therapy, 24*(9), 1686–1696.
62. Aldous, A. R., & Dong, J. Z. (2018). Personalized neoantigen vaccines: A new approach to cancer immunotherapy. *Bioorganic and Medicinal Chemistry, 26*(10), 2842–2849.
63. Rabinovich, G. A., Gabrilovich, D., & Sotomayor, E. M. (2007). Immunosuppressive strategies that are mediated by tumor cells. *Annual Review of Immunology, 25*, 267–296.
64. Montgomery, D. L., Donnelly, J. J., Shiver, J. W., Liu, M. A., & Ulmer, J. B. (1994). Protein expression in vivo by injection of polynucleotides. *Current Opinion in Biotechnology, 5*(5), 505–510.
65. Rinaldi, M., Fioretti, D., Iurescia, S., Signori, E., Pierimarchi, P., Seripa, D., Tonon, G., & Fazio, V. M. (2008). Anti-tumor immunity induced by CDR3-based DNA vaccination in a murine B-cell lymphoma model. *Biochemical and Biophysical Research Communications, 370*(2), 279–284.
66. Dean, D. A., Strong, D. D., & Zimmer, W. E. (2005). Nuclear entry of nonviral vectors. *Gene Therapy, 12*(11), 881–890.

67. Weide, B., Garbe, C., Rammensee, H. G., & Pascolo, S. (2008). Plasmid DNA-and messenger RNA-based anti-cancer vaccination. *Immunology Letters, 115*(1), 33–42.
68. Neelapu, S. S., & Kwak, L. W. (2007). Vaccine therapy for B-cell lymphomas: Next-generation strategies. *ASH Education Program Book, 2007*(1), 243–249.
69. Morgan, D. J., Kreuwel, H. T., & Sherman, L. A. (1999). Antigen concentration and precursor frequency determine the rate of CD8+ T cell tolerance to peripherally expressed antigens. *The Journal of Immunology, 163*(2), 723–727.
70. Sandberg, J. K., Franksson, L., Sundbäck, J., Michaelsson, J., Petersson, M., Achour, A., Wallin, R., Sherman, N. E., Bergman, T., Jörnvall, H., & Hunt, D. F. (2000). T cell tolerance based on avidity thresholds rather than complete deletion allows maintenance of maximal repertoire diversity. *The Journal of Immunology, 165*(1), 25–33.
71. Berzofsky, J. A. (1993). Epitope selection and design of synthetic vaccines molecular approaches to enhancing immunogenicity and cross-reactivity of engineered vaccines. *Annals of the New York Academy of Sciences, 690*(1), 256–264.
72. Lu, S., Wang, S., & Grimes-Serrano, J. M. (2008). Current progress of DNA vaccine studies in humans. *Expert Review of Vaccines, 7*(2), 175–191.
73. Chan, R. C., Gutierrez, B., Ichim, T. E., & Lin, F. (2009). Enhancement of DNA cancer vaccine efficacy by combination with anti-angiogenesis in regression of established subcutaneous B16 melanoma. *Oncology Reports, 22*(5), 1197–1203.
74. Stopeck, A. T., Hersh, E. M., Akporiaye, E. T., Harris, D. T., Grogan, T., Unger, E., Warneke, J., Schluter, S. F., & Stahl, S. Phase I study of direct gene transfer of an allogeneic histocompatibility antigen, HLA-B7, in patients with metastatic melanoma. *Journal of Clinical Oncology, 15*(1), 341–349.
75. Drape, R. J., Macklin, M. D., Barr, L. J., Jones, S., Haynes, J. R., & Dean, H. J. (2006). Epidermal DNA vaccine for influenza is immunogenic in humans. *Vaccine, 24*(21), 4475–4481.
76. Egan, M. A., Megati, S., Roopchand, V., Garcia-Hand, D., Luckay, A., Chong, S. Y., Rosati, M., Sackitey, S., Weiner, D. B., Felber, B. K., & Pavlakis, G. N. (2006). Rational design of a plasmid DNA vaccine capable of eliciting cell-mediated immune responses to multiple HIV antigens in mice. *Vaccine, 24*(21), 4510–4523.
77. Trimble, C., Lin, C. T., Hung, C. F., Pai, S., Juang, J., He, L., Gillison, M., Pardoll, D., Wu, L., & Wu, T. C. (2003). Comparison of the CD8+ T cell responses and antitumor effects generated by DNA vaccine administered through gene gun, biojector, and syringe. *Vaccine, 21*(25-26), 4036–4042.
78. Luckay, A., Sidhu, M. K., Kjeken, R., Megati, S., Chong, S. Y., Roopchand, V., Garcia-Hand, D., Abdullah, R., Braun, R., Montefiori, D. C., & Rosati, M. (2007). Effect of plasmid DNA vaccine design and in vivo electroporation on the resulting vaccine-specific immune responses in rhesus macaques. *Journal of Virology, 81*(10), 5257–5269.
79. Ahlén, G., Söderholm, J., Tjelle, T., Kjeken, R., Frelin, L., Höglund, U., Blomberg, P., Fons, M., Mathiesen, I., & Sällberg, M. In vivo electroporation enhances the immunogenicity of hepatitis C virus nonstructural 3/4A DNA by increased local DNA uptake, protein expression, inflammation, and infiltration of CD3+ T cells. *The Journal of Immunology, 179*(7), 4741–4753.

80. Murtaugh, M. P., & Foss, D. L. (2002). Inflammatory cytokines and antigen presenting cell activation. *Veterinary Immunology and Immunopathology, 87*(3-4), 109–121.
81. Liu, J., Kjeken, R., Mathiesen, I., & Barouch, D. H. (2008). Recruitment of antigen-presenting cells to the site of inoculation and augmentation of human immunodeficiency virus type 1 DNA vaccine immunogenicity by in vivo electroporation. *Journal of Virology, 82*(11), 5643–5649.
82. Bins, A. D., Jorritsma, A., Wolkers, M. C., Hung, C. F., Wu, T. C., Schumacher, T. N., & Haanen, J. B. (2005). A rapid and potent DNA vaccination strategy defined by in vivo monitoring of antigen expression. *Nature Medicine, 11*(8), 899–904.
83. Lu, S., Wang, S., & Grimes-Serrano. J. M. (2008). Current progress of DNA vaccine studies in humans. *Expert Review of Vaccines, 7*(2), 175–191.
84. Kelleher, A. D., Puls, R. L., Bebbington, M., Boyle, D., Ffrench, R., Kent, S. J., Kippax, S., Purcell, D. F., Thomson, S., Wand, H., & Cooper, D. A. (2006). A randomized, placebo-controlled phase I trial of DNA prime, recombinant fowlpox virus boost prophylactic vaccine for HIV-1. *Aids, 20*(2), 294–297.
85. Webster, D. P., Dunachie, S., McConkey, S., Poulton, I., Moore, A. C., Walther, M., Laidlaw, S. M., Peto, T., Skinner, M. A., Gilbert, S. C., & Hill, A. V. (2006). Safety of recombinant fowlpox strain FP9 and modified vaccinia virus Ankara vaccines against liver-stage P. falciparum malaria in non-immune volunteers. *Vaccine, 24*(15), 3026–3034.
86. Egan, M. A., Chong, S. Y., Megati, S., Montefiori, D. C., Rose, N. F., Boyer, J. D., Sidhu, M. K., Quiroz, J., Rosati, M., Schadeck, E. B., & Pavlakis, G. N. (2005). Priming with plasmid DNAs expressing interleukin-12 and simian immunodeficiency virus gag enhances the immunogenicity and efficacy of an experimental AIDS vaccine based on recombinant vesicular stomatitis virus. *AIDS Research & Human Retroviruses, 21*(7), 629–643.
87. Lu, Y., Ouyang, K., Fang, J., Zhang, H., Wu, G., Ma, Y., Zhang, Y., Hu, X., Jin, L., Cao, R., & Fan, H. (2009). Improved efficacy of DNA vaccination against prostate carcinoma by boosting with recombinant protein vaccine and by introduction of a novel adjuvant epitope. *Vaccine, 27*(39), 5411–5418.
88. Wang, R., Epstein, J., Charoenvit, Y., Baraceros, F. M., Rahardjo, N., Gay, T., Banania, J. G., Chattopadhyay, R., de la Vega, P., Richie, T. L., & Tornieporth, N. (2004). Induction in humans of CD8+ and CD4+ T cell and antibody responses by sequential immunization with malaria DNA and recombinant protein. *The Journal of Immunology, 172*(9), 5561–5569.
89. Wang, S., Kennedy, J. S., West, K., Montefiori, D. C., Coley, S., Lawrence, J., Shen, S., Green, S., Rothman, A. L., Ennis, F. A., & Arthos, J. Cross-subtype antibody and cellular immune responses induced by a polyvalent DNA prime–protein boost HIV-1 vaccine in healthy human volunteers. *Vaccine, 26*(31), 3947–3957.
90. Schneider, J., Gilbert, S. C., Hannan, C. M., Dégano, P., Prieur, E., Sheu, E. G., Plebanski, M., Hill, A. V. (1999). Induction of CD8+ T cells using heterologous prime-boost immunisation strategies. *Immunological Reviews, 170*(1), 29–38.
91. Schneider, J., Gilbert, S. C., Blanchard, T. J., Hanke, T., Robson, K. J., Hannan, C. M., Becker, M., Sinden, R., Smith, G. L., & Hill, A. V. (1998). Enhanced immunogenicity for CD8+ T cell induction and complete protective efficacy of malaria DNA

vaccination by boosting with modified vaccinia virus Ankara. *Nature Medicine, 4*(4), 397–402.

92. Estcourt, M. J., Ramsay, A. J., Brooks, A., Thomson, S. A., Medveckzy, C. J., & Ramshaw, I. A. (2002). Prime–boost immunization generates a high frequency, high-avidity CD8+ cytotoxic T lymphocyte population. *International Immunology, 14*(1), 31–37.
93. Dégano, P., Schneider, J., Hannan, C. M., Gilbert, S. C., & Hill, A. V. (1999). Gene gun intradermal DNA immunization followed by boosting with modified vaccinia virus Ankara: enhanced CD8+ T cell immunogenicity and protective efficacy in influenza and malaria models. *Vaccine, 18*(7-8), 623–632.
94. Wang, R., Doolan, D. L., Le, T. P., Hedstrom, R. C., Coonan, K. M., Charoenvit, Y., Jones, T. R., Hobart, P., Margalith, M., Ng, J., & Weiss, W. R. (1998). Induction of antigen-specific cytotoxic T lymphocytes in humans by a malaria DNA vaccine. *Science, 282*(5388), 476–480.
95. Calarota, S., Bratt, G., Nordlund, S., Hinkula, J., Leandersson, A. C., Sandström, E., & Wahren, B. (1998). Cellular cytotoxic response induced by DNA vaccination in HIV-1-infected patients. *The Lancet, 351*(9112), 1320–1325.
96. Greenland, J. R., & Letvin, N. L. (2007). Chemical adjuvants for plasmid DNA vaccines. *Vaccine, 25*(19), 3731–341.
97. Stevenson, F. K., & Rice, J. (2006). Optimizing cancer immunotherapies trials: Back to basics. *European Journal of Immunology, 36*(5), 1070–1073.
98. Keene, J. A., & Forman, J. (1982). Helper activity is required for the in vivo generation of cytotoxic T lymphocytes. *The Journal of Experimental Medicine, 155*(3), 768–782.
99. Homann, D., Tishon, A., Berger, D. P., Weigle, W. O., von Herrath, M. G., & Oldstone, M. B. (1998). Evidence for an underlying CD4 helper and CD8 T-cell defect in B-cell-deficient mice: Failure to clear persistent virus infection after adoptive immunotherapy with virus-specific memory cells from μMT/μMT mice. *Journal of Virology, 72*(11), 9208–9216.
100. Wolff, J. A., Ludtke, J. J., Acsadi, G., Williams, P., & Jani, A. (1992). Long-term persistence of plasmid DNA and foreign gone expression in mouse muscle. *Human Molecular Genetics, 1*(6), 363–369.
101. Rock, K. L., & Clark, K. (1996). Analysis of the role of MHC class II presentation in the stimulation of cytotoxic T lymphocytes by antigens targeted into the exogenous antigen-MHC class I presentation pathway. *Journal of Immunology, 156*(10), 3721–3726.
102. Rock, K. L., Gamble, S., & Rothstein, L. (1990). Presentation of exogenous antigen with class I major histocompatibility complex molecules. *Science, 249*(4971), 918–921.
103. Lindencrona, J. A., Preiss, S., Kammertoens, T., Schüler, T., Piechocki, M., Wei, W. Z., Seliger, B., Blankenstein, T., & Kiessling, R. (2004). CD4+ T cell-mediated HER-2/neu-specific tumor rejection in the absence of B cells. *International Journal of Cancer, 109*(2), 259–264.
104. Amici, A., Venanzi, F. M., & Concetti, A. (1998). Genetic immunization against neu/erbB2 transgenic breast cancer. *Cancer Immunology, Immunotherapy, 47*, 183–190.
105. Schüler, T., Qin, Z., Ibe, S., Noben-Trauth, N., & Blankenstein, T. (1999). T helper cell type 1–associated and cytotoxic T lymphocyte–mediated tumor immunity is

impaired in interleukin 4–deficient mice. *The Journal of Experimental Medicine, 189*(5), 803–810.

106. von Herrath, M. G., Yokoyama, M., Dockter, J., Oldstone, M. B., & Whitton, J. L. (1996). CD4-deficient mice have reduced levels of memory cytotoxic T lymphocytes after immunization and show diminished resistance to subsequent virus challenges. *Journal of Virology, 70*(2), 1072–1079.
107. Dyer, C. M., Zhan, Y., Brady, J. L., Carbone, F. R., Smyth, M. J., & Lew, A. M. (2004). Unexpectedly, induction of cytotoxic T lymphocytes enhances the humoral response after DNA immunization. *Blood, 103*(8), 3073–3075.
108. Albert, M. L., Sauter, B., & Bhardwaj, N. (1998). Dendritic cells acquire antigen from apoptotic cells and induce class I-restricted CTLs. *Nature, 392*(6671), 86–89.
109. Davis, H. L., Millan, C. L., & Watkins, S. C. (1997). Immune-mediated destruction of transfected muscle fibers after direct gene transfer with antigen-expressing plasmid DNA. *Gene Therapy, 4*(3), 181–188.
110. Zhang, L., Widera, G., Bleecher, S., Zaharoff, D. A., Mossop, B., & Rabussay, D. (2003). Accelerated immune response to DNA vaccines. *DNA and Cell Biology, 22*(12), 815–822.
111. Otten, G., Schaefer, M., Doe, B., Liu, H., Srivastava, I., zur Megede, J., O'Hagan, D., Donnelly, J., Widera, G., Rabussay, D., & Lewis, M. G. (2004). Enhancement of DNA vaccine potency in rhesus macaques by electroporation. *Vaccine, 22*(19), 2489–2493.
112. Kaur, R., Rauthan, M., & Vrati, S. (2004). Immunogenicity in mice of a cationic microparticle-adsorbed plasmid DNA encoding Japanese encephalitis virus envelope protein. *Vaccine, 22*(21-22), 2776–2782.
113. Kim, R., Emi, M., Tanabe, K., & Arihiro, K. (2006). Tumor-driven evolution of immunosuppressive networks during malignant progression. *Cancer Research, 66*(11), 5527–5536.
114. Zou, W. (2005). Immunosuppressive networks in the tumour environment and their therapeutic relevance. *Nature Reviews Cancer, 5*(4), 263–274.
115. Toka, F. N., Pack, C. D., & Rouse, B. T. (2004). Molecular adjuvants for mucosal immunity. *Immunological Reviews, 199*(1), 100–112.
116. Niethammer, A. G., Xiang, R., Becker, J. C., Wodrich, H., Pertl, U., Karsten, G., Eliceiri, B. P., & Reisfeld, R. A. (2002). A DNA vaccine against VEGF receptor 2 prevents effective angiogenesis and inhibits tumor growth. *Nature Medicine, 8*(12), 1369–1375.
117. Xiang, R., Lode, H. N., Chao, T. H., Ruehlmann, J. M., Dolman, C. S., Rodriguez, F., Whitton, J. L., Overwijk, W. W., Restifo, N. P., & Reisfeld, R. A. (2000). An autologous oral DNA vaccine protects against murine melanoma. *Proceedings of the National Academy of Sciences, 97*(10), 5492–5497.
118. Xiang, R., Silletti, S., Lode, H. N., Dolman, C. S., Ruehlmann, J. M., Niethammer, A. G., Pertl, U., Gillies, S. D., Primus, F. J., & Reisfeld, R. A. (2001). Protective immunity against human carcinoembryonic antigen (CEA) induced by an oral DNA vaccine in CEA-transgenic mice. *Clinical Cancer Research, 7*(3), 856s–864s.
119. Berzofsky, J. A., Ahlers, J. D., & Belyakov, I. M. (2001). Strategies for designing and optimizing new generation vaccines. *Nature Reviews Immunology, 1*(3), 209–219.

120. Eriksson, K., & Holmgren, J. (2002). Recent advances in mucosal vaccines and adjuvants. *Current Opinion in Immunology, 14*(5), 666–672.
121. Lauterbach, H., Gruber, A., Ried, C., Cheminay, C., & Brocker, T. (2006). Insufficient APC capacities of dendritic cells in gene gun-mediated DNA vaccination. *The Journal of Immunology, 176*(8), 4600–4607.
122. Trimble, C., Lin, C. T., Hung, C. F., Pai, S., Juang, J., He, L., Gillison, M., Pardoll, D., Wu, L., & Wu, T. C. (2003). Comparison of the CD8+ T cell responses and antitumor effects generated by DNA vaccine administered through gene gun, biojector, and syringe. *Vaccine, 21*(25-26), 4036–4042.
123. Mendiratta, S. K., Thai, G., Eslahi, N. K., Thull, N. M., Matar, M., Bronte, V., & Pericle, F. (2001). Therapeutic tumor immunity induced by polyimmunization with melanoma antigens gp100 and TRP-2. *Cancer Research, 61*(3), 859–863.
124. Quaglino, E., Iezzi, M., Mastini, C., Amici, A., Pericle, F., Di Carlo, E., Pupa, S. M., De Giovanni, C., Spadaro, M., Curcio, C., & Lollini, P. L. (2004). Electroporated DNA vaccine clears away multifocal mammary carcinomas in her-2/neu transgenic mice. *Cancer Research, 64*(8), 2858–2864.
125. Klinman, D. M., Currie, D., Gursel, I., & Verthelyi, D. (2004). Use of CpG oligodeoxynucleotides as immune adjuvants. *Immunological Reviews, 199*(1), 201–216.
126. Krieg, A. M. (2002). CpG motifs in bacterial DNA and their immune effects. *Annual Review of Immunology, 20*(1), 709–760.
127. Prud'homme, G. J. (2005). DNA vaccination against tumors. *The Journal of Gene Medicine,* 7(1), 3–17.
128. Meng, W. S., Butterfield, L. H., Ribas, A., Dissette, V. B., Heller, J. B., Miranda, G. A., Glaspy, J. A., McBride, W. H., & Economou, J. S. (2001). α-Fetoprotein-specific tumor immunity induced by plasmid prime-adenovirus boost genetic vaccination. *Cancer Research, 61*(24), 8782–8786.
129. Pasquini, S., Peralta, S., Missiaglia, E., Carta, L., & Lemoine, N. R. (2002). Prime-boost vaccines encoding an intracellular idiotype/GM-CSF fusion protein induce protective cell-mediated immunity in murine pre-B cell leukemia. *Gene Therapy, 9*(8), 503–510.
130. McConkey, S. J., Reece, W. H., Moorthy, V. S., Webster, D., Dunachie, S., Butcher, G., Vuola, J. M., Blanchard, T. J., Gothard, P., Watkins, K., & Hannan, C. M. (2003). Enhanced T-cell immunogenicity of plasmid DNA vaccines boosted by recombinant modified vaccinia virus Ankara in humans. *Nature Medicine, 9*(6), 729–735.
131. Dhiman, N., Bonilla, R., & Poland, G. A. (2001). Gene expression microarrays: A 21st century tool for directed vaccine design. *Vaccine, 20*(1-2), 22–30.
132. Villaret, D. B., Wang, T., Dillon, D., Xu, J., Sivam, D., Cheever, M. A., & Reed, S. G. (2000). Identification of genes overexpressed in head and neck squamous cell carcinoma using a combination of complementary DNA subtraction and microarray analysis. *The Laryngoscope, 110*(3), 374–381.
133. Sturniolo, T., Bono, E., Ding, J., Raddrizzani, L., Tuereci, O., Sahin, U., Braxenthaler, M., Gallazzi, F., Protti, M. P., Sinigaglia, F., & Hammer, J. (1999). Generation of tissue-specific and promiscuous HLA ligand databases using DNA microarrays and virtual HLA class II matrices. *Nature Biotechnology, 17*(6), 555–561.

134. Alizadeh, A. A., & Staudt, L. M. (2000). Genomic-scale gene expression profiling of normal and malignant immune cells. *Current Opinion in Immunology, 12*(2), 219–225.
135. Miller, J. C., Zhou, H., Kwekel, J., Cavallo, R., Burke, J., Butler, E. B., Teh, B. S., & Haab, B. B. (2003). Antibody microarray profiling of human prostate cancer sera: Antibody screening and identification of potential biomarkers. *Proteomics, 3*(1), 56–63.

CHAPTER 10

Cancer Immunotherapy Using a DNA Vaccination

ABSTRACT

By allowing the patient's body's immune system to recognize and eliminate tumor cells, cancer immunotherapy has emerged as a cutting-edge technique for treating malignancies. Among the several methods used in this area, DNA vaccination has drawn a lot of interest due to its potential to trigger powerful and focused antitumor immune responses. The concept, underlying processes, and present status of DNA vaccination as an effective cancer immunotherapy technique are briefly summarized in this chapter. Plasmid DNA containing tumor-specific antigens is injected into the body as part of a DNA vaccination procedure. Once produced by host cells, these antigens trigger an immune response targeting cancer cells. The capacity to stimulate both cellular and humoral immunological reactions, improved antigen presentation, and simplicity of customization to target a variety of cancer types are just a few benefits of this strategy. In addition, DNA vaccines demonstrate a favorable safety profile and are more affordable than conventional vaccine delivery methods. To combat tumor-induced immunosuppression, cytotoxic T lymphocyte (CTL) production that is specific for an antigen, activation of antigen-presenting cells (APCs), along activation of immune checkpoints are required and important factors behind the effectiveness of DNA vaccination for cancer immunotherapy. Neoantigens, tumor-associated antigens, or viral oncoproteins produced by cancer cells can all be the targets of DNA vaccines.

DNA- and m-RNA-Based Vaccines: An Immunotherapeutic Approach to Cancer.
Sonali Sundram and Rishabha Malviya (Authors)

DOI: 10.1201/9781774919613-10

10.1 INTRODUCTION

For the immune system's adaptive response, which comprises CD4+ helper T lymphocytes, B lymphocytes, along CD8+ T lymphocytes that are cytotoxic, for activation, antigen-presenting cells (APCs) are required for the formal presentation of antigens. The adaptive type of immune system initiates the generation of T- and B-cell lymphocytes with antigen specificity [1]. We now have a better understanding of the complex interaction between tumor cells as well as the immune system [2]. It is now recognized that an improper innate immune response, plus an inappropriate adaptive immune reaction, contributes to the development of tumors by favoring aggressive clones, bringing about immunosuppression, and fostering the proliferation plus spread of cancer cells [3]. Immune checkpoint inhibitors (ICIs), including anti-cytotoxic T lymphocyte antigen-4 (CTLA4), anti-programmed death protein-1 (PD-1), and anti-programmed death ligand 1 (PDL1), which alter the patient's natural immune system, have produced long-lasting remissions in a range of cancer types [4]. Additionally, compelling evidence has shown that chronic inflammation is crucial for the emergence of pancreatic and colon cancers, both in human tumors and in animal tumor models [5]. Because they exhibit tumor antigens during cancerous immune editing, the immunological system of the body can identify and eradicate the most immunologically susceptible cancer cells, resulting in their eradication [6]. In addition to actively evading the immune system, tumors are capable of controlling several immunological functions. The tumor's alteration of the tumor stroma is a key mediator of this process of co-optation. The extracellular matrix (ECM), endothelial cells, fibroblasts, immune cells, nerve cells, and endothelial cells are some of the cell types that make up the stroma and contribute to tissue homeostasis. It typically maintains tissue homeostasis by regulating the ratio of cell death to proliferation through interactions with fibroblasts and the ECM [7]. When compared to tumors where tumor-infiltrating lymphocytes are absent, active lymphocytes that infiltrate tumors being present in initial melanoma portend a survival benefit. The immune system occasionally prompts tumors to spontaneously shrink. For instance, partial regression is frequently observed in primary cancer lesions, whereas complete remission of metastatic melanoma has very occasionally been reported. The increased prevalence of malignancies in immunosuppressed and immunodeficient people is a proof that the critical immune system's involvement is important in avoiding cancer [8]. A novel type of cancer immunotherapy that precisely prevents immune effector suppression has been developed in response to the identification of tumor-associated T-cell suppressive signals, including PD-L1. This therapy reactivates and may even expand preexisting anticancer immune reactions [9]. The actions of cancer cells are modified by tumor-infiltrating immune cells (TIICs), and they have a significant role in the tumor microenvironment (TME). Due to their tremendous plasticity and heterogeneity, TIICs can either stimulate the growth of tumors or repress malignancy. Numerous studies have clarified the roles played by tumor-associated mast cells, macrophages, and natural killer cells. Preclinical research and clinical trials have shown the safety and effectiveness of neutrophils and lymphocytes in the development of several characteristics of cancer that served as the foundation for effective immunotherapies [10].

10.2 IMMUNE SYSTEM AND CANCER

Tumor immunology has seen a renaissance thanks to immunotherapy, which has transformed cancer treatment. The ways that cancer evades the immune system would be clarified by the thorough profile of immune cells that are invading tumors, opening up possibilities for the creation of novel therapeutic approaches [11]. Immunosurveillance relies heavily on the immune system; immune cells that originate from both the adaptive and innate immune systems contribute to the regulation of cancer growth as they enter the TME [12–15]. Through a process known as cancer immunoediting, several immune system elements safeguard the host against the emergence of primary tumors, enhance tumor cell escape, or both. They accomplish this either by modifying tumor immunogenicity or by reducing antitumor immune responses [16]. On the one hand, stimulating the body's immune system is necessary for stopping the spread of cancer, but it also results in autoimmune disease [17]. The main downsides of immunotherapies are typically immune-related adverse effects, an immune activation alongside a response of inflammation to the host's tissue health [18].

10.3 STRATEGIES INVOLVED IN CANCER IMMUNOTHERAPY

Many cancer immunotherapy techniques are being researched. A few of them have been authorized for the treatment of cancer [19].

10.3.1 CELLULAR MECHANISM

Cellular immunotherapies have made great strides toward moving through the "bench to bedside" stage during the past ten years, with the Food and Drug Administration's (FDA's) 2010 approval of Sipuleucel-T (Provenge), a DC vaccination [20]. Giving a patient living cells is referred to as "cellular immunotherapy." This sort of immunotherapy could be active, like a dendritic cell (DC) vaccine, wherein the cells can cause the patient to have an antitumor response, or it could be passive, like adoptive cell transfer (ACT), in which the cells had intrinsic antitumor activity [21]. T cells are important immune response orchestrators and effectors that use the T-cell receptor (TCR) to detect peptide antigens displayed on MHC molecules, which are produced by APCs. Between a naive T cell and an APC, the TCR–peptide–MHC complex creates an immunological junction that recruits coreceptors like CD28 and starts a signaling cascade that increases T-cell activation [22]. Co-stimulatory and co-inhibitory receptor interactions using peptide–MHC complex (pMHC) influence how the TCR interacts with it; molecules like CD28 and 4-IBB TCR signaling and CD134 work together to enhance T-cell proliferation and increase the immune system's resilience response [23]. Adoptive therapy with T cells is a treatment method that involves reinfusing patient-derived T lymphocytes, which have been expanded *in vitro* to target tumor antigens. In numerous therapeutic trials, the adoptive transmission of TIL has demonstrated potential in patients having metastatic melanoma. However, because there are so few TILs, it could be challenging and time-consuming to produce enough TIL cells for adaptive T-cell treatment [24, 25]. Similar in concept to previous ACTs, particularly TCR-T cell therapy, CAR-T-cell therapy uses collected lymphocytes for expressing a chimeric antigen receptor (CAR), rather than *TCR* genes specific to cancer antigens [26]. Targeting MAGE-A3, a cancer-testis antigen, TCR T cells can also have catastrophic cardiotoxicity and neurotoxicity. Alternatively, TCR T cells that target the cancer-testis antigen NY-ESO-1 show therapeutic benefit with no overt toxicity in phase I/II trials for individuals with multiple myeloma [27]. In the realm of cellular immunotherapies, natural killer T (NKT) cells, another special subtype of T cells, are becoming more significant [28]. Figure 10.1 shows the role of immunotherapy in treating cancer.

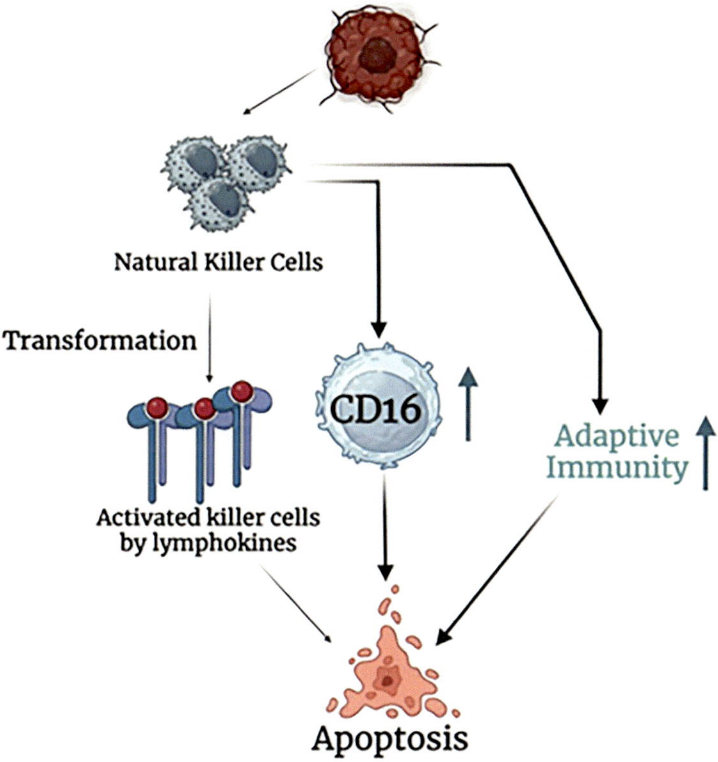

FIGURE 10.1 Immunotherapy in the treatment of cancer.

10.3.2 MOLECULAR THERAPY

Numerous molecularly targeted therapeutic drugs have been employed in cancer treatment to this point. Small-molecule kinase inhibitors (SMKIs) along with monoclonal antibodies (mAbs) are the two main forms of molecular targeted therapy [29]. The cytokine IL-2 encourages the expansion of various T cells. For the therapy of metastatic renal cell cancer (RCC) as well as metastatic melanoma, IL-2 has FDA approval [30]. Resistance to drugs is a significant barrier to effective cancer treatment. Primary (intrinsic) resilience is characterized as an inability to respond to initial therapy as a result of cellular, genetic, and epigenetic abnormalities that are intrinsic. Hyperactivation of reversible signaling pathways, such as reduced HER2 expression (p95HER2), contributes to resistance against HER2 monoclonal antibodies (mAbs) [31]. Molecular targeted approaches are cutting-edge treatments that interfere with particular molecules to obstruct the development, progression, and metastasis of cancer. The FDA has given its approval for numerous molecular targeted medicines that have shown significant clinical effectiveness in treating several cancer types, like lung, breast, leukemia, colorectal, and ovarian malignancies [32]. Abnormal DNA methylation and histone modification, the two most common epigenetic silencing mechanisms, are being used as targets for molecular treatments that are therapeutically effective in the therapy of cancer [33]. Chemotherapy is a vital component of cancer care, but its efficacy is severely constrained due to a lack of selectivity, which causes insufficient tumor cell clearance and systemic toxicity [34]. Molecularly targeted therapy is thus gaining popularity since it specifically targets tumor cells while protecting healthy cells. Molecular targeted treatments include creating medications that suppress cancer's unmistakable signs [35].

10.3.3 NONSPECIFIC IMMUNOTHERAPY

Although the identification and elimination of malignant cells are ultimately necessary for the success of immunotherapy, some treatments put more emphasis on causing widespread changes that, in the constantly changing conflict between cancer and the immune system of the host, aim to tip the scales in the immune system's favor. Although not antigen-specific, these treatments are also referred to as immunomodulatory therapy and frequently engage the immune systems, both innate and adaptive [36]. Blockers of essential enzymes like cyclo-oxygenase or IDO, antagonists, and agonists of crucial immune-regulatory substances like CD40 or PD-1, in addition to vaccination approaches that are capable of covering a wide range as well as the heterogeneity of tumor antigens like syngeneic whole-cell vaccine as well as *in situ* vaccines, are among the many instances of these kinds of therapies [37]. By depriving tumor cells of vital development signals or causing the intracellular buildup of arachidonic acid, inhibiting cyclo-oxygenase may cause tumor cells to die immediately. It can also reverse immunological suppression by preventing the synthesis of PGE2 [38–41]. To attack the immunosuppressive TME, numerous strategies have been devised. A well-researched element of tumor-induced suppression is regulatory T (Treg)-cells that can prevent effector T-cells from functioning as well as APCs [42]. Immunosuppressive enzyme IDO inhibition is a different tactic being investigated in clinical trials. IDO, an inducible enzyme that catabolizes tryptophan, has been demonstrated to diminish T-cell-mediated fetal indifference in mice, indicating that it can be used to promote tolerance to alloantigens [43]. Initiating both adaptive and innate cell-mediated immunity, APC, which includes DCs, can be activated by CpGs via toll receptor-9 signaling. Presentation of the antigen, co-stimulation, and cytokine production during inflammation all rise as a result of this activation [44].

10.3.4 IMMUNE CHECKPOINT INHIBITORS

mAbs called ICIs combat immunological inhibitory pathways called checkpoints. The anti-cytotoxic T lymphocyte antigen-4 (CTLA-4) anti-PD-1 and anti- PD-L1 antibodies are the most frequently utilized ICIs [45, 46]. mAbs called ICIs target immunological inhibitory mechanisms. A higher overall survival rate for cancer patients is achieved as a result of the administration of ICIs, which increases immune responses mediated by T cells against tumors [47]. Both TILs and many cancer cells express a variety of inhibitory receptors and ligands. There are thus numerous options to increase antitumor immunity through various immune checkpoint blockades [48]. Eight ligands of the B7 family, comprising PD-L1, PD-L2, B7-H3, B7-H4, and B7-H6 (also called NCRLG1), as well as ICOS-L (also known as ICOSLG), CD80, CD86, have been discovered to date. These ligands are discussed in Greaves and Gribben [49]. Although the receptors for other molecules that inhibit the B7 family, like B7-H3 and B7-H4, have not yet been identified, mice knockout investigations suggest that these ligands have an immune-inhibitory function [50]. A recent work demonstrating successful ACT in the mouse leukemia model by simultaneously inhibiting CTLA4, PD-1, along LAG-3 offered more evidence underlining the significance of various immune checkpoint pathways in cancer [51]. Designing efficient immunotherapy plans for patients will require a thorough understanding of the primary immune checkpoint pathways that are activated in various cancer types as the disease progresses [48]. The coordinated action of numerous inhibitory B7-related molecules on primary human leukemia (upregulated CD200, PD-L 1, B7-H3, and HVEM) along with lymphoma cells (CLL, FL,

DLBCL, MM, and HL) has been demonstrated to cause resistant adaptive immunity (malfunction of T cells caused by tumors) through this research methodology [52].

10.4 DNA VACCINES IN CANCER IMMUNOTHERAPY

Cancer vaccines based on DNA have become a potential method for boosting the body's defenses against the disease. In preclinical along with early-phase clinical investigations, immunizations with plasmid DNA demonstrated a favorable safety profile resulting in the production of both generalized and targeted immune responses [53]. DNA vaccinations can be repeated for ongoing protection and are also very cost-effective. Despite all the advantages in terms of application, immunological tolerance to endogenous self-antigens in tumors makes it difficult for DNA vaccines to trigger powerful antigen-specific cellular immune responses [54]. Cancer vaccines contain tumor antigens that cause antitumor immunity when administered as whole peptides, the cells, nucleic acids, and so on. Both humoral and cellular immunity would be stimulated by the ideal cancer vaccines, which would also overcome tumor-induced immune suppression [55]. The effective administration of antigens and adjuvants to trigger a regulated yet potent tumor-specific T-cell response is a significant problem in cancer vaccination treatment. APCs can unlock the vaccine in lysosomes thanks to the inclusion of DNA "locking strands" out of the nanostructures that respond to low pH, exposing adjuvants as well as antigens and triggering a potent immune response [56]. Figure 10.2 demonstrates the mechanism of cancer DNA vaccines for tumor apoptosis.

10.5 IMMUNE MECHANISMS OF DNA VACCINES

TME contains stromal cells and other immune cells, regulatory proteins, ECM, as well as blood vessels. Myeloid-derived stem cells (MDSCs), as well as regulatory T cells (Tregs), are two ideal examples of immune cells. MDSCs are the immunosuppressive, tumor-infiltrating macrophages that participate in anti-inflammatory actions [57]. Tregs can reduce the immune reactivity to tumors by releasing suppressive cytokines such as IL-35 along with transforming growth factor

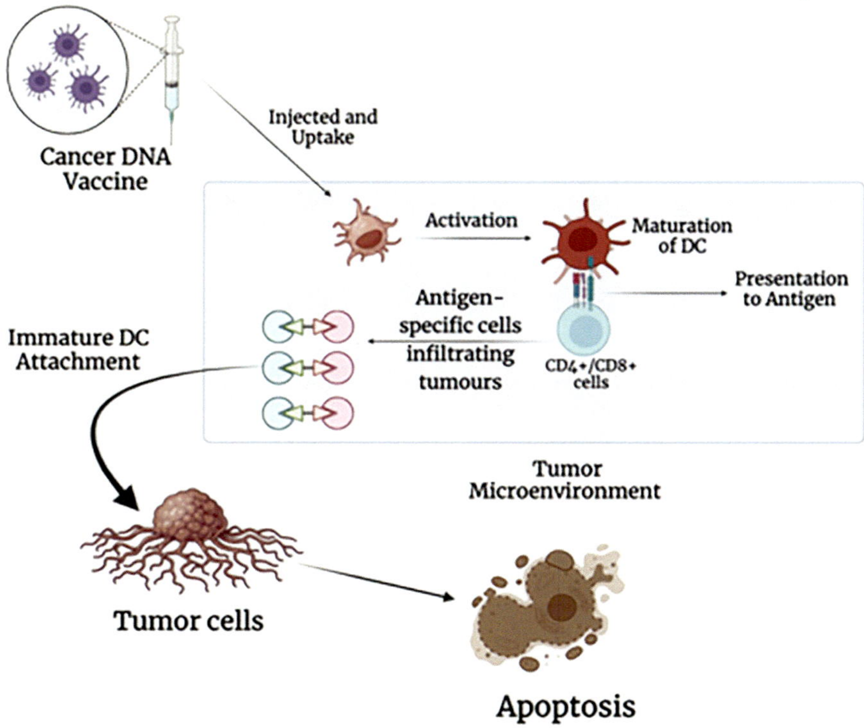

FIGURE 10.2 Mechanism of cancer DNA vaccines in the destruction of tumor.

(TGF) [58]. The tumor increases the activity of Tregs and broadens its tolerance toward the lymph nodes that drain it. By releasing soluble molecules like TGF-, IL-10, and vascular endothelium growth factor, tumors impair the APCs' maturation and differentiation [59]. The two fundamental characteristics of DNA vaccines are the plasmid DNA composition as well as the fast onset of immunity [60]. Plasmid DNA is introduced, allowing the immune to choose which material it should react to and determine the antigen. The antigens are produced, attached to the APCs by the immunological processes aroused, and then delivered to the T cells. The vaccine's DNA plasmid's genetic information is processed either with the help of its natural adjuvant characteristics or by the expression of Tas [53]. Figure 10.3 shows plasmid DNA vaccines' mechanism of action.

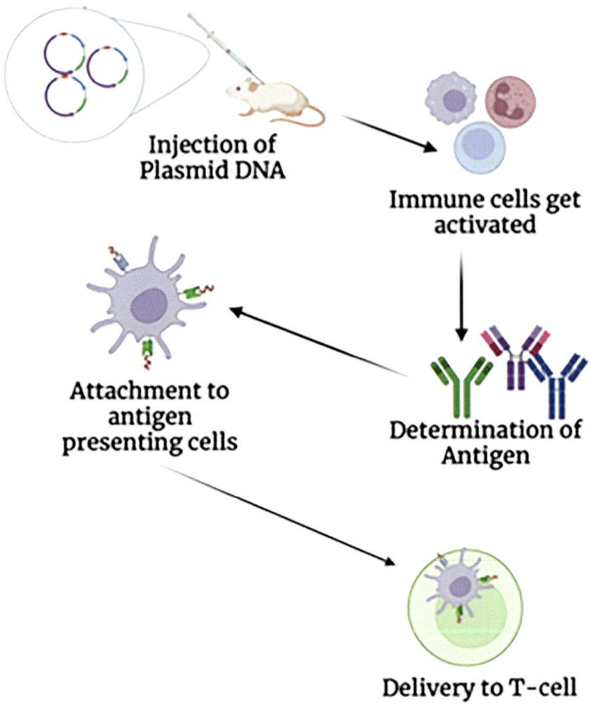

FIGURE 10.3 Plasmid DNA vaccinations' mechanism of action.

The tumor-specific antibodies, which recognize the epitopes onto the surfaces of cancerous cells—have Fc receptors that enable the innate immune responses, which are composed of phagocytose the malignant cells by recognizing the cancer antigens on NK cells, neutrophils, and macrophages [61]. These vaccinations can be given topically or systemically. Topical methods include intramuscular, subcutaneous, transdermal, and intradermal, whereas there are oral, pulmonary, and intravenous systemic routes. According to reports, the method of administration affects the mechanism of action. Systemic pathways are more likely than topical ones to activate more APCs throughout secondary lymphoid organs [62]. Although clinical experiments using naked DNA vaccines may produce specific antibody and CTL responses via the intramuscular route or intradermal route, substantial dosages of DNA were required to produce measurable immune reactions [63]. To marginally improve immunogenicity, large dosages (5–10 mg) are required [64]. Changing the microenvironment at the location of vaccination with the concurrent delivery of genetic, or DNA-based plasmids that contain protein, immunostimulatory particles, the limited immunogenicity of DNA immunizations, or chemical adjuvants can be increased [65, 66]. Due to the ease of plasmid DNA development and production utilized to combat specific cancer, the use of biological adjuvants is modified as well as within the identical DNA vector and encoded [67]. Granulocyte-macrophage colony-stimulating factor (GM-CSF) is one of the cytokines commonly used in plasmid DNA vaccinations, which can improve immune responses by promoting DC proliferation, development, as well as migrating B- and T-cell development and differentiation are also involved [68]. The CD4+ Th cell, which is essential to the immune system's reaction and can produce elevated levels of immunity as well as maintaining the efficiency of the response, has been the subject of extensive investigation by Stevenson and colleagues [69]. The theory was used to create DNA fusion gene vaccines that encode a tumor antigen paired with a tetanus toxin-derived antigen by concentrating on the range of antimicrobials. The fusing of the tetanus toxin's Fragment C (FrC) boosted the immune reactions to many tumor antigens, which led to the reduction of tumor expansion [70]. Immunization protocols that combine regimens for prime-boost with various vector systems that provide the required antigen appear to have successfully improved the DNA vaccine technology [71]. In actuality, prime-boost routines have demonstrated the potential to elicit a human immunological response that is greater when compared to DNA immunization alone [72]. The approach of DNA-prime-viral vector-boost main purpose is to activate immunological reactions of T cells. In this approach, the same booster vaccination contains an antigen that is identical to that of the prior immunization [73, 74]. On the one hand, a homologous prime-boost method using DNA vaccines and EP could produce antibody responses similar to those caused by Complete Freund Adjuvant's protein, as well as magnified CTL responses [75].

10.6 CHALLENGES AND LIMITATIONS OF DNA VACCINES

The goal of a DNA-based cancer vaccine is nearly achieved. It features a clear design and the ability to provide long-term protection. Compared to live-attenuated vaccinations, it is safer and more economically produced.

Additionally, it has a strong solubility profile and maintains stability at room temperature [76]. A few minor but significant negatives outweighed these benefits in preventing the application of human DNA-based cancer vaccinations. The main downside of DNA vaccines is their possible inability to elicit the necessary immunogenicity, and the primary culprits here are insufficient DNA transfection as well as immune stimulation [77]. Because each person's cellular and nuclear membranes are complex, these vaccines' ability to transfect DNA yields uneven outcomes [78]. These vaccines frequently result in systemic inflammatory reactions by elevating cytokine production, which might result in a persistent fever, raising safety concerns. We need to use techniques that limit cytokine storms (as demonstrated via adjuvant-encoded plasmids) and demonstrate the inflammatory immune systems that DNA vaccines activate [79, 80]. In addition to the safety concerns, there is a chance that vaccines will be released into the environment and disseminated by predatory creatures. Additionally, the possibility exists that DNA vaccinations will integrate with the host's genome, which would obstruct the host genome's ability to express itself. The regulations' criteria depend on what species is being investigated. Animals that have received DNA vaccinations must be identified as genetically modified organisms (GMOs) to prevent their widespread use [81]. Additionally, the immunosuppressive environment that tumor cells create hinders the effectiveness of these vaccines [82]. It is still difficult to create vaccinations for nonviral malignancies brought on by genetic changes in healthy tissues. If vaccines are created that specifically target cell antigens that demonstrate driver mutation signals for cell survival, this issue can be resolved [83]. Finding patterns in tumor antigen distribution at critical times when tumor cells are most receptive in the premalignant stage is one of the main problems in the science of cancer immunotherapy [84].

10.7 CONCLUSION AND FUTURE PERSPECTIVES

DNA vaccination for cancer immunotherapy has become a potential and ground-breaking method of cancer treatment. By delivering DNA encoding particular tumor antigens, the idea of using the immune system for the goal of getting rid of cancer cells has shown a lot of promise. Numerous clinical and preclinical investigations conducted over the last few decades have shed important light on the security and effectiveness of DNA vaccination for the treatment of cancer. Even if there are obstacles and restrictions, the advancements gained so far are positive and portend an encouraging future for this immunotherapeutic strategy. The adaptability of DNA vaccination for cancer immunotherapy is one of its main advantages. Encoding antigens particular to a patient's tumor enables the formulation of personalized treatment plans, improving the ability to customize medicines for individual patients. Clinical trial outcomes have demonstrated that DNA vaccinations can trigger strong immune responses targeting cancer cells, leading to tumor shrinkage and, in some circumstances, persistent responses, although being mixed in some situations. These results highlight DNA vaccination's potential to have a big impact in the expanding field of cancer immunotherapies. For patient selection as well as treatment stratification, the identification of accurate indicators to forecast patient's reaction to the DNA vaccine is essential. The goal of this research is to minimize potential negative effects while maximizing the advantages of DNA immunization. The potential future of DNA vaccines presents the possibility of more efficient, individualized, and secure cancer therapy alternatives as research advances and novel strategies are investigated.

KEYWORDS

- **antigens**
- **DNA vaccination**
- **immunotherapy**
- **metastasis**
- **TCR-T cell**

REFERENCES

1. Oiseth, S. J., & Aziz, M. S. (2017). Cancer immunotherapy: A brief review of the history, possibilities, and challenges ahead. *Journal of Cancer Metastasis and Treatment, 3*, 250.
2. Moskovitz, J., Moy, J., & Ferris, R. L. (2018). Immunotherapy for head and neck squamous cell carcinoma. *Current Oncology Reports, 20*, 22.

3. Palucka, A. K., & Coussens, L. M. (2016). The basis of oncoimmunology. *Cell, 164*, 1233–1247.
4. Hiam-Galvez, K. J., Allen, B. M., & Spitzer, M. H. (2021). Systemic immunity in cancer. *Nature Reviews Cancer, 21*(6), 345–359.
5. Grivennikov, S. I., Greten, F. R., & Karin, M. (2010). Immunity, inflammation, and cancer. *Cell, 140*(6), 883–899.
6. Dunn, G. P., Old, L. J., & Schreiber, R. D. (2004). The three Es of cancer immunoediting. *Annual Review of Immunology, 22*, 329–360.
7. Nelson, C. M., & Bissell, M. J. (2006). Of extracellular matrix, scaffolds, and signaling: tissue architecture regulates development, homeostasis, and cancer. In *Annual review of cell and development biology* (Vol. 22, pp. 287–309).
8. Hastings, K. T., & Rausch, M. P. (2013). Innate and adaptive immune responses to cancer. In *Fundamentals of cancer prevention* (pp. 81–121). Springer Berlin Heidelberg.
9. Chen, D. S., & Mellman, I. (2013). Oncology meets immunology: The cancer-immunity cycle. *Immunity, 39*(1), 1–10.
10. Costa, A. C., Santos, J. M., da Costa, R. M., & Medeiros, R. (2021). Impact of immune cells on the hallmarks of cancer: A literature review. *Critical Reviews in Oncology/Hematology, 168*, 103541.
11. Zhang, Y., & Zhang, Z. (2020). The history and advances in cancer immunotherapy: Understanding the characteristics of tumor-infiltrating immune cells and their therapeutic implications. *Cellular & Molecular Immunology, 17*(8), 807–821.
12. Vesely, M. D., Kershaw, M. H., Schreiber, R. D., & Smyth, M. J. (2011). Natural innate and adaptive immunity to cancer. *Annual Review of Immunology, 29*, 235–271.
13. Schreiber, R. D., Old, L. J., & Smyth, M. J. (2011). Cancer immunoediting: Integrating immunity's roles in cancer suppression and promotion. *Science, 331*, 1565–1570.
14. Seager, R. J., Hajal, C., Spill, F., Kamm, R. D., & Zaman, M. H. (2017). Dynamic interplay between tumour, stroma and immune system can drive or prevent tumour progression. *Convergent Science Physical Oncoloy, 3*, 034002.
15. Grivennikov, S. I., Greten, F. R., & Karin, M. (2010). Immunity, inflammation, and cancer. *Cell, 140*, 883–899.
16. O'Donnell, J. S., Teng, M. W. L., & Smyth, M. J. (2019). Cancer immunoediting and resistance to T cell-based immunotherapy. *Nature Reviews Clinical Oncology, 16*, 151–167.
17. Esfahani, K., Roudaia, L., Buhlaiga, N., Del Rincon, S. V., Papneja, N., & Miller, W. H. Jr. (2020). A review of cancer immunotherapy: from the past, to the present, to the future. *Current Oncology, 27*(Suppl 2), S87–S97.
18. Hodi, F. S., Chiarion-Sileni, V., Gonzalez, R., & et al. (2018). Nivolumab plus ipilimumab or nivolumab alone versus ipilimumab alone in advanced melanoma (CheckMate 067): 4-year outcomes of a multicentre, randomised, phase 3 trial. *Lancet Oncology, 19*, 1480–1492.
19. Liu, M., & Guo, F. (2018). Recent updates on cancer immunotherapy. *Precision Clinical Medicine, 1*(2), 65–74.
20. FDA. (2019). "PROVENGE (sipuleucel-T)." https://www.fda.gov/ vaccines-blood-biologics/cellular-gene-therapy-products/ provenge-sipuleucel-t (accessed November 10, 2019)

21. Armstrong, A. C., Eaton, D., & Ewing, J. C. (2001). Cellular immunotherapy for cancer. *BMJ, 323*(7324), 1289–1293.
22. Gaud, G., Lesourne, R., & Love, P. E. (2018). Regulatory mechanisms in T cell receptor signalling. *Nature Reviews Immunology, 18*(8), 485–497.
23. Chen, L., & Flies, D. B. (2013). Molecular mechanisms of T cell costimulation and co-inhibition. *Nature Reviews Immunology, 13*(4), 227–242.
24. June, C. H., O'Connor, R. S., Kawalekar, O. U., & et al. (2018). CAR T cell immunotherapy for human cancer. *Science, 359*, 1361–1365.
25. June, C. H., Riddell, S. R., & Schumacher, T. N. (2015). Adoptive cellular therapy: A race to the finish line. *Science Translational Medicine, 7*, 280ps7.
26. Gross, G., Waks, T., & Eshhar, Z. (1989). Expression of immunoglobulin-T-cell receptor chimeric molecules as functional receptors with antibody-type specificity. *Proceedings of the National Academy of Science of the United States of America, 86*(24), 10024–10028.
27. Rapoport, A. P., Stadtmauer, E. A., & Binder-Scholl, G. K, et al. (2015). NY-ESO-1-specific TCR-engineered T cells mediate sustained antigen-specific antitumor effects in myeloma. *Nature Medicine, 21*, 914–921.
28. Nair, S., & Dhodapkar, M. V. (2017). Natural killer T cells in cancer immunotherapy. *Frontiers in Immunology, 8*, 1178.
29. Lee, Y. T., Tan, Y. J., & Oon, C. E. (2018). Molecular targeted therapy: Treating cancer with specificity. *European Journal of Pharmacology, 834*, 188–196.
30. Rosenberg, S. A. (2014). IL-2: The first effective immunotherapy for human cancer. *Journal of Immunology, 192*, 5451–5458.
31. Ellis, L. M., & Hicklin, D. J. (2009). Resistance to targeted therapies: Refining anticancer therapy in the era of molecular oncology. *Clinical Cancer Research, 15*, 7471–7478.
32. Lee, Y. T., Tan, Y. J., & Oon, C. E. (2018). Molecular targeted therapy: Treating cancer with specificity. *European Journal of Pharmacology, 834*, 188–196.
33. Pavlovic, S., Ugrin, M., Gasic, V., & Rakic, V. (2023). Using genetics for enhancement (liberal eugenics). In *Clinical ethics at the crossroads of genetic and reproductive technologies* (pp. 347—379). Academic Press.
34. Xu, G., McLeod, H. L. (2001). Strategies for enzyme/prodrug cancer therapy. *Clinical Cancer Research, 7*(11), 3314–3324.
35. Padma, V. V. (2015). An overview of targeted cancer therapy. *Biomedicine (Taipei), 5*(4), 19. DOI: 10.7603/s40681-015-0019-4
36. Monjazeb, A. M., Hsiao, H. H., Sckisel, G. D., & Murphy, W. J. (2012). The role of antigen-specific and non-specific immunotherapy in the treatment of cancer. *Journal of Immunotoxicology, 9*(3), 248–258.
37. Monjazeb, A. M., Zamora, A. E., Grossenbacher, S. K., Mirsoian, A., Sckisel, G. D., & Murphy, W. J. (2013). Immunoediting and antigen loss: Overcoming the achilles heel of immunotherapy with antigen non-specific therapies. *Frontiers in Oncology, 3*, 197.
38. Monjazeb, A. M., High, K. P., Connoy, A., Hart, L. S., Koumenis, C., & Chilton, F. H. (2006). Arachidonic acid-induced gene expression in colon cancer cells. *Carcinogenesis, 27*(10), 1950–1960.

39. Monjazeb, A. M., High, K. P., Koumenis, C., & Chilton, F. H. (2005). Inhibitors of arachidonic acid metabolism act synergistically to signal apoptosis in neoplastic cells. *Prostaglandins Leukot Essent Fatty Acids, 73*(6), 463–474.
40. Yaqub, S., Henjum, K., Mahic, M., Jahnsen, F. L., Aandahl, E. M., Bjørnbeth, B. A., & et al. (2008). Regulatory T cells in colorectal cancer patients suppress anti-tumor immune activity in a COX-2 dependent manner. *Cancer Immunology Immunotherpy, 57*(6), 813–821.
41. Ahmadi, M., Emery, D. C., & Morgan, D. J. (2008). Prevention of both direct and cross-priming of antitumor CD8+ T-cell responses following overproduction of prostaglandin E2 by tumor cells in vivo. *Cancer Research, 68*(18), 7520–7529.
42. Shevach, E. M. (2009). Mechanisms of foxp3+ T regulatory cell-mediated suppression. *Immunity, 30*(5), 636–645.
43. Munn, D. H., & Mellor, A. L. (2007). Indoleamine 2,3-dioxygenase and tumor-induced tolerance. *Journal of Clinical Investigation, 117*(5), 1147–1154.
44. Klinman, D. M., Yi, A. K., Beaucage, S. L., Conover, J., & Krieg, A. M. (1996). CpG motifs present in bacteria DNA rapidly induce lymphocytes to secrete interleukin 6, interleukin 12, and interferon gamma. *Proceedings of the National Academy of Sciences of the United States of America, 93*(7), 2879–2883.
45. Wolchok, J. D., Kluger, H., Callahan, M. K., Postow, M. A., Rizvi, N. A., Lesokhin, A. M., & et al. (2013). Nivolumab plus ipilimumab in advanced melanoma. *New England Journal of Medicine, 369*(2), 122–133.
46. Brahmer, J. R., Tykodi, S. S., Chow, L. Q., Hwu, W. J., Topalian, S. L., Hwu, P., & et al. (2012). Safety and activity of anti-PD-L1 antibody in patients with advanced cancer. *New England Journal of Medicine, 366*(26), 2455–265.
47. Hayase, E., & Jenq, R. R. (2021). Role of the intestinal microbiome and microbial-derived metabolites in immune checkpoint blockade immunotherapy of cancer. *Genome Medicine, 13*(1), 107.
48. Ramsay, A. G. (2013). Immune checkpoint blockade immunotherapy to activate anti-tumour T-cell immunity. *British Journal of Haematology, 162*(3), 313–325.
49. Greaves, P., & Gribben, J. G. (2013). The role of B7 family molecules in hematologic malignancy. *Blood, The Journal of the American Society of Hematology*, *121*(5), 734–744.
50. Yi, K. H., & Chen, L. (2009). Fine tuning the immune response through B7-H3 and B7-H4. *Immunological Reviews, 229*(1), 145–151.
51. Berrien-Elliott, M. M., Jackson, S. R., Meyer, J. M., Rouskey, C. J., Nguyen, T. L., Yagita, H., Greenberg, P. D., DiPaolo, R. J., & Teague, R. M. (2013). Durable adoptive immunotherapy for leukemia produced by manipulation of multiple regulatory pathways of CD8+ T-cell tolerance. *Cancer Research, 73*(2), 605–616.
52. Ramsay, A. G., Clear, A. J., Fatah, R., & Gribben, J. G. (2012). Multiple inhibitory ligands induce impaired T-cell immunologic synapse function in chronic lymphocytic leukemia that can be blocked with lenalidomide: Establishing a reversible immune evasion mechanism in human cancer. *Blood, The Journal of the American Society of Hematology, 120*(7), 1412–1421.
53. Pandya, A., Shah, Y., Kothari, N., Postwala, H., Shah, A., Parekh, P., & Chorawala, M. R. (2023). The future of cancer immunotherapy: DNA vaccines leading the way. *Medical Oncology, 40*(7), 200.

54. Yang, B., Jeang, J., Yang, A., Wu, T. C., & Hung, C. F. (2014). DNA vaccine for cancer immunotherapy. *Human Vaccines and Immunotherapeutics, 10*(11), 3153–3164.
55. Liu, J., Fu, M., Wang, M., Wan, D., Wei, Y., & Wei, X. (2022). Cancer vaccines as promising immuno-therapeutics: Platforms and current progress. *Journal of Hematology & Oncology, 15*(1), 28.
56. Liu, S., Jiang, Q., Zhao, X., Zhao, R., Wang, Y., Wang, Y., Liu, J., Shang, Y., Zhao, S., Wu, T., & Zhang, Y. (2021). A DNA nanodevice-based vaccine for cancer immunotherapy. *Nature Materials, 20*(3), 421–430.
57. Sica, A., & Bronte, V. (2007). Altered macrophage differentiation and immune dysfunction in tumor development. *Journal of Clinical Investigation, 117*(5), 1155–1166.
58. Collison, L. W., Workman, C. J., Kuo, T. T., Boyd, K., Wang, Y., Vignali, K. M., & et al. (2007). The inhibitory cytokine IL-35 contributes to regulatory T-cell function. *Nature, 450*(7169), 566–569.
59. Hiam-Galvez, K. J., Allen, B. M., & Spitzer, M. H. (2021). Systemic immunity in cancer. *Nature Reviews Cancer, 21*(6), 345–359.
60. Gordy, J. T., Luo, K., Zhang, H., Biragyn, A., & Markham, R. B. (2016). Fusion of the dendritic cell-targeting chemokine MIP3α to melanoma antigen Gp100 in a therapeutic DNA vaccine significantly enhances immunogenicity and survival in a mouse melanoma model. *Jurnal of Immunotherpy of Cancer, 4*, 96.
61. Souza-Fonseca-Guimaraes, F., Cursons, J., & Huntington, N. D. (2019). The emergence of natural killer cells as a major target in cancer immunotherapy. *Trends Immunology, 40*(2), 142–158.
62. Hobernik, D., & Bros, M. (2018). DNA vaccines—how far from clinical use?. *International Journal of Molecular Sciences, 19*(11), 3605.
63. Wang, R., Doolan, D. L., & Le, T. P., & et al. (1998). Induction of antigen-specific cytotoxic T lymphocytes in humans by a malaria DNA vaccine. *Science, 282*(5388), 476–480.
64. Calarota, S., Bratt, G., Nordlund, S., & et al. (1998). Cellular cytotoxic response induced by DNA vaccination in HIV-1-infected patients. *Lancet, 351*(9112), 1320–1325.
65. Graham, B. S., Koup, R. A., Roederer, M., & et al. (2006). Phase 1 safety and immunogenicity evaluation of a multiclade HIV-1 DNA candidate vaccine. *Journal of Infectious Diseases, 194*(12), 1650–1660.
66. Anderson, R. J., & Schneider, J. (2007). Plasmid DNA and viral vector-based vaccines for the treatment of cancer. *Vaccine, 25*(supplement 2), B24–B34.
67. Lowe, D. B., Shearer, M. H., Jumper, C. A., & Kennedy, R. C. (2007). Towards progress on DNA vaccines for cancer. *Cellular and Molecular Life Sciences, 64*(18), 2391–2403.
68. Perales, M.-A., Yuan, J., Powel, S., & et al. (2008). Phase I/II study of GM-CSF DNA as an adjuvant for a multipeptide cancer vaccine in patients with advanced melanoma. *Molecular Therapy, 16*(12), 2022–2029.
69. Stevenson, F. K., & Rice, J. (2006). Optimizing cancer immunotherapy trials: back to basics. *European Journal of Immunology, 36*(5), 1070–1073.

70. Stevenson, F. K., Rice, J., Ottensmeier, C. H., Thirdborough, S. M., & Zhu, D. (2004). DNA fusion gene vaccines against cancer: from the laboratory to the clinic. *Immunological Reviews*, *199*, 156–180.
71. Fioretti, D., Iurescia, S., Fazio, V. M., & Rinaldi, M. (2010). DNA vaccines: Developing new strategies against cancer. *BioMed Research International*, *2010*.
72. Lu, S., Wang, S., & Grimes-Serrano, J. M. (2008). Current progress of DNA vaccine studies in humans. *Expert Review of Vaccines*, *7*(2), 175–191.
73. Webster, D. P., Dunachie, S., McConkey, S., & et al. (2006). Safety of recombinant fowlpox strain FP9 and modified vaccinia virus Ankara vaccines against liver-stage P. falciparum malaria in non-immune volunteers. *Vaccine*, *24*(15), 3026–3034.
74. Egan, M. A., Chong, S. Y., Megati, S., & et al. (2005). Priming with plasmid DNAs expressing interleukin-12 and simian immunodeficiency virus gag enhances the immunogenicity and efficacy of an experimental AIDS vaccine based on recombinant vesicular stomatitis virus. *AIDS Research and Human Retroviruses*, *21*(7), 629–643.
75. Buchan, S., Grønevik, E., Mathiesen, I., King, C. A., Stevenson, F. K. , & Rice, J. (2005). Electroporation as a "prime/boost" strategy for naked DNA vaccination against a tumor antigen. *Journal of Immunology*, *174*(10), 6292–6298.
76. Paston, S. J., Brentville, V. A., Symonds, P., & Durrant, L. G. (2021). Cancer vaccines, adjuvants, and delivery systems. *Frontiers in Immunology*, *12*, 627932.
77. McNamara, M. A., Nair, S. K., & Holl, E. K. (2015). RNA-based vaccines in cancer immunotherapy. *Journal of Immunology Research*, *2015*.
78. Tretiakova, D. S., & Vodovozova, E. L. (2022). Liposomes as adjuvants and vaccine delivery systems. *Biochemistry (Moscow), Supplement Series A: Membrane and Cell Biology*, *16*(1), 1–20.
79. Suschak, J. J., Williams, J. A., & Schmaljohn, C. S. (2017). Advancements in DNA vaccine vectors, non-mechanical delivery methods, and molecular adjuvants to increase immunogenicity. *Human Vaccines and Immunotherapeutics*, *13*(12), 2837–2848.
80. Hobernik, D., & Bros, M. (2018). DNA vaccines—how far from clinical use?. *International Journal of Molecular Sciences*, *19*(11), 3605.
81. Myhr, A. I. (2017). DNA vaccines: Regulatory considerations and safety aspects. *Current Issues in Molecular Biology*, *22*(1), 79–88.
82. Shimizu, K., Iyoda, T., Okada, M., Yamasaki, S., & Fujii, S. I. (2018). Immune suppression and reversal of the suppressive tumor microenvironment. *International Immunology*, *30*(10), 445–454.
83. What are some challenges in developing vaccines for immunotherapy? https://www.beckman.com/support/faq/research/vaccine-challenges-for-immunotherapy
84. Ventola, C. L. (2017). Cancer Immunotherapy, Part 3 Challenges and Future Trends. *P T.*, *42*(8), 514–521.

CHAPTER 11

Cancer Vaccine Based on Plasmid DNA and Messenger RNA

ABSTRACT

Innovative ways of therapy and prevention are still required for cancer, which continues to be among the most difficult diseases in contemporary medicine. The creation of cancer vaccines has grown significantly in recent years as a viable area for immunotherapy. This chapter provides a summary of a cutting-edge cancer vaccination approach that uses messenger RNA (mRNA) and plasmid DNA to activate powerful immune responses specifically against cancers. Plasmid DNA and mRNA have special properties that can be used in the vaccine to deliver adjuvants and antigens that are particular to certain types of cancer to the immune system. Plasmid DNA provides a durable, long-lasting platform for the expression of antigens, whereas mRNA provides a momentary but incredibly effective means of protein synthesis. The effectiveness of the vaccination is eventually increased by a combination of both of these modalities, which enable persistent antigen presentation and quick immune activation. Additionally, this cancer vaccine employs personalized cancer immunotherapy, in which the encoded antigens are tailored to each patient's unique tumor mutations to target a variety of cancer types. The vaccination may be able to avoid problems with immune tolerance and considerably improve the immune system's capability of recognizing tumor cells by making use of this patient-specific strategy. According to encouraging preclinical and early clinical results, this innovative strategy has a great deal of promise for treating different cancer types with few side effects and strong immuno genicity. A successful development of such a vaccine would revolutionize

DNA- and m-RNA-Based Vaccines: An Immunotherapeutic Approach to Cancer.

Sonali Sundram and Rishabha Malviya (Authors)

DOI: 10.1201/9781774919613-11

the field of oncology and mark a big step toward more efficient and individualized cancer therapy. This abstract highlights the promise of plasmid DNA as well as vaccines based on mRNA in the battle against cancer and offers a glimpse into the exciting future of cancer immunotherapy.

11.1 INTRODUCTION

The development of DNA vaccines containing specific tumor antigens as well as molecules that control and amplify the intended effector pathways is made possible by genetic technology [1]. DNA vaccines give a rare chance to direct specified antigens, followed by certain activator molecules, via a patient's weakened immune system in addition to their inherent capacity to activate several innate immunity pathways. Many intracellular antigens need cytotoxic T cells as well as cell surface molecules that are sensitive to antibody attack as possible target antigens. The molecular structure of the antigen can be changed during vaccine design to choose the intended effector pathway [2]. A small quantity of antigen, seemingly enough for efficient priming, is produced by DNA vaccines. However, these vaccinations frequently cause potent CD8+ T-cell reactions that can eliminate antigen-presenting cells after booster injections. Due to this, "prime/boost" procedures have been developed to raise antigen levels [3]. The delivery of particular antigens using vaccines made from DNA at least enables an objective evaluation of immune reactions elicited as opposed to the particular target as well as the analysis of what truly is significant, the impact on tumor cells of the patients [1]. Reports of preventative DNA vaccinations in humans that can trigger antibodies along with CD4+ T-cell reactions and may be effective as opposed to many harmful viruses are mounting [4, 5]. DNA vaccines have various potential benefits over traditional immunization, including enhanced stability, increased safety, and ease of fabrication. They are capable of inducing both efficient humoral along cellular immune responses [6]. DNA vaccines are effective at inducing both humoral and cell-regulated immune reactions in the host in addition to innate immunological responses [7, 8]. In 1990, Wolff et al. [9] published their findings on the protein expression after intramuscular injection of plasmid in mice, which was the first to demonstrate DNA vaccines. Although undeviating gene transfer through the plasmid DNA in the muscular cells of the mice did not need a special route of delivery, it was established that intramuscular injection containing the gene-encoding plasmid DNA induced protein expression in myocytes. These vaccines are novel subunit vaccines that express a protein after plasmid or virus delivery to mammalian cells carrying an antigenic gene [10, 11]. Combining DNA vaccines with plasmids that encode cytokines or other immune-stimulating molecules also enhances and changes immune reactions to coded antigens. Because these vaccinations are heat resistant, they do not require special handling or upkeep [12, 13]. To manufacture many specific antigens from various infectious agents in the host cell, the DNA vaccine might be genetically modified. Despite the tiny number of antigens produced by transfected cells with DNA vaccines (between a picogram and a nanogram), the immune reactions are powerful [14, 15]. DNA-based treatments have made considerable use of plasmid DNA vectors. These vectors can be broken down into two parts: the transcription unit, which contains the therapeutic gene and its eukaryotic promoter, and the backbone of bacteria, which is needed by it for amplification and consists of the replication origin as well as selection markers (like genes for resistance to antibiotics) [16]. The intrinsic benefit production ease, which approaches the finest traditional vaccine manufacturing methods now available, builds therapeutic tumor vaccines that utilize messenger RNA (mRNA) an appealing alternative for cancer immunotherapy. These vaccinations are tolerated well and could be effective cancer prevention strategies. Numerous clinical trials researching mRNA vaccine treatment are currently recruiting patients having diverse tumor diagnoses. Technological advancements have enhanced the reliability, structure, and delivery techniques of mRNA-based vaccines [17, 18]. Vaccines made of mRNA are readily destroyed, well tolerated, and do not incorporate into the host's genome [19]. Due to the presence of RNAs, mRNA is temporary, which may be advantageous for the procedure by which organisms maintain the creation of desirable proteins [20]. Numerous immunostimulatory processes in mRNA may be advantageous or harmful for mRNA utilized in vaccinations or cancer immunotherapies [21]. Which cell in a vaccine constructs the protein concealed by the plasmid DNA or mRNA could be crucial as, unlike in the case of antibodies, wherein the protein must likely be secreted, in the case of cellular immune responses like Cytolytic T lymphocytes, the kind of cell making the protein (thus the kind of cell that produces it transduced via plasmid DNA or mRNA) is significant [22, 23].

TABLE 11.1 Difference Between Vaccines Based on DNA and RNA.

Sr. No.	DNA-Based Vaccines	RNA-Based Vaccines	Reference
1	Genetic info of virus transmitted to another mol	Genetic info transmitted by DNA vaccine into mRNA vaccine	[24]
2	Creates an immunological response by transfecting a certain DNA sequence into an infected organism	Creates an immunological response by copying the messenger RNA (mRNA) molecule	[25]
3	DNA vaccines must go from the cytoplasm up to the nucleus to create the essential bacterial or viral proteins	mRNA vaccines demand a more direct path	[26]
4	DNA vaccines use specialized equipment to transfer the pathogen's genetic code into the cell via a brief electrical pulse	Injections are used to give mRNA vaccinations	[26]
5	They might combine with the host's native genome	They do not merge with the host genome and enter the cell nucleus	[27]
6	In a laboratory setting, DNA is more stable and less prone to degradation than RNA	Many scientists also think RNA vaccines are less dangerous than DNA vaccines because they would not have to alter the DNA of the host or even enter the host cell's nucleus since the mRNA was previously created	[27]
7	A plasmid is used as the DNA vaccine's delivery system	An RNA vaccine is administered via liquid nanoparticles	[28]

11.2 mRNA VACCINES

A subcategory of nucleic acid vaccinations is the mRNA vaccination. Self-amplifying RNA (siRNA) along with nonreplicating mRNA are the two kinds [29]. saRNA vaccinations are replicons that are genetically modified and made from viruses with single-stranded RNA that can replicate themselves [30, 31]. Enveloped proteins are given in trans-like faulty helper constructions when manufacturing to produce replication-defective VRPs. After an initial infection, the ensuing VRPs are consequently not able to produce infectious viral particles; only the RNA can undergo further amplification [32]. Self-amplifying mRNA vaccination given nonvirally has the potential of being very adaptable, powerful, efficient, scalable, and affordable. Self-amplifying mRNA imitates a viral infection by amplification of its genome along with the mRNA that encodes the antigen in the host cell. As a result, sustained amounts of the targeted protein and innate immunological responses that act as adjuvants are produced, which in turn trigger powerful and persistent humoral along with cellular immune reactions that are specific for the antigen [33]. Self-amplifying (sa) RNA vaccines need less RNA at the start since the mRNA is amplified inside the cells. For instance, 5 g saRNA was effectively employed in a clinical experiment and a dosage of just 10 ng saRNA could trigger an immune system-specific reaction to SARS-CoV-2 in mice [34]. The internal innate-multiplication characteristics of several positive-sense RNA viruses served as the inspiration for the self-amplifying mRNA (saRNA) vaccinations, a very beneficial category of mRNA vaccines. Such vaccination platforms offer both self-adjuvanticity capabilities and significantly increased levels of vaccination antigen(s) expression [35]. Numerous nonreplicating virus vectors were developed and created for utilization in gene treatment along with developing the vaccine. The alphavirus genome is where the saRNA vaccine was developed. One transgene that controls viral RNA replication along with another that encodes the therapeutic antigen is included in such a vaccine [36]. Dannull et al. [37] injected RNA-transfected DCs into renal cell carcinoma (RCC) patients, and they also decreased the amount of regulatory T cells. The recombinant IL-2 diphtheria toxin combination DAB389IL-2 (ONTAK), which specifically kills regulatory T cells that are CD25-positive, was utilized to lessen the amount of Tregs. When compared to injections using DC vaccines alone, the notable, combination treatment increased CD8 specific to tumor as well as CD4 T-cell reactions [37]. Mice with lymphoproliferative conditions that do not express CTLA-4 offer additional proof of the significance of the regulation of T-cell reactions [38, 39]. Increased T-cell reactions could come from the suppression of CTLA-4. Anti-CTLA-4 inhibitory antibodies that are humanized include tremelimumab and ipilimumab. Patients receiving treatment responded more favorably clinically as a result of their use in melanoma trials [40]. Combining RNA vaccination alongside the administration of tyrosine kinase inhibitors (TKIs) is a different option to improve effects against cancer. Sorafenib and sunitinib, TKIs, block intracellular signaling networks that promote cellular proliferation and angiogenesis. Hepatocellular carcinoma (HCC) and RCC are both cured with sorafenib. In the treatment of RCC and gastrointestinal tumors (GIST), sunitinib is used. Recent mice studies demonstrated that sunitinib had no such effect while sorafenib pretreatment inhibited the production of antigen-specific T cells [41].

11.3 PLASMID DNA VACCINE

Plasmids, which are tiny circular molecules initially procured from bacteria, are the majorly popular DNA-based therapeutic vectors for cancer and DNA vaccines. In addition to plasmids, several systems based on DNA for delivery of genes, other than plasmids, have been identified recently. Instances of this kind of platform include Doggybone DNA (linear, covalently shut, double-stranded molecules), Minicircle DNA (the redundant plasmid foundation that is eliminated by recombination), MIDGE DNA, and linear DNA amplicons generated by polymerase chain reaction (PCR) [42–45]. A minimum of a single-expression cassette which regulates a protein's expression which will cause the clinical effect must be included in all plasmids utilized in cancer gene therapy/DNA vaccination. After being absorbed through the cell, the DNA should make it to the nucleus, wherein the gene can control the production of the beneficial protein in a way similar to how the cell makes its very own proteins [46]. The plasmid must be well-designed and optimized for treatment to be successful [47]. For example, if several important genes must be declared on a single plasmid, we may accomplish so independently (with every gene having its own promoter), in a multicistronic system (in which two or more genes are regulated by identical promoter), or by using a fusion protein (as well as a linker sequence among the two sequences). A virus-derived T2A sequence or an internal ribosome entry site (IRES) must be positioned in between many genes in the multicistronic system [48–50]. Even though direct gene exchange between the plasmid DNA in the mice's muscle cells did not need a special delivery route, it was established that intramuscular injection containing the gene-encoding plasmid DNA induced protein expression in myocytes. These vaccines are novel subunit vaccines that express a protein after plasmid or virus delivery to mammalian cells carrying an antigenic gene [51, 52]. Immune reactions to coded antigens are also improved or altered when DNA vaccines are combined with plasmids which encode cytokines and other immune stimulant molecules. Because these vaccinations are heat resistant, they do not require special handling or upkeep [53, 54]. Because they solely contain genetic information of the antigen, are much stable as well as simpler to create, also can elicit both humoral and cellular immune reactions, plasmid DNA vaccinations are frequently safer compared to conventional vaccinations [55]. Plasmid DNA sequences inside the plasmid, the produced products (antigen) of genes, the formulation, the delivery mechanism, administration routes, and the kind of exposed cells toward the plasmid are only a few instances of the several variables that can influence how frequently plasmid DNA vaccinations integrate inside host cellular DNA [56]. These DNA platforms, known as plasmids, typically contain a viral promoter gene, a gene encoding antibiotic resistance, a gene encoding bacterial origin of replication, as well as a multiple cloning site (MCS) to form a transgenic region, wherein one or more genes of antigenic relevance can be introduced. By using these recombinant vectors for vaccination, the molecular as well as cellular machinery of cells that are transfected can express the encoded antigens intracellularly, inducing an immune response that is unique to the antigen. This procedure offers efficient defense against a variety of infections, tumor cells, and even autoimmune and allergic illnesses. The development of a potent humoral along with cellular immune response depending on B and T cells results in protective effectiveness. Plasmid-based immunization has evolved into a secure method for the prevention of numerous diseases thanks to the immunity created through these DNA vaccines, as well as their simplicity in manufacture, administration, stability of genes, and safety [57].

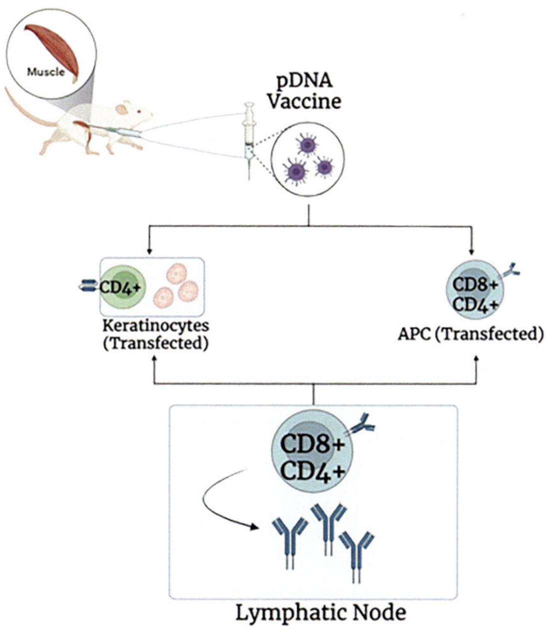

FIGURE 11.1 pDNA vaccine and its fate in the biological environment.

11.4 CLINICAL SETTINGS OF PDNA VACCINES

By delivering the genes encoding vaccine antigens, DNA plasmids may be utilized for stimulating a protective (or curative) immune reaction. Given how sophisticated the immune system is at avoiding pathogen invasion, it is especially amazing that bare DNA (with no sophistication of coated proteins and host evasion systems) may penetrate the cell from the outside and be produced inside the nucleus. DNA vaccines hold out the tantalizing potential of the upcoming vaccine technology upswing due to the simplicity, cheap cost, and speed of custom genome synthesis, providing either particular designer vaccinations for tumors or bulk immunizations by a quick timing of responses to looming pandemics. There is a lot of enthusiasm for the strategy of DNA vaccination, though this zeal needs to be restrained given the repeated inability of therapeutic trials to elicit a strong immune reaction [58]. Toll-like receptor (TLR) 9 is a natural adjuvant used to stimulate innate immunity because plasmid DNA (pDNA) obtained from bacteria naturally includes a significant warning sign in the form of CG sequences without methylation. When resident APCs like dendritic cells are triggered by the pDNA through activation of TLR9, the protein that is encoded will be expressed immediately at that location. When such APCs are activated, there is a localized inflammatory response, improved antigen processing, as well as immune cell presentation and location via blood, and APC go toward lymphoid organs. Consequently, despite the lack of additional adjuvants, injection of raw pDNA provides an effective immunization strategy. However, modifications to transfected reagents or physical methods can enhance pDNA's penetration into cells, increasing the effectiveness of pDNA-based vaccinations. The main disadvantage of pDNA vaccinations is their ability to remain *in vivo* as well as change the genetic makeup of the host cells of some by incorporation in chromosomes. Their benefits are simple to manufacture and consistent *in vitro* and *in vivo* [59]. Patients with stage IV melanoma were examined using an improved technique that involved intranodal administration of tyrosinase-coding pDNA weighing up to 800 g at intervals of 2 weeks [60]. During this treatment, which also turned out to be safe, 11 of the 26 patients generated cytotoxic T-lymphocytes (CTLs) specifically opposed to tyrosinase epitopes. Although no relapse was seen, the overall rate of survival in the treated group appeared to be quite high, particularly in individuals who had a stronger immune response following vaccination.

Seven out of twelve patients received a T-cell but also a B-cell immune response after receiving monthly needle-free (projector: intramuscular administration) of up to 1.8 mg of pDNA coding the idiotype of B-cell lymphoma in a patient-specific environment [61]. Because these viral proteins are intolerable to the immune system, immunization against oncogenes released by viruses is advantageous as a substitute for self-tumor antigens. Two oncogenes, E6 and E7, are encoded by the human papillomavirus-16 (HPV-16). Patients with HPV-16-related anal dysplasia who were HLA-A2-positive received an intramuscular injection of a pDNA build coding for a few HLA-A2 epitopes [62]. pDNA immunization using DNA is becoming the method of choice for preventing crippling diseases. Quality control is essential in the production of pharmaceutical-grade pDNA to meet regulatory agency standards for purity, potency, safety, and efficacy. Full consistency in the sequence of DNA that is to be injected is one of the requirements that pDNA must achieve. There are currently several proven analytical techniques available to control this parameter [63]. Understanding of host processes is limited. Over time, limitations in antigen production *in vivo* from plasmid DNA vaccination arise, even though plasmid-based DNA immunogens are being explored as potential vaccines for protection against these infections [64].

11.5 CLINICAL SETTINGS OF mRNA VACCINES

The use of mRNA in therapeutic cancer vaccines makes them an appealing option to conventional cancer immunotherapy due to the inherent benefit of ease of manufacture, which is comparable to the best conventional vaccine manufacturing techniques now available. These vaccinations are tolerated well and could be effective cancer prevention strategies. Patients with various cancer diagnoses are being enrolled in many clinical trials investigating the use of an mRNA vaccine. Technological advancements have optimized the stability, structure, and administration techniques of mRNA-based vaccines. Results from early clinical trials utilizing mRNA vaccinations as a solo and in combination with checkpoint inhibitors have been positive, although therapeutic mRNA-based vaccines for cancer are not yet licensed for routine treatment [65]. In a few studies, mRNA-based vaccination therapy led to long-lasting objective responses in cancer patients without uncontrollable toxicities [66–69]. Future cancer therapies may benefit from the use of mRNA vaccines, particularly when combined with other immunotherapies [70]. Autologous dendritic cells that have been *ex vivo* modified to express synthetic mRNA that encodes tumor-associated or tumor-specific antigens can also deliver synthetic mRNA, as can injections of formulated or unformulated mRNA [71]. mRNA is delivered to the cytoplasm, where it is processed to produce antigen as well as enters the MHC-presenting cascade after vaccination along with cellular uptake according to antigen-presenting cells [72]. To activate CD8+ and CD4+ T lymphocytes, antigen-presenting cells deliver tumor-related antigens on both MHC class I and class II. Furthermore, CD4+ T cells may coactivate B cells that are specific for an antigen and trigger a humoral immune response. After internalizing external proteins and presenting them to MHC class II of B cells, antigen-presenting B cells can also activate CD4+ T cells [73]. mRNA molecules are contained in a buffer solution in mRNA vaccines that are unformulated or naked. In the past 5 years, there have been a few clinical trials that have used nonformulated mRNA vaccines for treating cancer patients. In a phase 1 clinical trial, non-formulated mRNA vaccines were administered intravenously to 13 patients with stage III or stage IV melanoma who had stable disease, an incomplete response, or an entire response to prior therapy. All patients produced T-cell responses against a range of vaccine-encoded neoepitopes, and two (40%) of the five patients with stage IV melanoma experienced vaccine-related clinical responses [74]. Peptides that are positively charged and cationic called protamines join mRNA that is negatively charged to form complexes that shield the molecules from deterioration [69]. RNActive vaccines, which are mRNA vaccines made with protamine, have undergone evaluation in numerous clinical trials [75]. RNActive vaccines use protamine-complexed mRNA molecules modified by nucleotides to boost protein expression as well as immunogenicity [76]. The mRNA lipoplex vaccine is a hybrid delivery system made of a lipid shell, an mRNA complex, and a polycationic component [77]. An mRNA lipoplex vaccine (BNT111), carrying four melanoma tumor-associated antigens, was tested for safety and efficacy in a Phase 1 dose-escalation study (NCT02410733) involving patients with advanced melanoma who expressed at least one of the four antigens [78]. The first of an array of fixed blends of common antigens linked to malignancy (FixVac) mRNA vaccines, BNT111, included a predetermined combination of common tumor-related antigens. Out of 50 patients, 39 (75%) had immune reactions targeting one or more tumor-associated antigens, and BNT111 generated both CD4+ and CD8+ T-cell reactions. BNT111 was administered to 17 individuals in addition to the traditional anti-PD-1 therapy; 6 (35%) of these individuals experienced a partial response, while two (12%) experienced steady illness. Twenty-five patients received a single dose of BNT111, and three (12%) of them saw a partial response while seven (28%) experienced steady illness [79]. mRNA tumor vaccine platforms beat other conventional vaccination platforms because of their excellent efficacy, safe administration, speedy development potentials, and low cost of production. The application of mRNA vaccines has been constrained, nevertheless, by instability, intrinsic immunogenicity, and inefficient *in vivo* administration. These problems have been researched, and suitable mRNA structural changes (such as codon optimizations, self-amplifying mRNA, nucleotide alterations (etc.) as well as formulation techniques (such as lipid nanoparticles (LNPs), polymer compounds, peptides, etc.) are being explored. The possibility of eliminating tumor cells has risen thanks to the administration routes being adjusted as well as the co-delivery of several mRNA vaccinations alongside additional immunotherapeutic drugs (such as checkpoint inhibitors) [78].

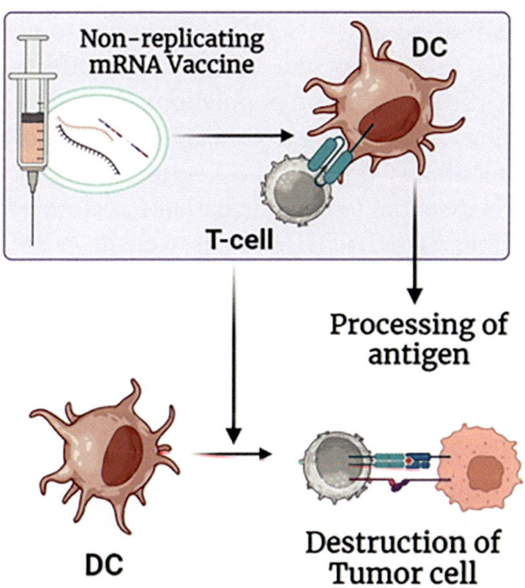

FIGURE 11.2 In vivo fate of mRNA vaccine.

11.6 CONCLUSION AND FUTURE PERSPECTIVES

A promising research focus in the battle against tumors is the creation of cancer vaccines that utilize plasmid DNA along with mRNA. Numerous clinical and preclinical studies have produced hopeful findings, and over the past several years, this field has made substantial development. The creation of DNA along with mRNA-based cancer vaccines will be improved with continued investigation into the discovery of tumor-specific antigens as well as neoantigens. Personalized vaccines may become more common, increasing their efficacy because they are made specifically for each patient's genetic profile and cancer profile. These vaccinations can encourage a patient's immune system to identify and combat tumor cells, providing a cutting-edge and focused method of treating and preventing cancer. The flexibility of DNA along with mRNA-based vaccines for cancer is one of their main advantages. These vaccines, in contrast to conventional cancer therapies, can be made to target certain antigens linked to different cancer types, thus rendering them extremely customizable and perhaps useful against a variety of malignancies. Additionally, they are often well accepted by patients and have a favorable safety profile, which lessens the load of unfavorable side effects that frequently come along with conventional chemotherapy as well as radiation therapy. It will be necessary to conduct extensive therapeutic trials to confirm the security and effectiveness of these vaccinations on a scale of patient populations. Guidelines for acceptance and incorporation into accepted cancer treatment regimens will be established by regulatory organizations, which will play a crucial role in this process. It is essential to educate patients and medical professionals about the possible benefits of DNA as well as mRNA-based cancer vaccines. Patients who are well-informed about the possibilities for treatment can choose the best course of action and push for the inclusion of these medicines in the healthcare system. In conclusion, the creation of cancer vaccines using mRNA and plasmid DNA has enormous potential for the continued fight against cancer. These cutting-edge medicines have the potential to greatly improve cancer prevention and treatment, giving patients and their families fresh hope, with sustained research, and clinical trials, along with a focus on enhancing vaccine design and administration.

KEYWORDS

- **antigens**
- **DNA**
- **immunotherapy**
- **plasmid**
- **RNA**
- **T cells**

REFERENCES

1. Stevenson, F. K., Ottensmeier, C. H., & Rice, J. (2010). DNA vaccines against cancer come of age. *Current Opinion in Immunology, 22*(2), 264–270.
2. Rice, J., Ottensmeier, C. H., & Stevenson, F. K. (2008). DNA vaccines: Precision tools for activating effective immunity against cancer. *Nature Reviews Cancer, 8*(2), 108–120.
3. Gilbert, S. C., Moorthy, V. S., Andrews, L., Pathan, A. A., McConkey, S. J., Vuola, J. M., Keating, S. M., Berthoud, T., Webster, D., McShane, H., & Hill, A. V. (2006). Synergistic DNA–MVA prime-boost vaccination regimes for malaria and tuberculosis. *Vaccine, 24*(21), 4554–4561.
4. Jin, X., Newman, M. J., De-Rosa, S., Cooper, C., Thomas, E., Keefer, M., Fuchs, J., Blattner, W., Livingston, B. D., McKinney, D. M., & Noonan, E. (2009). A novel HIV T helper epitope-based vaccine elicits cytokine-secreting HIV-specific CD4+ T cells in a Phase I clinical trial in HIV-uninfected adults. *Vaccine, 27*(50), 7080–7086.
5. Martin, J. E., Sullivan, N. J., Enama, M. E., Gordon, I. J., Roederer, M., Koup, R. A., Bailer, R. T., Chakrabarti, B. K., Bailey, M. A., Gomez, P. L., & Andrews, C. A. (2006). A DNA vaccine for Ebola virus is safe and immunogenic in a phase I clinical trial. *Clinical and Vaccine Immunology, 13*(11), 1267–1277.
6. Huang, T., Liu, L., Lv, Z., Zhao, K., Yi, Q., & Zhang, J. (2022). Recent advances in DNA vaccines against lung cancer: A mini review. *Vaccines, 10*(10), 1586.
7. Huang, T., Zhao, K., Song, X., Song, T., Wang, X., Zhang, X., Yue, B., & Chu, Y. (2022). Heterologous prime-boost immunization with DNA vaccine and modified recombinant proteins enhances immune response against Trueperella pyogenes in mice. *Vaccines, 10*(6), 839.
8. Rezaei, T., Davoudian, E., Khalili, S., Amini, M., Hejazi, M., de la Guardia, M., & Mokhtarzadeh, A. (2021). Strategies in DNA vaccine for melanoma cancer. *Pigment Cell & Melanoma Research, 34*(5), 869–891.

9. Wolff, J. A., Malone, R. W., Williams, P., Chong, W., Acsadi, G., Jani, A., & Felgner, P. L. (1990). Direct gene transfer into mouse muscle in vivo. *Science, 247*(4949 Pt 1), 1465–1468.
10. Bhopale, G. M. (2003). Development of a vaccine for toxoplasmosis: Current status. *Microbes and Infection, 5*(5), 457–462.
11. Kofta, W., & Wedrychowicz, H. (2001). c-DNA vaccination against parasitic infections: advantages and disadvantages. *Vetrinary Parasitology, 100*(1-2), 3–12.
12. Letscher-Bru, V., Pfaff, A. W., Abou-Bacar, A., & et al. (2003). Vaccination with Toxoplasma gondii SAG-1 protein is protective against congenital toxoplasmosis in BALB/c mice but not in CBA/J mice. *Infection and Immunity, 71*(11), 6615–6619.
13. Tighe, H., Corr, M., Roman, M., & Raz, E. (1998). Gene vaccination: Plasmid DNA is more than just a blueprint. *Immunology Today, 19*(2), 89–97.
14. Saade, F., & Petrovsky, N. (2012). Technologies for enhanced efficacy of DNA vaccines. *Expert Review of Vaccines, 11*(2), 189–209.
15. Shedlock, D. J., & Weiner, D. B. (2000). DNA vaccination: antigen presentation and the induction of immunity. *Journal of Leukocyte Biology, 68*(6), 793–806.
16. Eusébio, D., Neves, A. R., Costa, D., Biswas, S., Alves, G., Cui, Z., & Sousa, Â. (2021). Methods to improve the immunogenicity of plasmid DNA vaccines. *Drug Discovery Today, 26*(11), 2575–2592.
17. Lorentzen, C. L., Haanen, J. B., Met, Ö., & Svane, I. M. (2022). Clinical advances and ongoing trials on mRNA vaccines for cancer treatment. *The Lancet Oncology, 23*(10), e450-8
18. Karikó, K., Muramatsu, H., Welsh, F. A., Ludwig, J., Kato, H., Akira, S., & Weissman, D. (2008). Incorporation of pseudouridine into mRNA yields superior nonimmunogenic vector with increased translational capacity and biological stability. *Molecular Therapy, 16*(11), 1833–1840.
19. Thess, A., Grund, S., Mui, B. L., Hope, M. J., Baumhof, P., Fotin-Mleczek, M., & Schlake T. (2015). Sequence-engineered mRNA without chemical nucleoside modifications enables an effective protein therapy in large animals. *Molecular Therapy, 23*(9), 1456–1464.
20. Houseley, J., & Tollervey, D. (2009). The many pathways of RNA degradation. *Cell, 136*(4), 763–776.
21. Liu, M. A. (2019). A comparison of plasmid DNA and mRNA as vaccine technologies. *Vaccines, 7*(2), 37.
22. Deck, R. R., DeWitt, C. M., Donnelly, J. J., Liu, M. A., & Ulmer, J. B. (1997). Characterization of humoral immune responses induced by an influenza hemagglutinin DNA vaccine. *Vaccine, 15*(1), 71—78.
23. Hajj, K. A., & Whitehead, K. A. (2017). Tools for translation: Non-viral materials for therapeutic mRNA delivery. *Nature Reviews Materials, 2*(10), 1–7.
24. https://www.verywellhealth.com/rna-vs-dna-vaccine-5082285#:~:text=by%20the%20FDA.-,Recap,potential%20risk%20with%20DNA%20vaccines.
25. https://byjus.com/biology/difference-between-dna-and-rna-vaccines/
26. https://info.gbiosciences.com/blog/dna-and-mrna-vaccines-a-side-by-side-comparison
27. https://testbook.com/key-differences/difference-between-dna-and-rna-vaccines
28. http://www.differencebetween.net/science/difference-between-rna-and-dna-vaccines/

29. Wang, Y., Zhang, Z., Luo, J., Han, X., Wei, Y., & Wei, X. (2021). mRNA vaccine: A potential therapeutic strategy. *Molecular Cancer, 20*(1), 33.
30. Lundstrom, K. (2018). Self-replicating RNA viruses for RNA therapeutics. *Molecules, 23*, 3310.
31. Tews, B. A., & Meyers, G. (2017). Self-replicating RNA. *Methods in Molecular Biology, 1499*, 15–35.
32. Maruggi, G., Ulmer, J. B., Rappuoli, R., & Yu, D. (2022). Self-amplifying mRNA-based vaccine technology and its mode of action. *Current Topic in Microbiology and Immunology, 440*, 31–70.
33. Maruggi, G., Mallett, C. P., Westerbeck, J. W., Chen, T., Lofano, G., Friedrich, K., Qu, L., Sun, J. T., McAuliffe, J., Kanitkar, A., & Arrildt, K. T. (2022). A self-amplifying mRNA SARS-CoV-2 vaccine candidate induces safe and robust protective immunity in preclinical models. *Molecular Therapy, 30*(5), 1897–1912.
34. Pollock, K. M., Cheeseman, H. M., Szubert, A. J., Libri, V., Boffito, M., Owen, D., Bern, H., McFarlane, L. R., O'Hara, J., Lemm, N. M., & McKay, P. (2022). Safety and immunogenicity of a self-amplifying RNA vaccine against COVID-19: COVAC1, a phase I, dose-ranging trial. *EClinicalMedicine, 44*.
35. Pourseif, M. M., Masoudi-Sobhanzadeh, Y., Azari, E., Parvizpour, S., Barar, J., Ansari, R., & Omidi, Y. (2022). Self-amplifying mRNA vaccines: mode of action, design, development and optimization. *Drug Discovery Today,* 103341.
36. Lundstrom, K. (2020). Self-amplifying RNA viruses as RNA vaccines. *International Journal of Molecular Sciences, 21*, 5130.
37. Dannull, J., Su, Z., Rizzieri, D., Yang, B. K., Coleman, D., Yancey, D., Zhang, A., Dahm, P., Chao, N., Gilboa, E., & Vieweg, J. (2005). Enhancement of vaccine-mediated antitumor immunity in cancer patients after depletion of regulatory T cells. *The Journal of Clinical Investigation, 115*(12), 3623–3633.
38. Tivol, E. A., Borriello, F., Schweitzer, A. N., Lynch, W. P., Bluestone, J. A., & Sharpe, A. H. (1995). Loss of CTLA-4 leads to massive lymphoproliferation and fatal multiorgan tissue destruction, revealing a critical negative regulatory role of CTLA-4. *Immunity, 3*(5), 541–547.
39. Waterhouse, P., Penninger, J. M., Timms, E., Wakeham, A., Shahinian, A., Lee, K. P., Thompson, C. B., Griesser, H., & Mak, T. W. (1995). Lymphoproliferative disorders with early lethality in mice deficient in Ctla-4. *Science, 270*(5238), 985–988.
40. Ribas, A., Camacho, L. H., Lopez-Berestein, G., Pavlov, D., Bulanhagui, C. A., Millham, R., Comin-Anduix, B., Reuben, J. M., Seja, E., Parker, C. A., & Sharma, A. (2005). Antitumor activity in melanoma and anti-self responses in a phase I trial with the anti-cytotoxic T lymphocyte-associated antigen 4 monoclonal antibody CP-675,206. *Journal of Clinical Oncology, 23*(35), 8968–8977.
41. Hipp, M. M., Hilf, N., Walter, S., Werth, D., Brauer, K. M., Radsak, M. P., Weinschenk, T., Singh-Jasuja, H., & Brossart, P. (2008). Sorafenib, but not sunitinib, affects function of dendritic cells and induction of primary immune responses. *Blood, The Journal of the American Society of Hematology, 111*(12), 5610–5620.
42. Almeida, A. M., Eusébio, D., Queiroz, J. A., Sousa, F., & Sousa, Â. (2021). Minicircle DNA vaccine purification and E7 antigen expression assessment. In *DNA vaccines: Methods in molecular biology* (Vol. 2197, pp. 207–222). Humana Press.

43. Conforti, A., Salvatori, E., Lione, L., Compagnone, M., Pinto, E., Shorrock, C., Hayward, J. A., Sun, Y., Liang, B. M., Palombo, F., & et al. (2022). Linear DNA amplicons as a novel cancer vaccine strategy. *Journal of Experimental and Clinical Cancer Research, 41*, 195.
44. Kobelt, D., Aumann, J., Schmidt, M., Wittig, B., Fichtner, I., Behrens, D., Lemm, M., Freundt, G., Schlag, P. M., & Walther, W. (2014). Preclinical study on combined chemo- and nonviral gene therapy for sensitization of melanoma using a human TNF-alpha expressing MIDGE DNA vector. *Molecular Oncology, 8*, 609–619.
45. Short, C., & Savelyeva, N. (2021). Doggybones, DNA vaccines and skin-penetrating fluids: Whatever it takes to win the fight against cancer. *Biochemist, 43*, 22–25.
46. Martínez-Puente, D. H., Pérez-Trujillo, J. J., Zavala-Flores, L. M., García-García, A., Villanueva-Olivo, A., Rodríguez-Rocha, H., Valdés, J., Saucedo-Cárdenas, O., Montes de Oca-Luna, R., & Loera-Arias, M. D. (2022). Plasmid DNA for therapeutic applications in cancer. *Pharmaceutics, 14*(9), 1861.
47. Kutzler, M. A., & Weiner, D. B. (2008). DNA vaccines: Ready for prime time?. *Nature Reviews Genetics, 9*(10), 776–788.
48. Chen, X., Zaro, J. L., & Shen, W. C. (2013). Fusion protein linkers: Property, design and functionality. *Advanced Drug Delivery Reviews, 65*(10), 1357–1369.
49. Klein, J. S., Jiang, S., Galimidi, R. P., Keeffe, J. R., & Bjorkman, P. J. (2014). Design and characterization of structured protein linkers with differing flexibilities. *Protein Engineering, Design & Selection, 27*(10), 325–330.
50. Renaud-Gabardos, E., Hantelys, F., Morfoisse, F., Chaufour, X., Garmy-Susini, B., & Prats, A. C. (2015). Internal ribosome entry site-based vectors for combined gene therapy. *World Journal of Experimental Medicine, 5*(1), 11.
51. Bhopale, G. M. (2003). Development of a vaccine for toxoplasmosis: current status. *Microbes and Infection, 5*(5), 457–462.
52. Kofta, W., & Wedrychowicz, H. (2001). c-DNA vaccination against parasitic infections: advantages and disadvantages. *Veterinary Parasitology, 100*(1-2), 3–12.
53. Tighe, H., Corr, M., Roman, M., & Raz, E. (1998). Gene vaccination: Plasmid DNA is more than just a blueprint. *Immunology Today, 19*(2), 89–97.
54. Letscher-Bru, V., Pfaff, A. W., Abou-Bacar, A., Filisetti, D., Antoni, E., Villard, O., Klein, J. P., & Candolfi, E. (2003).Vaccination with toxoplasma gondii SAG-1 protein is protective against congenital toxoplasmosis in BALB/c mice but not in CBA/J mice. *Infection and Immunity, 71*(11), 6615–6619.
55. Eusébio, D., Neves, A. R., Costa, D., Biswas, S., Alves, G., Cui, Z., & Sousa, Â. (2021). Methods to improve the immunogenicity of plasmid DNA vaccines. *Drug Discovery Today, 26*(11), 2575–2592.
56. Manam, S., Ledwith, B. J., Barnum, A. B., Troilo, P. J., Pauley, C. J., Harper, L. B., Griffiths, T. G. 2nd, Niu, Z., Denisova, L., Follmer, T. T., Pacchione, S. J., Wang, Z., Beare, C. M., Bagdon, W. J., & Nichols, W. W. (2000). Plasmid DNA vaccines: tissue distribution and effects of DNA sequence, adjuvants and delivery method on integration into host DNA. *Intervirology, 43*(4-6), 273–281.
57. Gómez, L. A., & Oñate, A. A. (2018). Plasmid-based DNA vaccines. *Plasmid.*
58. Tregoning, J. S., & Kinnear, E. (2015). Using plasmids as DNA vaccines for infectious diseases. In *Plasmids: Biology and impact in biotechnology and discovery* (pp. 651–668).

59. Weide, B., Garbe, C., Rammensee, H. G., & Pascolo, S. (2008). Plasmid DNA-and messenger RNA-based anti-cancer vaccination. *Immunology Letters, 115*(1), 33–42.
60. Tagawa, S. T., Lee, P., Snively, J., Boswell, W., Ounpraseuth, S., Lee, S., & et al. (2003). Phase I study of intranodal delivery of a plasmid DNA vaccine for patients with stage IV melanoma. *Cancer, 98*, 144–154.
61. Timmerman, J. M., Singh, G., Hermanson, G., Hobart, P., Czerwinski, D. K., Taidi, B., & et al. (2002). Immunogenicity of a plasmid DNA vaccine encoding chimeric idiotype in patients with B-cell lymphoma. *Cancer Research, 62*, 5845–5852.
62. Klencke, B., Matijevic, M., Urban, R. G., Lathey, J. L., Hedley, M. L., Berry, M., & et al. (2002). Encapsulated plasmid DNA treatment for human papillomavirus 16- associated anal dysplasia: a phase I study of ZYC101. *Clinical Cancer Resarch, 8*, 1028–1037.
63. Salim, B., Zghal, M., Salem-Bekhit, M., Jamous, Y., Al-Anazi, F., Al Sarra, I., Bayomi, M., & Fathallah, M. D. (2012). Introducing plasmid DNA fingerprinting in the quality control of pDNA vaccine. *International Journal of Biotechnology and Biochemistry, 8*(2), 87–100.
64. Greenland, J. R., Geiben, R., Ghosh, S., Pastor, W. A., & Letvin, N. L. (2007). Plasmid DNA vaccine-elicited cellular immune responses limit in vivo vaccine antigen expression through Fas-mediated apoptosis. *The Journal of Immunology, 178*(9), 5652–5658.
65. Lorentzen, C. L., Haanen, J. B., Met, Ö., & Svane, I. M. (2022). Clinical advances and ongoing trials on mRNA vaccines for cancer treatment. *The Lancet Oncology, 23*(10), e450–e458.
66. Sahin, U., Derhovanessian, E., Miller, M., & et al. (2017). Personalized RNA mutanome vaccines mobilize poly-specific therapeutic immunity against cancer. *Nature, 547*, 222–226.
67. Papachristofilou, A., Hipp, M. M., Klinkhardt, U., & et al. (2019). Phase Ib evaluation of a self-adjuvanted protamine formulated mRNA-based active cancer immunotherapy, BI1361849 (CV9202), combined with local radiation treatment in patients with stage IV non-small cell lung cancer. *Journal for Immunotherpy of Cancer, 7*, 38.
68. Mackensen, A., Koenecke, C., Haanen, J., & et al. (2021). BNT211: A phase I/II trial to evaluate safety and efficacy of CLDN6 CAR-T cells and vaccine-mediated in vivo expansion in patients with CLDN6-positive advanced solid tumors. *Journal for Immunotherpy of Cancer, 9*
69. Burris, H. A., Patel, M. R., Cho, D. C., & et al. (2019). A phase I multicenter study to assess the safety, tolerability, and immunogenicity of mRNA-4157 alone in patients with resected solid tumors and in combination with pembrolizumab in patients with unresectable solid tumors. *Journal of Clinical Oncology, 37.*
70. De Keersmaecker, B., Claerhout, S., Carrasco, J., & et al. (2020). TriMix and tumor antigen mRNA electroporated dendritic cell vaccination plus ipilimumab: link between T-cell activation and clinical responses in advanced melanoma. *Journal for Immunotherpy of Cancer, 8*(1), e000329.
71. Beck, J. D., Reidenbach, D., Salomon, N., & et al. (2021). mRNA therapeutics in cancer immunotherapy. *Molecular Cancer, 20*, 69.

72. Hollingsworth, R. E., & Jansen, K. (2019). Turning the corner on therapeutic cancer vaccines. *NPJ Vaccines, 4*, 7.
73. Hong, S., Zhang, Z., Liu, H., & et al. (2018). B cells are the dominant antigen-presenting cells that activate naive $CD4^+$ T cells upon immunization with a virus-derived nanoparticle antigen. *Immunity, 49*, 695–708.e4.
74. Zeng, C., Zhang, C., Walker, P. G., & Dong, Y. (2020). Formulation and delivery technologies for mRNA vaccines. *Current Topics in Microbiology and Immunology, 2*, 1–40.
75. Stenzl, A., Feyerabend, S., Syndikus, I., & et al. (2017). Results of the randomized, placebo-controlled phase I/IIB trial of CV9104, an mRNA based cancer immunotherapy, in patients with metastatic castration-resistant prostate cancer (mCRPC). *Annal of Oncology, 28*, v408–v409.
76. Kallen, K.-J., Heidenreich, R., Schnee, M., & et al. (2013). A novel, disruptive vaccination technology: self-adjuvanted RNActive(®) vaccines. *Human Vaccines and Immunotherapeutics, 9*, 2263–2276.
77. Persano, S., Guevara, M. L., Li, Z., & et al. (2017). Lipopolyplex potentiates anti-tumor immunity of mRNA-based vaccination. *Biomaterials, 125*, 81–89.
78. Sahin, U., Oehm, P., Derhovanessian, E., & et al. (2020). An RNA vaccine drives immunity in checkpoint-inhibitor-treated melanoma. *Nature, 585*, 107–112.
79. Miao, L., Zhang, Y., & Huang, L. (2021). mRNA vaccine for cancer immunotherapy. *Molecular Cancer, 20*(1), 1–23.

Index

E

G

V

X